For Bonnie

May you have a Long,

Happy, Healthy Life

YOU ARE WHAT YOU EAT

HUMAN

BODY

FUNCTION

IN RELATION

TO FOOD

SALLY F. JACKSON

WESTBOW
PRESS®
A DIVISION OF THOMAS NELSON
& ZONDERVAN

Written by
Sally F. Jackson RN, CLNC, CPT, Pt. Adv.
CEO/ Owner: Proactive Health Education LLC.

WestBow Press books may be ordered through booksellers or by contacting:

WestBow Press
A Division of Thomas Nelson & Zondervan
1663 Liberty Drive
Bloomington, IN 47403
www.westbowpress.com
1 (866) 928-1240

ISBN: 978-1-9736-3387-7 (sc)
ISBN: 978-1-9736-3388-4 (hc)
ISBN: 978-1-9736-3386-0 (e)

Library of Congress Control Number: 2018908285

Print information available on the last page.

WestBow Press rev. date: 10/19/2018

Sincere thanks to the physicians and researchers
who were the major inspiration for this book;

Dr. Robert Lusting; Pediatric obesity, UCSF,
Bonnie Bassler; Bio Research, Princeton University,
Dr Joseph Mercola; Renowned advocate
for 'practical health solutions',
Stephanie Seniff; Bio Physics and Research at MIT,
Fred A. Kummerow PHD; Biochemist, University of Illinois.

Contents

So You Ask Yourself; Why Read This Book?

No matter what your age, we all grew up, learning the same way.

We all learned to eat three meals a day and drink plenty of liquids, simply through the influences of our parents. In school, we learned basic science and sex education, but unless you took a cooking class, you learned nothing about nutrition—and neither did your parents. The government attempts nutritional education by using outdated and flawed science as its basis for teaching and never connects the simple **function of the body** with the effects of food.

In order to understand the whys and wherefores of the foods we eat, we must be able to connect those foods directly to the body's functions. Otherwise, the statement that "vitamin D is good for you" has no meaning.

Years ago, the food pyramid was devised in an attempt to guide the general public in food consumption. Today, it's the 'food plate', but the science that backed these theories of eating was severely flawed. As a result, this country slowly began seeing destructive changes in health. The very first premise we need to understand is that your health is not affected by when you eat, how much you eat or how little you eat, but by **what you eat!**

Nutrition, is not calorie counting, chemical reactions, or metabolism.

Nutrition is proper and effective **body function**, as a result of **what you eat!** If you don't understand how your body uses or misuses foods for function and what that function is, how can you know what foods to eat or avoid in order to remain healthy?

Sixty years ago, this country began altering our foods through chemistry with artificial flavors, chemical vitamins, synthetics, preservatives, chemical flavor enhancers, processed oils, and excessive use of sugars. Today, a large portion of foods around the world are anywhere from 50 percent to 80 percent artificial or chemical, and as a result, these foods provide no nutritional value to the body. Our bodies can't use them for survival. So what was once food, is no longer, it has been replaced by a look-alike, that provides only malnutrition and disease. We need to learn, once again, what **real food** is and return to its proper use.

Let's make a quick comparison and see where we are headed.

The average healthy cow lives twenty-one to twenty-three years. They are grass-eating animals, which means their primary and only food source should be grass. These are hearty animals, that have high disease resistance and remain healthy under a wide variety of conditions as long as they remain on their primary food source. We learned from science that cows produce more milk and heavier meat when they are forced to eat processed grains, corn, soy, GMOs (genetically modified organisms), and chemicals. This increased their production, which resulted in milk—and meat—that is full of toxins. Since we changed their diets, they now suffer from disease, infections, and illness, and their life spans are now six to seven years.

If we look at our diets, there is a good comparison. Our diets should be comprised of healthy protein and fats and very small amounts of sugar. Today, we consume large quantities of sugars, GMOs, corn, soy, unhealthy fats and proteins, and a sizable amount of chemicals, which we were 'never' designed to eat. In other words, **we are not synthetic.** And each year that passes, the chemical content of our foods continues to grow at ever increasing rates.

The American diet has fostered illness, disease, and even death, resulting in ever-decreasing life spans. What was once one hundred or more years of human life span, is now seventy to eighty years—and it will soon become forty to fifty years as our ratio of illness and disease continues to climb. There is no end in sight—unless we make the changes that return us to our natural, real foods. If you look at it from this perspective, you can see that **we truly are what we eat.**

This book is not a weight loss book, but it does advocate a healthy weight and waist size for overall health improvement. This is the first step that everyone needs to cover since improved health does not occur when excess weight and waist size are present.

So, why read this book?

To learn, what we all should have been taught eighty years ago. And in doing so, we can give the next generations the advantage that we didn't have. In the process, we can reduce the disease rate, regain true health, and live longer, healthier lives, ourselves.

No more medical bills—only vacation bills!

Know your body, and be prepared.

The days of the relaxed and informative conversations with your doctor have long since passed. You will probably spend more time in the waiting room than you will in the examination room, and most patients never see their doctor's desk—let alone his office. Your doctor will spend the minimum required time with you in his frantic rush to see as many as fifty patients per day.

In this era of lower insurance payouts and higher demand for services, modern medicine has unfortunately become **revolving-door therapy**. Doctors are financially forced to see an increasing number of patients, which leads to increased episodes of diagnostic mistakes and errors. They also have little or no time to research their patients' problems. They tend to rely on the information provided by the FDA (Food and Drug Administration) and the pharmaceutical industry, which is often biased and severely lacking in actual research. Almost every drug placed on the market in the past five years has only the minimum required research (six weeks). The studies are extremely small, and the FDA often completely ignores the testing and clinical results provided by their own teams of scientists when making judgments that will affect public health. Today's conventional medicine is at the very least, overburdened. With fewer physicians entering the field, it is stretched far beyond its limits. It is up to you to get your doctor's eyes off of his computer screen and onto you.

Hence the statement; Be prepared!

Learn the basics of body function, listen to what your body has to say, and respect its needs.

In this book, you will find discussions on body function in relation to the three basic elements of a healthy diet. These **three elements** are bondable versus non-bondable or **sugars,** healthy versus unhealthy, **proteins** and **fats.** We will cover all the other elements that work with the basic ones to improve and maintain healthy body function. These include biologics or probiotics, cholesterol, CoQ-10, vitamins, and minerals. You will learn about all the organs, that are directly and indirectly connected to these elements, their functions, and how they are influenced by these elements. The goal here is to change the way you look at food, which will result in improved overall body function and a longer happier, healthier life.

You will notice that the word carbohydrate is not used anywhere in this book.

This word is simply an overused term that describes sugars, starches, non-bondable, and nonessential nutrients that are simply not healthy and do not contribute to healthy body function. The body does not recognize what—up until now—has been classified as carbohydrates.

Bondable versus non-bondable encompasses the entire spectrum that utilizes the flow of insulin in the body.

To change the way you look at these terms, think of **carbohydrates as non-bondable** and **vegetables that contain natural sugars (glucose) as**

bondable. Keep in mind that fructose is a natural sugar found in fruit, but here it is classified as a non-bondable.

The human body knows exactly what to do.

The body has been doing its job for thousands of years. Of the one trillion cells that make up the human body, each and every cell works with its neighbor, communicates, and functions by performing its specific job in coordination with all the surrounding cells as a community effort for survival. **And survival is the key word here**. The body will do whatever is necessary to maintain its very survival—no matter what you throw at it. Unfortunately, we do not listen to our bodies, and as a result, what we throw at it can ultimately create our own demise. And that monkey wrench that we use can be anything from the types of foods we eat to the pharmaceuticals we use.

We are the sum of everything we put into our bodies, and that includes food, water, and exercise. The risk of illness, debilitating disease, and early death is always present. As long as we work to promote good health and eating habits, resulting in a strong foundation and a healthier body, then that risk will remain very low. If we are to build a strong healthy body that is able to fight off disease and give us a long, healthy, and active life, then we must start with the basics.

Before we begin, please be informed that this author is an independent researcher. Who holds, no direct ties to, nor is influenced by, any organized group. This includes the American Medical Association, the Academy of Nutritional Dietetics, the American Dairy Association, the FDA, or the pharmaceutical industry. The information provided is derived from sound logic mixed with aggressive scientific work and research from around the world. Leading respected scientists, doctors, and researchers have provided the basis for these teachings. Proactive health education will not advocate for any product, company, or organization that has not earned profound respect for its work at providing high-quality, sound science.

This book is designed to teach you the basics of body function.

The following pages contain only **basic, simple material** that is easy to understand and utilize. You will understand exactly how your body works, how you can make changes to improve your overall health, and how to prevent—and in some cases even eliminate—a variety of diseases. Most importantly, the disease of the twenty-first century: metabolic syndrome or syndrome X. This syndrome is a series of diseases (obesity, diabetes, heart disease, hypertension, and renal failure) that seem to occur together, but according to the medical establishment, these diseases or 'medical problems' have no known common cause. The ultimate goal is the prevention and eventual elimination of metabolic syndrome or syndrome X in this country. And with this teaching, you will learn how your body **can prevent and even reverse metabolic syndrome or syndrome X.**

The following chapters are based on research gathered from independent scientists and respected researchers from around the world. The most important discoveries have only surfaced in the last four or five years. The theories for the chapters in this book are extrapolated logically from this research. Amazingly enough, your body knows how to solve most of your health problems. You just need to know how to assist the body in its job. While standing on the shoulders of scientists, we fit the pieces of the puzzle together. The entire picture cannot be seen, unless **all the pieces fit properly.**

CHAPTER 1
Keeping It Simple

In order to understand the reasoning behind the information provided in these guides, we must first understand how the body works at the cellular level. Not to worry, this information is not terribly complicated. This is your only class in biochemistry, and it will make everything else seem simple and clear.

Biochemistry 101

Our bodies are made up of one trillion cells, give or take a few thousand.

Understanding their basic function is vital for understanding the unique and different talents that each cell possesses. As humans, we all eat, drink, and sleep the same way, but we have unique and different jobs to perform. The same can be said for the communities of cells that make up our bodies. All cells eat, drink, and sleep the same way, but their unique talents are very different.

All cells live in a densely packed fluid bed.

This extracellular fluid contains nutrients in the form of poly-glucose (derived from sugars), amino acids and essential fatty acids (derived from protein and fats), water (H_2O), vitamins, sodium, potassium, sulfur, and at least ten other minerals. These are the nutrients that cells "eat" or utilize to maintain their healthy function. Also floating within this rich nutrient bed we find cholesterol, enzymes, heavy metals, toxins, and fat cells.

Within each cell, we find energy factories called mitochondria.

The number of mitochondria will vary wildly with any given tissue. For example, immature red blood cells have few mitochondria and mature red blood cells have no mitochondria, but high-function tissues like liver cells have two thousand mitochondria per cell. This is where the cell produces ATP (adenosine triphosphate), otherwise known as energy. All cells have an exterior protective coating made of cholesterol (lipid bi-layer), which supports electrical activity, repairs damage, and—with the aid of stimulants and antioxidants—allows glucose and other nutrients (including cholesterol) to pass into the cell.

Water (H_2O), along with sodium and potassium, creates a positive electrical charge outside the cell and a negative charge inside the cell.

The process is simple yet effective. The **sodium inside the cell** is forced out of the cell with production of ATP (cellular energy). This flow of negative charge to the outside of the cell actually causes an influx or flow of positively charged ions back into the cell. And like a little pump, the sodium is pushed out to pull in potassium. These **positively charged ions are seen in potassium**, which is an element the cell needs to balance its neurological charge, resulting in **cellular relaxation**. If you get a muscle cramp, it's very likely that your cells are attempting to retrieve more potassium that is not available in that cellular bed (extracellular fluid). The cells continue to pump out sodium without retrieving the needed potassium, and the muscle remains contracted. The result is a muscle cramp.

The movement of ions back and forth across this cellular wall is the **main form of nutrient transport for all cells.** This is how nutrients are carried into the cell and by-products are carried out of the cell. This electrical exchange back and forth (positive/negative), in and out of the cell is called the **sodium pump.**

Fat cells are neutral.

They do not utilize the sodium pump mechanism, and like little sponges, they soak up the leftover poly-glucose that the muscle and other tissue cells can't utilize at the time. Fat cells not only store excess energy (poly-glucose), but actively produce hormones, absorb toxins and heavy metals.

If the positive/negative charge is altered, as seen in vitamin and mineral deficiencies with a loss of muscle activity and decreased metabolism (loss of ATP), then the fat cells get fatter while the muscle and other tissue cells starve.

This sodium pump, in conjunction with sulfa and cholesterol, facilitates the transport of by-products (substances the cells create), such as hormones and insulin, for function of the community of cells (the body) as a whole.

What about sleep?

The continuous supply of nutrients keeps the cells alive, but each community of cells performs a different function and will rest or 'sleep' until called upon. When active, they will grow, divide, and multiply throughout the body. We notice this particularly in skin, muscle, and bone growth.

Some cells that are exposed to toxins and carcinogens (cancer-causing substances) will be stimulated to grow inappropriately and become malformed or damaged; this includes damage to our mitochondria and our precious DNA (our genetic blueprint). If the immune system does not recognize and destroy these cells, they can become cancer.

If completely inactive (no sodium pump exchange) or damaged, cells will eventually shrivel and die.

No, cells do not live forever. Natural cell death is seen as necrobiosis. Specialized cells throughout the body have different life spans. For example, brain cells live only three to four days, and skin cells (including nails and hair) live fifteen to thirty days. As a result, we are continually triggering the process of cell life, growth, activity, and death by merely eating food, drinking water, and remaining active. This means we **literally are what we eat.**

If our diet is poor, it will cause changes that will affect our health. After all, health maintenance and improvement are the goals here.

You have just completed your basic biochemistry lesson. Although there are hundreds of other chemical actions that occur in the body, knowing the basics gives you a firm foundation for what comes next.

The basis of all normal body functions evolve around proper **insulin production and control of its circulating levels within the body.** It has been found—and most scientists agree—that the frequency and intensity of insulin production within the human body is the main culprit to address for health improvement. As a result, you will find a new form of instruction that involves the reduction of free insulin production within the body and the nutrition that revolves around it.

If we look closely, we will see that the foods that bond with insulin, are readily used by the body. Foods that do not bond, must be processed by the liver, which dramatically increases the liver's workload and results in damaging by-products. Insulin works directly with a fuel, otherwise known as simple glucose, and known in this book as bondable sugar, and is also best known, as the fuel of life.

CHAPTER 2
How Our Body Uses Fuel

What do we see when we look at terms like:

Insulin resistance and insulin sensitivity? This is modern medicine's terminology for explaining insulin's role in diabetes. Quite - frankly, these terms complicate basic body functions. They are misleading and extremely confusing. As a result, we are left in the dark.

Now, let's turn on the lights!

Your body and the chemistry involved in insulin and its relationship to diabetes and weight gain are very simple. Let's stop stumbling over terminology and use basic, direct, and simple terms.

When we see the terms **sensitive or resistant**, modern medicine should be referring to the foods we eat and not the insulin itself. So, **sensitive foods** (glucose) bond with insulin, and **resistant foods** (non-bondable) do not bond with insulin. Without reference to those foods, the words sensitive and resistant are meaningless, which adds to our confusion.

Your insulin does not change, it does not get stronger or weaker. Your insulin capabilities are set for life with development and function of your pancreas at birth. **It never changes, your pancreas can only make more or**

less insulin, that's all it can do. So, now let's look realistically at the body's functions and the digestion and function of bondable natural dietary foods.

Bondable Fuel

Bondable natural dietary fuels are forms of glucose (sugars).

Glucose is also known as the fuel of life, and literally every living thing on this earth needs glucose to survive.

Some forms of glucose are simple molecular chains, and some are complex molecular chains (monosaccharides and disaccharides). The one thing they have in common is their outer shell of electrons can **actually bond** with the

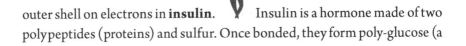

outer shell on electrons in **insulin.** Insulin is a hormone made of two polypeptides (proteins) and sulfur. Once bonded, they form poly-glucose (a

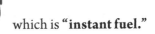

glucose molecule with a sulfur bond), which is **"instant fuel."**

Sulfur is a unique molecule since it has the ability to travel throughout the body without restrictions. The presence of sulfur in poly-glucose gives the glucose mobility. Now it is able to travel throughout the entire body—to literally every cell. Bondable natural dietary sugars can be found in such foods as organic vegetables, unrefined grains, organic brown rice, beans, unpasteurized raw honey, unpasteurized raw milk, raw organic cacao, and 100 percent maple syrup. **These are all-natural, unprocessed, real foods.**

Let's look at what happens when we sit down to a meal of only bondable sugars (a plate of vegetables).

Bondable Fuel (Instant Fuel)   We Eat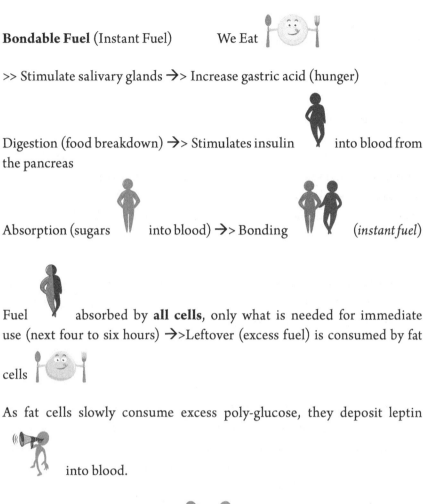

>> Stimulate salivary glands →> Increase gastric acid (hunger)

Digestion (food breakdown) →> Stimulates insulin   into blood from the pancreas

Absorption (sugars   into blood) →> Bonding   (*instant fuel*)

Fuel   absorbed by **all cells**, only what is needed for immediate use (next four to six hours) →>Leftover (excess fuel) is consumed by fat cells

As fat cells slowly consume excess poly-glucose, they deposit leptin

into blood.

Leptin accumulates in brain   →> Stimulates production of

ghrelin in the hypothalamus

Ghrelin stimulates the vagus nerve →   Signals shutdown of the stomach

Satiety 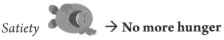 → **No more hunger**

Lasts approximately four to six hours (to next meal)

Non-bondable Fuel

We also get sugars (fuel) by a second process. Seen as **delayed food or complex chain- glucose production.** By this process, we produce glycogen, **a closed molecule with no ability to bond with insulin.** This process also produces other by-products that are not desirable. These sugars (fuel) are **non-bondable sugars** , some of, which (artificial sugars) do not cause an initial rise in the insulin response, and can be seen as low on the glycemic index. (We will learn why later.)

Such foods (**non-bondable fuels**) are found in fructose (fruit sugar), sucrose (table sugar; 50 percent fructose/50 percent glucose), all artificial sugars, all processed or refined foods and grains (containing sugars, chemical additives, and preservatives), pasteurized/homogenized milk products (including whey and whey protein), soy, white rice, potatoes, and all genetically altered foods. All of these molecular structures (fuels) are **too large or complex** to be utilized directly by the cells. These fuels, are the result of food processing, or they are recognized by the body as toxins.

Processing—the use of high heat (pasteurization) and/or the use of chemicals—renders the outer shell of electrons useless in these sugars (the outer shell is destroyed) like lactose found in milk. **When these outer shells are destroyed, they cannot bond with insulin, so they are sent straight to the liver for processing or molecular breakdown.**

Now let's look at what happens when we eat a **non-bondable fuel** like orange juice (processed fruit containing artificial sugars—with no fiber or quercetin to decrease absorption of fructose). Fiber and quercetin are bonding agents that are naturally found in whole fruit and work in the intestinal tract. They bond with sugars and prevent their absorption into the body.

We Eat >> Stimulate salivary glands →> Increased gastric acid

Digestion (food breakdown) -→ Stimulates insulin secretions into blood

 (from the pancreas)

Absorption into blood →> **No Bonding** = (free insulin)

 + a molecule (sugar) filtered out of the blood and >> **processed by the liver**

(all non-bondable sugars, processed grains, toxins, and alcohol use the same pathway in the liver)

End products of processing:

1. Uric Acid (hypertension, heart disease)

2. VSLDL (hardening of arteries, plaque), very small, dense lipoprotein

3. Glycogen (<u>closed molecule</u>, cannot bond), but **still stimulates insulin secretions**

Glycogen (most is pushed - out around liver) goes directly to fat storage (belly fat). **While it stimulates free insulin production, this form of glycogen cannot bond with insulin (no sulfur), has no mobility, and cannot travel.** As a result, it floats around the liver, where it is consumed by fat cells (the spare tire).

Fat cells consume glycogen 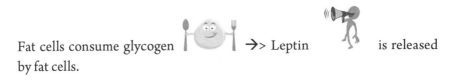 →> Leptin is released by fat cells.

Stimulated **free** **insulin spikes** (no bonding) →> Insulin accumulates in brain and clouds brain (brain fog)

Multiple insulin spikes occur one to three hours after digestion

Accumulated free insulin spikes in the brain →>

Blocks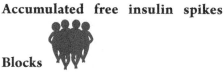

- any leptin reception = (brain fog)

- poly-glucose absorption = (brain damage)

Hypothalamus absorbs **no leptin** →> **no** ghrelin is produced (the brain thinks you are starving)

ghrelin absent →> **no vagus nerve stimulation** →> stomach continues to function

→> **End Result = Hunger** →> 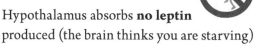 eat—eat—eat

We need to look closely at the end- products of processing since these are **the main contributors to metabolic syndrome or syndrome X.** The liver is our toxic waste processing plant, and all non-bondable foods (including alcohol and processed grains) are treated as toxins and use the same processing pathway.

Uric acid is a natural waste product made by the liver when processing toxins. Uric acid is the primary culprit in the formation of gout. When uric acid accumulates, it forms crystals that block tiny blood vessels (where veins and arteries meet), causing damage with swelling and pain (usually seen in fingers and toes). It also causes the same problem in kidneys, damaging the renal tubules (our tiny filtering system). In small quantities, it remains dilute and causes no problems, but an 80 percent non-bondable diet causes large accumulations. These accumulations also block the formation of nitric oxide in the blood. Nitric oxide keeps the walls of arteries soft, allowing them to expand, thereby lowering blood pressure. When uric acid is present, nitric oxide cannot form. As a result, the arteries stiffen, resulting in hypertension (high blood pressure).

Very small dense lipoprotein (VSLDL) 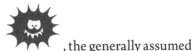 , the generally assumed *bad cholesterol,* but this is not the only LDL cholesterol in your body. There are two kinds of LDL. One is large, fluffy, and buoyant and serves as a carrier for nutrients such as CoQ-10 and vitamins. It floats through the bloodstream effortlessly as a necessary transporter. The other is small and dense (VSLDL). It cannot float, and it tends to get lodged or embedded in the inner lining of artery walls, blocking off the circulation to that lining, which slowly becomes hard and dry with dead cells that flake off and become plaque. Plaque aids in the natural formation of clots and is necessary in small amounts. Most blood tests do not measure these LDLs separately. Normally, the body has a higher percentage of large LDLs than small dense LDLs. But with increased consumption of non-bondable foods, the percentage of VSLDLs is dramatically increased, resulting in peripheral artery disease (hardening of the arteries) and a cascade of other heart problems.

Glycogen ; a closed molecule, the outer electrons in this element are balanced and cannot bond with other substances. The presence of glycogen stimulates the pancreas to produce insulin, but the insulin cannot bond with this end- product, so there is no sulfur to give it mobility. The glycogen is pushed out of the liver wall and floats around the major organs of the body, where it is consumed by fat cells. This is the formation of **belly fat.**

As this cycle continuously repeats itself over time (years), the end products of liver processing of non-bondable fuels accumulate dramatically. Increasing pressure from accumulated fat stores in the core of the body (belly fat) causes increased pressure on vital organs, resulting in decreased function of those organs, especially the liver.

Keep in mind; the volume of substances entering the liver for processing does not decrease, and in some instances, it actually increases. With increased pressure, the liver's ability to process toxins - is dramatically slowed. As a result, two things happen:

- The unprocessed toxins remain in the bloodstream and circulate causing a wide variety of damage, including cancers.
- Processing by the liver slows to a point of **causing multiple, almost**

continuous insulin spikes, resulting in permanent brain fog and brain damage (Alzheimer's). Over time, continued, increasing pressure from belly fat will cause the vital organs, including the liver and pancreas, to fail.

We are discussing the use of bondable versus non-bondable fuels (sugars). If we take a close look at the above scenario, we can see **how type 2 diabetes develops**.

Type 2 diabetes is the end-result of pancreatic failure.

The pancreas is unable to produce sufficient quantities of insulin to bond with sugars that cross the intestinal wall into the bloodstream, which can occur in two ways.

The repeated high production of insulin (insulin spikes), which is triggered

by the closed glycogen molecule produced by the liver (non-bondable) after digestion, which causes forced pancreatic fatigue. **Think of it as too much wattage into the light bulb, burning out the circuit.**

When the response to leptin from the hypothalamus is gone,

ghrelin cannot be produced. Hunger remains, which feeds a vicious cycle. Eating more creates an endless process of insulin spikes. This repeated dietary increase causes an increased demand for insulin to meet the bondable as well as non-bondable stimulus during digestion. Again, we see the light bulb effect and pancreatic failure. **In both instances, we see multiple, repeated, forced pancreatic fatigue (the 'light bulb effect').**

When the production of insulin is lost, glucose cannot bond, allowing

bondable glucose to float free in the system. **Free-floating bondable**

glucose behaves much like a free radical. It is an extremely - strong oxidizer, that can damage cells throughout the body with **oxidation (the theft of electrons from stable structures to balance the structure of that free radical).** This oxidative damage, creates damage to very-small blood vessels throughout the body, resulting in the multiple symptoms, seen in diabetes; which includes; the loss of nerve sensation in the hands and feet (peripheral neuropathy), loss of renal tubule structure (renal failure), and retinal nerve damage (blindness).

A small number of the closed molecules of non-bondable glycogen pass into the circulating bloodstream from the liver. This increase in free-floating

non-bondable glycogen—along with that free-floating bondable glucose—results in damage by falsely increasing the blood sugar, and it cannot be lowered with insulin. This is the cause of what is termed the brittle diabetic—the aggressive use of too much insulin to counter falsely increased blood sugars, resulting in rapid loss of bondable sugars to dangerously low levels.

To sum it up;

If we give a type 2 diabetic (a diabetic not totally dependent on injectable

insulin) a diet of bondable fuels only (using only the amount of fuel required for that body weight), this process will reverse itself. Removing the excessive load from the pancreas, while improving its function, allows the leptin and ghrelin signals to complete, creating satiety. Total body weight will decrease with no non-bondable glycogen for fat cells. And the liver will slowly recover. The type 2 diabetic will become a non-diabetic.

Now we can see why free insulin, and the end- products of non-bondable fuels are the culprits we need to control. They are not what the body needs for good health.

With the slow accumulation of these end- products, the body develops metabolic syndrome or syndrome X (hypertension, heart disease, diabetes, obesity, fatty liver disease, and renal failure, with eventual multisystem failure). The medical community classifies 'metabolic syndrome'; as a series of associated diseases with no known associated disease cause. Now we

see that this syndrome is **all simply due to** **overconsumption of non-bondable fuels**, and the resulting elevated end- products with

uncontrolled free insulin, —in other words, **what you eat.**

Bondable **Vs. Non-Bondable**

Eighty years ago, 80 percent of the American diet was consumed as bondable foods, with only 20 percent consumed as non-bondable. This was good. The liver maintained stable function and was not overburdened. The immune system was more active, and not only improved digestion of vital nutrients, but also protected us from a wide variety of diseases.

Today, the American diet consists of 80 percent non-bondable fuels and only 20 percent bondable. As a result; the liver is functioning far beyond its capacity and is overburdened, which eventually results in failure. The immune system has lost a large portion of its functional capacity, leaving us vulnerable to illness and disease.

Eighty years ago, the theory of "calories in, calories out" would have worked. Less calorie consumption using 80 percent bondable fuels and more energy production would yield weight loss. Today, this theory cannot work. Even if you could run like a mouse on a wheel, if you are still using non-bondable fuels, the end- result will be weight gain and a progressive move toward metabolic syndrome. An example is the skinny diabetic.

We need to look at food differently and change the way our bodies process fuels. This means we need to change the way we eat. Eliminate the non-bondable foods and increase the bondable foods, driving down the free insulin in the body, while maintaining optimum nutrition. And these foods should be organic, thus eliminating toxins (pesticides, herbicides, and GMOs).

Now you ask organic is expensive, won't my grocery bill go up?

No. In fact, for some people, the cost will decrease. Those people who follow bondable versus non-bondable teaching actually eat less food as a result. Think about it, sit down, and tabulate the cost of the processed foods in your cupboard. Now use that amount to replace those processed foods with organic vegetables (fresh and fresh-frozen). Your supply of healthy bondable fuels has just increased dramatically, and it didn't cost any more than before. Do the same for all the other non-bondable foods in your cupboard. Bingo!

You have just solved the cost factor. You are on your way to healthy, healthy, healthy, and it did not cost you an added penny!

There are lots of diets out there that can get you started, but only one controls insulin spikes. Bondable versus non-bondable teaching along with the BMI is a healthy start that you can do yourself. Mediterranean people have been using it for centuries. The Mediterranean diet is the closest to bondable versus non-bondable teaching available. It is not totally the same, but it is close.

If you just eat bondable foods and use the dietary guidelines provided in this book, you will return to a healthy weight that you can control for the rest of your healthy life. Imagine – **"no more medical bills— only vacation bills"**!

CHAPTER 3
The BMI and Why

Use this chapter as a guide for setting your goals.

This is your health! You make the decisions that will affect the outcome, and you need to set your own goals.

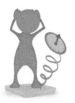

Now you ask; Why do I need to know this?

The answer is simple, if you know where you stand now, you will be able to determine how much weight you need to lose. Proactive health means you make the decisions and changes in your health with education. In the following pages, you will find frequent references to the vital organs of the body. Without full, active function of these organs (your liver in particular), your body **will not respond** to any changes you attempt to make.

All adverse pressure, needs to be removed from these organs before you can even attempt changes, such as removal of pharmaceuticals or treatments for chronic infections or disease.

Your BMI needs to be in a healthy range (19 to 22 for adults, and 23 to 28 for bodybuilders, depending on muscle mass development and waist measurement), and your waist measurements must be below the maximum numbers. The term **adverse pressure** refers to excess weight, and **weight loss is the very first step in recovery and control of your health.**

The foundation for the body's natural defense or built-in immunology, is based on the premise that nutrients can enhance the body's immune response. Studies performed by the National Institute on Ageing found a direct link between calorie intake and immune response. Without distinguishing between the types of calories, they found that excess calories suppressed T cell formation, which is the base indicator of the immune system's strength. They concluded that *"a weight gain of twenty pounds will lower your T cell count, thereby decreasing your immunity's strength"*. This alone indicates the importance of weight management. According to the Dietary Guidelines National Advisory Committee, healthy weight is measured by the BMI (body mass index) combined with your waist measurement or fat index.

If your BMI is between 19 and 23, you have a healthy body weight. With higher BMI readings, more stress is placed on the body's vital organs. Remember that a high percentage of weight gain is seen in the core of the body (in and around the vital organs), which means the increase in fat in these areas causes increased pressure on the heart, liver, spleen, pancreas, and lungs. As this pressure increases, the ability of these organs to function- normally, is progressively - decreased. Left unchecked, it will result in eventual organ failure (morbid obesity).

Find your height and weight on the chart below.

Body Mass Index Table

	Normal						Overweight					Obese										Extreme Obesity														
BMI	19	20	21	22	23	24	25	26	27	28	29	30	31	32	33	34	35	36	37	38	39	40	41	42	43	44	45	46	47	48	49	50	51	52	53	54
Height (inches)												Body Weight (pounds)																								
58	91	96	100	105	110	115	119	124	129	134	138	143	148	153	158	162	167	172	177	181	186	191	196	201	205	210	215	220	224	229	234	239	244	248	253	258
59	94	99	104	109	114	119	124	128	133	138	143	148	153	158	163	168	173	178	183	188	193	198	203	208	212	217	222	227	232	237	242	247	252	257	262	267
60	97	102	107	112	118	123	128	133	138	143	148	153	158	163	168	174	179	184	189	194	199	204	209	215	220	225	230	235	240	245	250	255	261	266	271	276
61	100	106	111	116	122	127	132	137	143	148	153	158	164	169	174	180	185	190	195	201	206	211	217	222	227	232	238	243	248	254	259	264	269	275	280	285
62	104	109	115	120	126	131	136	142	147	153	158	164	169	175	180	186	191	196	202	207	213	218	224	229	235	240	246	251	256	262	267	273	278	284	289	295
63	107	113	118	124	130	135	141	146	152	158	163	169	175	180	186	191	197	203	208	214	220	225	231	237	242	248	254	259	265	270	278	282	287	293	299	304
64	110	116	122	128	134	140	145	151	157	163	169	174	180	186	192	197	204	209	215	221	227	232	238	244	250	256	262	267	273	279	285	291	296	302	308	314
65	114	120	126	132	138	144	150	156	162	168	174	180	186	192	198	204	210	216	222	228	234	240	246	252	258	264	270	276	282	288	294	300	306	312	318	324
66	118	124	130	136	142	148	155	161	167	173	179	186	192	198	204	210	216	223	229	235	241	247	253	260	266	272	278	284	291	297	303	309	315	322	328	334
67	121	127	134	140	146	153	159	166	172	178	185	191	198	204	211	217	223	230	236	242	249	255	261	268	274	280	287	293	299	306	312	319	325	331	338	344
68	125	131	138	144	151	158	164	171	177	184	190	197	203	210	216	223	230	236	243	249	256	262	269	276	282	289	295	302	308	315	322	328	335	341	348	354
69	128	135	142	149	155	162	169	176	182	189	196	203	209	216	223	230	236	243	250	257	263	270	277	284	291	297	304	311	318	324	331	338	345	351	358	365
70	132	139	146	153	160	167	174	181	188	195	202	209	216	222	229	236	243	250	257	264	271	278	285	292	299	306	313	320	327	334	341	348	355	362	369	376
71	136	143	150	157	165	172	179	186	193	200	208	215	222	229	236	243	250	257	265	272	279	286	293	301	308	315	322	329	338	343	351	358	365	372	379	386
72	140	147	154	162	169	177	184	191	199	206	213	221	228	235	242	250	258	265	272	279	287	294	302	309	316	324	331	338	346	353	361	368	375	383	390	397
73	144	151	159	166	174	182	189	197	204	212	219	227	235	242	250	257	265	272	280	288	295	302	310	318	325	333	340	348	355	363	371	378	386	393	401	408
74	148	155	163	171	179	186	194	202	210	218	225	233	241	249	256	264	272	280	287	295	303	311	319	326	334	342	350	358	365	373	381	389	396	404	412	420
75	152	160	168	176	184	192	200	208	216	224	232	240	248	256	264	272	279	287	295	303	311	319	327	335	343	351	359	367	375	383	391	399	407	415	423	431
76	156	164	172	180	189	197	205	213	221	230	238	246	254	263	271	279	287	295	304	312	320	328	336	344	353	361	369	377	385	394	402	410	418	426	435	443

In the overweight and obese range, you will notice a lower level of energy, gradual elevations in blood pressure, more frequent episodes of illnesses like the flu, digestive disorders, and a weakened immune system, which can result in diabetes and increased cardiovascular disease.

Morbid obesity is life-threatening. In this range, every organ in the body is overtaxed, and the body cannot support the pressure or stress. This causes slow but progressive failure of each organ. The end- result of these failures; is seen as diabetes, renal failure (kidney failure), congestive heart failure, liver failure, and a higher risk of genetic damage, which can result in the formation of cancer.

Your BMI and waist measurement are the keys here.

The closer you are to the lower numbers, the happier your body will be— and you will feel that happiness. You will have more energy and vitality than you ever thought you could have. Your skin will be radiant and more youthful in appearance. Your blood pressure, blood cholesterol, and blood sugars will **normalize naturally.**

A BMI of less than 18.5 is indicative of illness, and unexplained weight loss may be an early clue to health problems. If you fall in this category, see your doctor for a thorough physical. Eat a diet with improved healthy proteins and saturated fats that are all organic, including raw milk for children. Raw milk for adults with a BMI below 18.5 may be necessary. Pasteurized, homogenized milk in any form for adults or children is not recommended.

Build up your stores of healthy foods before attempting any aggressive forms of detoxification, which is necessary for losing more than fifteen pounds. See chapter 16 for more detailed information on detoxification.

The **fat index** is a **waist measurement of the distance around the smallest area of your abdomen—below your rib cage and above your belly button—while standing.** This is the measurement of internal body fat and can place you at greater risk for health problems, such as diabetes and heart disease, even if your BMI is at a healthy level. For men, the measurement should be forty inches or less. For women, it should be thirty-five inches or less.

For men, between thirty-seven and forty inches is overweight, and more than forty inches is obese. Healthy is below thirty-seven inches. For women, 31.5–34.6 inches is overweight, and more than 34.6 inches is obese. Healthy is below 31.0 inches.

Your health risk increases as your waist size increases.

Elevated levels of abdominal fat cause **adverse pressure on the internal organs**, which decreases their function. Before attempting any changes in your health, read and thoroughly understand chapter 2.

Some people have difficulty losing abdominal fat. There are a few ways to enhance the loss of abdominal fat, along with applying bondable versus non-bondable. The simplest and quickest is using 80–90 percent bondable fuels along with healthy fats and limited protein to maintain necessary body nutrition. This will automatically decrease caloric intake and eliminate insulin spikes.

Incorporate mild exercise, especially abdominal wall exercises. This loosens the fat that clings to the muscles of the abdominal wall, giving it a chance to burn more readily.

Another simple trick is to stimulate central body metabolism by forcing an increase in core body temperature. This increased metabolism, can be accomplished by drinking 10–12 ounces of ice water thirty minutes before breakfast and dinner. The ice water (extreme cold induction) forces the body to increase the core temperature (metabolism) in an attempt to return the body to normal body temperature in that area. This demand for fuel will force core body fat cells to release their stored poly-glucose as ketones, the energy required to raise the body temperature.

The general stimulation of cardiac function and increased circulation will decrease all stores of body fat throughout the body. This increased circulation, can be accomplished with light to moderate exercise (without weights) daily for thirty to sixty minutes, preferably before breakfast.

Keep in mind, the BMI is a general guide. The **waist measurement is the more important of the two numbers.**

Where to Start?

Weight loss, can be accomplished in many ways. You could use progressive dietary changes done at home with the glycemic index guide or use diet assistance by groups such as Weight Watchers, Medi-Fast, or Jenny Craig. These are all good diet aids, but **none of them control your insulin levels, prevent insulin spikes, or reverse metabolic syndrome.** Using bondable versus non-bondable teaching, utilizing the Mediterranean type diet, or adopting an organic, vegetable-based diet, will. They work together to give you the specific desired results that you want—and losing has never been so easy.

There is no calorie counting or heavy exercise. Just follow the diet program

and watch the pounds fall off.

This is a lifestyle change, which means you don't go back to the foods you used to eat.

Start the program by making the changes in the foods you use at home. Eliminate all sugars. This means no sweetened drinks of any kind (including juices). Only drink water and small amounts of tea or coffee (sweetened with stevia only).

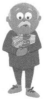

How to Detox from Sugar

There are only three major elements to a healthy diet: bondable versus non-bondable (sugars), proteins, and fats. Once you understand the function of each of these elements in the body, you will be able to make changes that will keep you healthy for life.

If we look at the dietary history of the United States, we find statistics that show we should have changed our eating habits a long time ago, but so far, nothing really has changed.

Among the thirty-five largest countries in the world, the United States has the third highest death rate from sugary beverage consumption with an estimated annual death rate of twenty-five thousand. In chapter 2, we saw that fructose is the number one problem, followed closely by a wide variety of sugar blends and artificial sweeteners. These multiple forms of sugar are all classified as non-bondable. They are the culprits that shut down your leptin-to-ghrelin signaling, leaving you with brain fog and hunger and producing damaging side effects in the liver.

Start with what you drink!

Whether your drink contains table sugar or cane sugar, which is also known as sucrose (fructose and glucose), fruit sugar (fructose), high-fructose corn syrup (fructose on steroids), crystalline fructose (fructose on speed), aspartame (NutraSweet), sucralose (Splenda), or any other artificial (chemically derived) sugar in it, then you are using a very damaging non-bondable. The problem lies in 'getting off' of these products. The leptin-to-ghrelin signaling is gone, and you continue to eat. The spell is decreased, but it is not completely lost by moving the sweetened drinks to water. There are several methods that can employed here.

In the United States, processed foods contain far more hidden sugars than any other country in the world. That hidden sugar can diminish or even destroy any efforts to detoxify from sugar in liquids alone. The removal of sugar from your diet may take up to six weeks, but it can be done, and you must start with what you drink.

For those who consume sugar-laden beverages daily, this includes coffee with sugar, the first step is switching your sugar content to something that is more natural. Stevia (100 percent pure) is the only natural sweetener that does not spike the insulin level in the body. It is safe, non-chemical and non-toxic, so it can be used in coffee or tea, in cooking, and even in baked goods. As for other sugary drinks, like sodas, the move to cane sugar or small amounts of table sugar, which is 50 percent fructose and 50 percent glucose, is advised. It can be found in the new natural sodas—**read your labels.** Making the switch to stevia and natural sodas cuts the damage from non-bondable sugars in half.

The next step is to replace one of those new more natural drinks every two or three days with filtered water (preferred reverse-osmosis filtration that takes out the chlorines and fluoride). You can taper off the sugary drinks one at a time over several weeks. When you get down to just one sugary drink a week, keep it in the refrigerator and put a note on the door: "Not till Saturday." After two weeks, the need for that drink will be gone.

Those hidden sugars are very important.

They are the culprits that still block your leptin-to-ghrelin signaling, and as you remove sugar from your drinks, you also need to slowly remove the hidden sugars from your foods. As you reduce your sweet drink consumption, go through your food cupboard each week and remove several items that contain sugar, replacing them with organic vegetables. Applying this consistent and progressive decrease in sugars, especially the artificial ones, will allow your leptin-to-ghrelin signals to connect, completing the cycle and resulting in satiety. **You'll have no more hunger and no more thirst.**

The types of sugars are important here.

Our bodies need glucose (the natural sugars found in vegetables) to function. This is the body's basic form of fuel. In later chapters, we will learn how the body can move easily from burning glucose to burning fat as fuel. The point here is the ability to **recognize, which types of sugars benefit body function and, which do not.** Just keep thinking about bondable versus non-bondable.

Natural sugars (glucose), are found in many foods, and a majority of these sugars (bondable) are found in plant-source foods such as vegetables. Some are found in animal-source foods, such as lactose in milk. Some foods are considered to be natural plant-source sugars and are actually fructose or fruit sugar, found in fruit. This is Mother Nature's desert and should be used sparingly since it is classified as a non-bondable (it does not bond with insulin). The most commonly confused **concentrated fruit sugars** are agave syrup, corn syrup or Karo syrup, and molasses. These concentrated fruit sugars should be avoided completely. Black strap molasses, cane syrup, and crystalline cane are **super-concentrated forms of sucrose or distilled sugars. These will double or even triple the fructose content and should not be a part of any diet.**

Product manufacturers will use all kinds of names to try to convince you that the sugar in a product is 'safe'. When it comes to sweeteners, we usually think of natural products, but name brands can be very deceiving. Please use only the 100 percent pure form of stevia as a sweetener.

There are several brand-name sweeteners on the market today, that only have minute amounts of stevia in them, but they lean heavily on the word *stevia* for sales purposes. The main ingredient in these stevia sweeteners is **erythritol**, a sugar alcohol derived from corn. **It is high-fructose corn syrup in disguise.**

Sugar alcohols are, basically - high-fructose corn syrup, and are not recommended as they defeat the very concept of health improvement. The use of stevia mixes can also be deceiving since they also contain fructose in the form of concentrated grape juice or maltodextrin (a corn-derived sweetener), which is not a recommended form of sweetener. These sweeteners are classified as natural, but caution must be employed here. Most of the market brands (Nuvia, Truvia, Sweet Leaf, Sweet Sensation, Xylitol, Luo Han or monk fruit, and Yacon syrup) contain mainly fructose in various forms and concentrations. **None of, which are classified as bondable forms of fuels, and even though they are natural, they all cause the non-bondable side effects in the liver to various degrees.** They only contain minute amounts of stevia. So, please read your labels and stick to 100 percent pure stevia for a healthier life.

Since the only safe sugar is a bondable one, the sugars found in vegetables are safe.

Organic maple syrup and unpasteurized honey are not fruit sugars and are classified, as bondable. Use them sparingly, especially if you are looking to keep or drive down your weight. We burn glucose first, and we need to deplete all of it in order to burn stored fat (chapter 5). If you pile on the glucose, even if it's bondable, you will not lose your stored fat.

With this teaching you will not count calories, but a basic knowledge of your body's caloric needs may help you in keeping your total intake (including sugars) below that basic number that your body requires for weight maintenance in order to decrease your weight and burn stored fats. You will see this calculation in the chapter on fats (chapter 11) as a tool for adjusting your total fat intake. Read your labels for caloric content and remember that **artificial sugars do not have a caloric value.** They are the most effective way of increasing your weight and waist at the same time (non-bondable). This calculation is only to be used as a general guide if you need it.

If you wish to measure the general caloric need of your body at your present or future weight, use this calculation:

- Women: Your weight (or desired weight) x 3.95 + 825 = caloric limit for that weight
- Men: Your weight (or desired weight) x 5.3 + 879 = caloric limit for that weight

We must also keep in mind that many vegetables are now, genetically altered. **GMO's** (see chapter 19) **are classified, as toxic to the body and non-bondable.** Foods like tomatoes, sugar beets, peas, yellow crookneck squash, zucchini, papaya, corn, some forms of sugarcane, and some forms of honey need to be USDA-certified organic before considering consumption. If any of these foods are a part of the processed food label without the word **organic,** put them back on the shelf.

Soy is not included in the above list.

No one knows if genetically modified soy, once fermented, losses its protein structural changes, which is what makes it even more deadly than organic soy, which is already a known toxin to body function. Dr. Kaalyla Daniel (author of *The Whole Soy Story*) president of the Hunt Gather Grow Foundation and former vice president of the Weston A. Price Foundation (nonprofit nutrition-education foundations) notes; "that no direct toxic symptoms appear to occur with the use of **naturally fermented organic soy**". This is the only form of soy that the body can safely handle.

If the label states **organic** cane or organic table sugar, then small amounts, can be used while removing sugar from your diet. The point here is removing as much sugar (non-bondable) from your diet as possible. We need bondable fuels, but this means vegetables—not breads, cereals, and processed foods that contain hidden sugars. In order to decrease weight, reach to a chosen BMI, improve overall liver function, improve intestinal function, prevent or reverse any or all the problems involving metabolic syndrome, and live a longer, healthier life, we need to start by removing sugar from the diet.

For adults, avoid all processed milk, juice, whey, and whey protein products (see chapter 7). These are not health foods. The liquid recommendation for children is water and raw milk only (no juices). And the recommendation is no fruit for adults and children in the first eight to twelve weeks.

Let's stop here for a moment to look at what we have just learned.

We can plainly see that sugar or non-bondable fuel is the culprit we need to control. Fructose is non-bondable and is found in fruit (Mother Nature's desert). Our bodies still operate extremely well on 20 percent or less non-bondable fuels. If you are doing well and have a weight and waist size that is acceptable (chapter 2), then the consumption of small amounts of fruit is perfectly fine. Eating the whole fruit gives you the added fiber and quercetin that limit the body's absorption of that fructose. If you are ill, overweight, or fighting disease, give yourself time to improve the liver's function (chapter 6) before embarking on the use of fruit. Fruit in its whole form is a powerhouse of vitamins and antioxidants (chapters 17 and 18) and can aid in healing and health improvement, but the liver needs to be at its peak (chapter 6) to handle the fructose that comes along with it. Stick to one piece of organic fruit per day and have plenty of organic vegetables.

Start sifting through all those items in your pantry. **Read all the labels**, eliminate all the sugars, including those hidden in your processed foods, and eliminate all chemical additives and gluten (chapter 7). Avoid breads, cereals, and other processed foods. Eliminate genetically altered foods,

especially corn and soy, and look for USDA organic labels. The USDA is your best protection until the United States has labeling laws.

Thirty-four thousand processed foods in this country (including supplements) have soy as an ingredient. **Soy is not a health food. If it is not fermented soy, don't put it in your mouth.** Avoid all foods that spike the insulin levels (non-bondable fuels) and go as organic as possible, eliminating herbicides, pesticides, and all GMOs.

Stick to a healthier supply of simple, 80 percent bondable foods, no more than twenty-five grams of protein (three or four ounces) in any one meal (chapter10), plenty of fish (wild-caught only) and poultry, grass-fed organic pork or beef (commercial pork is highly contaminated), and moderate-to-high amounts of organic saturated fats (chapter11), including raw nuts and seeds. Cold-processed butter, olive oil, and coconut oil should be your primary oils. Avoid hydrogenated oils and vegetable oils (trans fats – chapter13).

The entire family will be eating healthy foods. There will be no separate meals for other family members. Improved health is the goal—and that goes for the whole family. Once you have reached your desired BMI and waist size, improving your health will be even easier. Your body will respond to the changes you want to make, such as the removal of pharmaceuticals or treatment for chronic disease or infections. Any further diet and exercise adjustments will be much easier.

Now you ask; What about fasting?

In chapter 5, we will discuss the natural ketogenic effect of fasting between 7:00 p.m. and 9:00 a.m. This is a natural fasting period between dinner to breakfast. Studies show an increase in this ketogenic effect when the fast is extended or manipulated. Dr. Krista Varady, assistant professor at the University of Illinois, found a form of fast that she calls "the every-other-day fast." This involves using five hundred total calories of vegetable-based food, which includes forty grams of protein, as a part of a one-day fast. This food, is consumed in the early afternoon and increases the body's drive to utilize stored fats. This results in two short fasts, from 7:00 p.m. to 1:00 p.m. the next day (eighteen hours), then a five hundred-calorie meal, followed by another fast from 2:00 p.m. to 7:00 a.m. (another seventeen hours). The two fasts force the stored fats to be utilized as fuel, resulting in a more rapid and controllable weight loss. This also involves a larger water intake during those fasting periods. Since this fast is done every other day, the normal calorie intake (required for maintenance of body weight), using a vegetable-based diet (bondable fuels only) and healthy foods (fats and proteins), can be used on those opposite days.

This "every other day fast" could be used as a less stressful form of weight loss, but the sugars need to be removed first, including sugars in food and liquid forms. The only drawback to this form of dieting is headaches and initial periods of hunger, but these can be controlled with the use of water and small amounts of coconut oil as used in the ketogenic diet. And remember, you need to remove the sugars first.

Can I lose weight with portion control?

Yes it's true; you can eat small amounts of high-glycemic-index foods and still lose weight. The problem lies in portion sizes. High-glycemic-index foods (non-bondable fuels) **stimulate appetite by causing insulin spikes**. This results in more eating—with an end- result of no portion control.

Studies have repeatedly shown that the uncontrolled consumption of raw vegetables, will satisfy the hunger while still losing weight (chapter 2). Or the use of saturated fats during fasting periods will also satisfy hunger, as seen in the ketogenic diet and the use of 'bullet proof coffee'. (Chapter 5)

When you want that candy bar or super-sized drink, reach for the super-sized salad and a tall glass of unsweetened iced tea. Instead of breadsticks at the restaurant, eat the dinner salad. The entire theory behind this form of eating is the maintenance of a very low insulin level with no insulin spikes. The hunger will disappear—and you will still lose weight. Look for lower-glycemic alternatives (bondable fuels) that can help you reach that self-directed goal.

CHAPTER 4

Getting from Point A to Point B

All facets of health are important, we can change the function of our internal organs just by changing what we eat. We can also change the function of the digestive tract to improve the quality and quantity of absorbed nutrients and strengthen our first line of defense—our immune system—by **what we eat**.

Up to this point, we have concentrated on the internal body functions: the functions after digestion. It is just as important to look at the functions that create actual digestion. **What occurs from the time you put the food in your mouth to the time it actually enters your bloodstream.**

Before we embark on the subject of digestion and its intricate nature, keep in mind that we can consume large amounts of vitamins, protein, and fatty acids, and they will slip through our system without ever being recognized or utilized, if we do not have the proper balance of minerals in our system first. Minerals can supply some function in the body alone, without any other nutrient, **but vitamins, protein, and fatty acids cannot be absorbed or utilized without the presence of balanced minerals.**

Point A: The digestion of Foods

Food digestion begins with the stomach. When we eat, the glands in the mouth secrete enzymes that stimulate the production of hydrochloric acid in the stomach, which is a vital element for the initial breakdown of foods, especially the molecules that bind proteins (the major building blocks of life). Without enough hydrochloric acid in our stomachs, we cannot break down and digest proteins, this leads to a loss of muscle structure and literally every hormone and enzyme formation within the body.

The main components of hydrochloric acid are found in minerals, namely sodium, chloride and potassium.

These elements are the main constituents of sea salt. **Sea salt** is not table salt. These are two diversely different sets of elements. Sea salt is 85 percent sodium, chloride, potassium, magnesium and 15 percent other (trace) minerals, including sulfur, strangely enough, **this is exactly what we**

need and exactly in the right proportions for complete mineral balance of the entire body.

Table salt, on the other hand, is 100 percent sodium chloride with no balance for formation of stomach acids. When consumed in excess amounts, sodium chloride alone will put the rest of the body's minerals completely out of balance, causing a cascade of multiple problems: hypothyroidism, protein deficiencies, gastric disturbances, including constipation and GERD, depression, anxiety, migraines, and insomnia.

We need whole crystal, unprocessed sea salt (grind it as you use it) for proper production of gastric acids. In my opinion, sea salt should be used generously in the diet—with a grinder on the dining table for those who need more. Digestion problems—gas, bloating, constipation, or indigestion—indicate **mineral deficiencies** that will result in not enough stomach acid and incomplete digestion. These problems can easily be corrected with the use of sea salt.

Heartburn and GERD are the result of low stomach acid production (not excess stomach acid). **This is a mineral deficiency,** and the correction lies in the liberal use of sea salt. If these are long-term problems, then the recommend is hair and tissue analysis testing to pinpoint mineral imbalances and correct them. For those who want to use independant testing, go to

33

www.aurorahealthandnutrition.com for testing and consultation on the results.

The acid in the stomach breaks down proteins and fats, and the food progresses into the first portion (first ten inches) of the small intestine (the duodenum). This is where the common bile duct is located, and connects to the gallbladder containing digestive enzymes, waste products, and toxins. The bile and waste products are pushed into the digestive tract by the gallbladder (your toxic waste disposal plant), which is where these products are stored. The presence of fat in the food you eat is the stimulus for the gallbladder to contract. The bile found in this mixture will aid in the further breakdown of fats into fatty acids. The digestive enzymes will aid in the breakdown of proteins.

From this point on, the food is moved or pushed, by rhythmic contractions of the intestine, through twenty feet of small intestine, which is packed with bacteria (three to five pounds worth). These organisms are microscopic (can only be seen with a microscope). Beneficial bacteria —single-cell organisms only visible with a microscope—live off of the environment and multiply by dividing. Bacteria function only in large groups, performing specific tasks in large numbers or colonies.

Researchers at Princeton University recently learned that bacteria communicate with each other (quorum sensing) to work as a functional group. It has been estimated that, at any time, your body has ten trillion bacterial cells in or on you. If you compare this to the simple fact that your body is composed of about one trillion cells, then this means that, for every single cell in your body, at least ten beneficial bacterial cells are helping keep it alive. You could also look at it differently and say that the body is more bacterial than human. Either way, bacteria plays a primary role in our very survival. Beneficial bacteria have been lovingly called "your invisible body armor." These bacteria are found in your small and large intestine, which is approximately twenty-six feet long. **This is your fermentation plant, and it is the most important part of digestion.**

Now you ask; what do they do and how does it work ? ?

Without using the mechanics of microbiology, we can say the bacteria on your skin prevent most infections by keeping out most environmental toxins—as long as the skin remains unbroken. Large numbers of beneficial bacteria

inside the body also prevent the growth of harmful bacteria .
These large colonies can prevent toxins from getting past the intestinal wall.

The bacteria break down your food by fermentation (by literally eating the food) and produce absorbable nutrients (vitamins, fatty acids, and amino acids). These nutrients give each of our cells strength and structure, provide the basic elements for all hormone production throughout the body, and facilitate continued healthy function of all of our organs. Other benefits of beneficial bacteria or probiotics include; milk digestion and the production of lactase (bondable milk sugars), the production of intestinal antibiotic action in the form of acidity that prevents pathogenic growth (kills bad bacteria), anti-carcinogenic (anti-cancer) effects that prevent the growth of intestinal tumors and provide enzymes that help break down and control the absorption of cholesterol and toxic pollutants (keeping the toxins out), and the recycling of estrogen back to the body to aid in estrogen level balance.

At the same time, the bacteria in your gut are extremely sensitive.

They will die if they are exposed to chemicals, toxins, viruses, or antibiotics. The best way to control the amount of chemicals in your intestinal tract is to avoid processed foods and nonorganic fruits and vegetables. This automatically limits the amounts of herbicides, pesticides, and chemicals you eat.

Viruses and destructive bacteria are a problem.

Usually viruses are self-limiting (they die on their own after a short period of time), and the intestinal tract needs to be reseeded with a large colony count of probiotics after the virus has passed. So after the flu, use probiotics. As for bad bacteria , when too many unfriendly bacteria are present, antibiotics are the answer. After you complete a course of antibiotics, you need to reseed your intestinal tract with sufficient quantities of probiotics. Also, the use of steroids (cortisone, ATCH), prednisone, birth control pills, and Splenda (artificial sugar) will damage healthy intestinal flora (killing off the good bacteria). These products need to be countered by routine use of healthy live bacteria.

Recent studies have found that a high favorable bacterial count in the intestinal tract will prevent the growth of unfavorable bacteria (more good bacteria than bad). As a result, new dietary recommendations include the routine use of probiotics in all diets, including fermented foods, and the use of unpasteurized (raw) milk in children's diets.

As your food passes through this fermentation factory, the bacteria produce vitamins, proteins (amino acids), and fatty acids.

This process creates literal bubbles of nutrients that are forced up against the intestinal wall, where they cling, rupture, and eventually pass across its membranes to the blood vessels on the other side (**point B**), which is where bonding occurs with insulin, and those large non-bondable molecules are sent directly to the liver.

When the gas bubbles created by your bacteria press against the intestinal wall, they burst, leaving a film of nutrients on the lining of the intestinal wall. The gas from those bubbles will collect and continue through your system and be expelled. If you are passing gas every day, you know that your bacteria are functioning well (this is a good thing).

Once past the twenty feet of fermentation, your food still contains large amounts of liquefied nutrients and minerals. The last six feet of your digestive tract is called the large intestine or colon. This is where the semisolid and fully processed materials collect; the solid portions of food that bacteria do not break down and the remaining liquid, which still contains some nutrients. This liquid is extracted while in the colon, making the remaining material more solidified (otherwise known as stool or poop). At this point constipation can occur, simply because not enough water is consumed, the stomach or intestines are not functioning properly (sea salt and probiotics), or the products of digestion sit too long in the colon, causing the contents to become dry and hard.

If you are wondering how long is too long, the average meal should only last in the intestinal tract for no more than twenty-four hours. So, what goes in should come out within fifteen to twenty-four hours, be soft, formed, and easy to pass. If you eat three meals a day, you should pass a minimum of two stools a day.

Throughout the small and large intestine, peristalsis or rhythmic, functional muscle movement occurs.

This is the pushing of the digested contents through this system. When peristalsis slows or even stops, then we develop what is called an 'ileus' (otherwise known as intestinal colic). This can result in constipation or an actual bowel blockage, a problem seen frequently in newborns, who have little or no beneficial bacterial development. A majority of these occurrences are a result of pharmaceuticals, especially medications for pain and sleep (including antihistamines), which can pass through the nursing mother's milk. Excessive use of these medications leads to overuse of laxatives (laxative dependence) and bowel stimulants. Developing an ileus can be avoided with proper consumption of water, preferably filtered by reverse osmosis (no chlorine or fluorides). The recommended guideline includes one ounce of water for every two pounds of body weight and daily physical activity. Chapter 12.

This is the perfect reason why -

Babies with colic should be fed water between feedings (keeping the stool in the colon soft and preventing bowel blockage). Mothers, if you breastfeed your babies and take any muscle relaxants, pain relievers, antihistamines, or sleep medications, feed your baby at least two ounces of filtered water between feedings. When necessary, raw cow or goat's milk for babies is recommended (actually raw goat milk is almost identical to human breast milk). All forms of commercial baby formula are not recommended, but if you must use formula and colic occurs, give filtered water. **Never use soy formula.**

When you wake up in the morning, your body is on the dehydrated side.

The body normally consumes fluids during sleep, and this is normal fluid loss. The recommendation here is twelve ounces of water every morning before exercise. The water keeps the stool soft, and the physical activity stimulates peristalsis. If you take medications for pain, depression, antihistamines, or sleep issues, remember to drink extra water during this time—and always maintain a high count of beneficial bacteria in your intestinal tract. For those who have had problems with constipation and slow intestinal function, we will discuss detoxification and cleansing the colon of retained products of digestion in chapter 16.

Maintaining a healthy mineral balance and a high count of beneficial bacteria in the intestinal tract is the solution to many of our health problems—from basic immune defense to malabsorption syndrome (loss of essential mineral absorption through the intestinal wall), protein disturbances (bone and muscle diseases), multiple neurological disturbances, and even tumors.

What Do I Need to Correct or Change?

A majority of intestinal problems and resulting diseases stem from any one, or a combination of three things.

The lack of sufficient mineral balance; (sea salt) for proper gastric acid production, utilization of proteins, and overall body function (neurological as well as hormonal).

Lack of sufficient beneficial bacteria; , healthy active colonies in the intestinal tract allow the complete and proper absorption of nutrients through the intestinal wall. They protect the body from harmful and disease-causing agents (bacterial and chemical toxins).

Inappropriate food consumption The American diet contains excessive sugars of all types, excessive and inappropriate use of protein, insufficient fats, insufficient nutritional value, GMOs, and multiple toxins.

By addressing each of these problems, you can achieve your weight goals and improve your overall health.

First, and foremost, use **sea salt** liberally in your diet. Do not restrict its use like you did with table salt. Your body's minerals are in direct proportion to sea salt, and your body functions best when it is **balanced.** Sea salt comes in several forms. Its best to use the natural, **unprocessed crystal form.** Grind it as you use it. Pick **forms that have color—gray, black, pink, or red**—since the natural mineral content is still there. When it is white, it has been processed and the balance is lost. Use whole crystals to get all the minerals that are found in each crystal. When it is pre-ground, the minerals are separated and the balance is lost. Although you can buy unprocessed sea salt in other forms, its best to use the crystal form and a grinder.

Do not be misled.

Many commercial food companies are taking advantage of the health-improvement movement and sell products that are extremely expensive. Sea salt is not expensive, when purchasing sea salt, buy in **color** and buy in **bulk.**

When it comes to beneficial bacteria, the best forms are found in fermented foods:

- cultured vegetables, chutneys
- condiments (homemade salsa or homemade mayonnaise)

- cultured dairy (yoghurt, kefir, and sour cream—all unpasteurized)
- fish (mackerel and Swedish gravlax)

For those who are interested in culturing or fermenting your own foods, the recommended reading is; *Gut and Psychology Syndrome* by Dr. Campbell-McBride. On the internet, you may use www.immunitrition.com as a reference on cultured and fermented foods. Check www.culturedvegetables. net or www.culturednutrition.com for products to guide you in this venture. With fermented foods, start slowly and build your bacteria count up gradually. Moving too fast will result in diarrhea and excessive gas.

For those looking for something more convenient, probiotic supplements can be used.

Remember, you want live bacteria, and these multiple forms of bacteria are extremely sensitive to heat and trauma. **Any supplement should be cold-processed, freeze-dried, refrigerated or frozen, and preferably in powder form.** Packaging in the capsule form will kill delicate bacteria, and heat (above eighty-six degrees) will kill bacteria. Bacteria will become active and multiply at around seventy-two degrees.

If the bacteria are not in a medium or environment conducive to growth (in a culture or in your gut), the bacteria will live for two to three hours and then die. As a result, many packaged commercial room air products, with no control over heat exposure, are nothing more than dead bacteria.

Some forms of probiotic supplements come with an additive called FOS (fructooligosaccharides), this is a sugar-based medium in which bacteria can grow. Your bacteria have a sweet tooth and readily absorb sugars, which increases their growth rate. Look for FOS that is comprised of stevia, basic vegetable glucose, or trehalose and avoid those containing fructose or Splenda. Fructose is damaging to the liver, and Splenda will kill your bacteria. Splenda (sucralose) does not readily pass beyond the intestinal tract into the body. Other sugars do pass beyond the intestinal wall and into the bloodstream, which results in a wide variety of severe damage to your liver and brain.

The recommendations remain unchanged: no sugars. If you must sweeten your foods, use stevia (100 percent pure, no additives). If you want to add probiotics to your morning shake, do not add them in the blender (it will decapitate the little guys). Gently stir them into your blend mix after pouring into your glass.

Most supplements found on the market today contain lactobacilli (bacteria that colonize the small intestine) and bifidobacteria (bacteria that colonize the colon or large intestine). An acceptable blend of beneficial bacteria is lactobacilli, bifidobacteria, and streptococci. Other bacteria may include L casei, L plantarum, L sporogenes, L brevis, and saccharomyces boulardii. These bacteria should be processed by filtering only, since separation of bacteria by centrifuge or spinning causes damage. Also, they must be cold-processed since the application of heat in the processing of these bacteria into capsule or tablet form causes damage to the delicate organisms. The most effective form of probiotics is powdered and should be available in dark glass containers and refrigerated or stored in the freezer (microorganisms will activate and die within hours of exposure to heat). Other bacteria such as bacillus laterosporus and streptococcus facium are found in smaller quantities, in different regions (large intestine or colon) of the digestive tract. If needed, they may be taken in a capsule of vitamin E or wheat germ oil, which will prevent destruction as it travels to its destination.

The recommended dosage is between one billion and ten billion bacteria per day. Specific bacterial count should be present on the product label. If you use steroids, the dose of bacteria should be above ten billion per day. If you have finished a course of antibiotics, then re-colonizing the intestinal tract should start at fifteen to twenty billion bacteria per day for at least two weeks before tapering down.

Please note that re-colonizing your intestinal tract may cause loose stools and gas for the first few days. This is normal. Discontinue use if the symptoms continue for more than two weeks. It may be an indication that destructive or bad bacteria have over-colonized and overpowered the good bacteria. If this occurs, antibiotics may be necessary to clear the intestinal tract before re-colonizing.

When choosing supplemental products, please read your labels carefully.

If they contain added vitamins (usually derived from corn, a GMO) artificial sugars, wheat, or soy, that you do not need, put them back. If the label does not specify non-GMO, be careful. **Many of today's vitamins are derived from genetically altered foods.** Try to get all your vitamins from natural organic vegetables—eight to ten servings per day. For some, vegetable juicing may be the answer. If you must supplement, use naturally fermented, organic liquid vitamins. Then you get the entire vitamin chain instead of one small link. More about vitamins and what supplements may really be needed can be found in chapters 17 and 18.

Do not be deceived by commercial promotions for yogurt as a probiotic supplement.

Commercial yogurt has insufficient amounts of bacteria in a pasteurized medium (so it can't grow) and contains lots of sugars. It is not a health food.

The remaining chapters will show you the pitfalls of the American diet and guide you in the right direction to create improvement with healthy function throughout the body. We are **changing the way you look at food** by learning how the body's organs function in relation to the use of foods, thereby creating healthier functions. From the use of balanced whole nutrients found in natural foods for efficient, healthy weight loss, to maintenance of strong muscles and healthy organs that function the way they were designed, you can achieve an overall healthier body and a longer life—all without metabolic syndrome.

At Proactive Health, our motto is **"No more medical bills—only vacation bills!"**

CHAPTER 5
Cellular Metabolism

We have reviewed the major points of fuel consumption by the body with bondable versus non-bondable foods. We need to **understand some of the fine points of cellular function**, which is **sometimes referred to as metabolism**, in order to have a clear view of how we gain and lose weight and maintain optimum cellular health.

No chemistry or complicated molecular biology is necessary.

You only need a good understanding of body function at the cellular level.

Previously we learned that fat cells consume the leftover poly-glucose that is not readily used by muscles and other tissues for energy. These fat cells

 (including belly fat) consume the poly-glucose and grow larger—with increased production of fatty acids **inside the fat cell.**

When we exercise -

We increase the tissue's demand for energy (commonly called metabolism). If this is done early in the day (preferably before breakfast) when the body has little or no excess poly-glucose floating around the cells, then the tissues that need energy will force the fat cells (with enzyme signaling) to expel

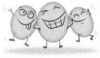

fatty acids, which convert to **ketone bodies** . The healthy cells in your body will consume these ketone bodies as fuel, converting

them inside the healthy cell back to **glucose** . As a result, we obtain fuel and lose weight and fat at the same time, while keeping the cells healthy and functional. If we exercise within that four-to-six-hour window of eating (between breakfast and lunch or before or after dinner), then our bodies

will utilize the remaining **bondable glucose** (excess poly-glucose floating around the cells) that have not yet been consumed by those fat cells. The result of this exercise will prevent increased weight gain, but it will not utilize those ketone bodies that decrease the size of our fat cells (no weight gain and no fat loss).

The use of ketone bodies for metabolism, is recognized by the body as 'starvation mode'.

Since there is no available excess poly-glucose in the tissues at the time, the body responds in 'starvation mode' to produce **ketone bodies**

from fat (fatty acids -from the fat cell) as **a secondary form of fuel** until more poly-glucose can be produced from food consumption. This is a normal body response.

Let's take a quick look at the normal human cell.

We see the lipid bilayer or cell wall, holding inside the fluid or cytoplasm, a nucleus (the brain and DNA), and mitochondria (the powerhouses that produce energy or ATP). The normal human cell is comprised of 50 percent mitochondria, hundreds of them, whereas cancer cells contain very small numbers of poorly functioning mitochondria.

Dr. Otto Warburg MD, PhD is known as the pioneer in cellular metabolism. He discovered the difference in cellular function and the use of fuels. He found that, in the presence of oxygen, cancer cells overproduce lactic acid. This is known as the 'Warburg effect'.

Tom Seyfried, physician and researcher, found that all cancer cells, having fewer and poorer functioning mitochondria, will overproduce lactic acid in the presence of ketones. Unable to release the large amounts of toxic lactic acid inside the cell, it self-destructs from the inside out.

If we take this one step further and replace our processed foods and all non-bondable foods (such as breads and grains) with fats (**only healthy fats**), we can create a continuous mild to moderate ketonic state (**the Ketogenic diet**) with those ketone bodies being utilized instead of glucose for fuel. Healthy cells can easily use this form of fuel, but abnormal or diseased cells (cancer and tumor cells) cannot. When glucose is not available, they die. This is an effective and safe way to stop cancer in its tracks—without damaging a single healthy cell in your body. Healthy fats consist only of organic butter, organic olive oil (cold-pressed), animal fat (beef, poultry from organically grown sources, and wild caught fish), raw nuts, nut meats, nut flours, sesame, walnut, and flaxseed oils (cold-pressed), avocado oil, and coconut oil or coconut cream (organic concentrate). **No vegetable oils**, and remember that **fat does not make you fat—sugars do.** If you would like to look further into this diet, the recommended starting points are; www.metabolicoptimization.com or ketogenic-diet-resource.com. See the charts and graphs section for further references and reading.

Forcing your fat cells to expel fatty acids as ketone bodies and utilizing them as fuel (starvation mode) is a natural body response and is perfectly healthy.

Stimulating metabolism with chemical concoctions and stimulants (caffeine, ginseng, chemical sugars, and herbal concoctions) is dangerous. These forms of stimulus force the body to increase the body functions with increased heart rate and increased neurological activity (commonly seen as a buzzed or wired feeling) without exercise. This increases the drive for large amounts of ketone bodies that cannot be rapidly consumed (metabolic ketoacidosis). At this point excess poly-glucose has not been completely consumed. If the muscles are not active as in exercise, they have no need for the rapidly developed, overwhelming amounts of ketone bodies that are present. The blood PH (acid-base balance) will rise (ketoacidosis), and the high amounts of stimulants present in tissues will result in damage to muscles and blood vessels. This could result in strokes due to elevated blood pressure, heart damage, and even cardiac arrest (heart attacks and death). The advice here; **no artificial stimulants—just mild to moderate exercise.**

Our bodies will continue to lose weight and not regain it as long as we eat bondable fuels.

As soon as we consume non-bondable fuels, we put that lost fat right back into those fat cells (yo-yo dieting). It is important to understand that we need to change the way we look at food since **this is a lifestyle change.**

People in the nutrition and fitness fields teach 'calories in, calories out' as a form of decreased calorie consumption and increased exercise to lose weight. They don't pay attention to the types of foods consumed—only the caloric content of those foods. This form of dieting works by building muscle, which increases the body's demand for fuel. By building muscle, you will gain weight, and that muscle requires even more fuel just for maintenance (thus more food). This form of dieting does not address metabolic syndrome since this diet still uses non-bondable fuels. The most important fuel that is emphasized here is **protein, which is actually not a fuel**. It is a building block for hormones and tissue structure (see chapter10). **The inappropriate use of protein can be <u>very dangerous</u>.**

We must remember that the body burns fuel in three steps.

First, it uses all available glucose. Once that is gone, it will burn all available fat (ketosis). Finally, it will burn protein, but it will not burn protein until all ketone bodies are utilized. This form of metabolism is only seen in extreme sports and extreme bodybuilding. Most people never exercise enough to force their bodies beyond ketosis (this involves extreme work, the results of, which can be dangerous). These people (extreme sports and body builders) require healthy protein replacement to correct **tissue damage.**

If you use 'calories in, calories out' with non-bondable fuels, calorie counting, and exercise, then getting to your goal will take longer and be twice as difficult. It's like running up the hill to get to the store on the other side, rather than walking around the hill in less time—with less effort, and you still achieve your goal (getting to the store). Additionally, you cannot see the muscles you are working on since they are covered in fat. Avoid weight-resistance training. Only do mild to moderate exercise (cardio), and do not build muscle until after you have removed the fat. Remove the fat first. And do not use non-bondable fuels to build that muscle, which includes corn, whey, gluten, wheat, soy.

With bondable versus non-bondable, you have just learned that **it's not the calories that truly make a difference but rather the type of foods.** If we eat bondable fuels, our caloric intake dramatically drops since vegetables have a very low caloric content and a low glycemic index (the sugar index used by most diet formula companies). Non-bondable fuels in the American diet generally have a high caloric and glycemic (sugars) index content. They also

spike insulin, which induces continued hunger and fat storage, generating the production of by-products directly associated with metabolic syndrome. A diet that only limits caloric content and still uses non-bondable fuels will not succeed. The weight will return, and metabolic syndrome will remain unaffected (ergo; the skinny diabetic).

Now let's put it all together.

If we consume bondable fuels at 80 percent or higher (20 percent or less of non-bondable fuels), we will **automatically** utilize 'calories in- calories out',

without ever counting a single calorie. We will lose weight at a higher rate because the leptin and ghrelin signals will complete—and satiety will be achieved after each meal. With fewer calories consumed (with bondable fuels), this leaves less excess poly-glucose to be stored in fat cells. And with consistent, simple, twenty-minute exercise each morning before breakfast, ketone bodies will be produced and fat cells will decrease in size. **This is not just weight loss, it is fat loss.**

When anyone is considering illness, the cancer factor must be included. When looking at the hundreds of cases of full ketosis (80–90 percent healthy fat diet) as part of a treatment for cancer, most of those cases cited were cancer-free in four to six months. The time it takes for sick cells to die and are eventually replaced by healthy growth from stem cells. Not enough studies have been completed to see a comparison for health when stem cell cancer is involved. This is an area in cancer studies that has yet to be fully researched. The present theory is that the longer the ketogenic diet is maintained, the risk of cancer reoccurrence shrinks. That being said, if cancer is not yet present, then a bondable versus non-bondable diet will help you to achieve the weight you want and sometimes even reverse the problems that come from metabolic syndrome including the risk of cancer. This will keep you healthy for the rest of your life.

CHAPTER 6
It Takes a Community

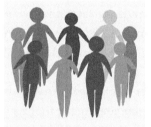

The most important organ in the human body!

It's sad to say, but we take the function of the human body for granted.

Stop and think?   **What is the most important organ?**

You cannot live without your heart or the basic functions of your brain, but there is one overlooked organ, that actually regulates and **maintains function of all the other organs**, including the heart and brain.

The Liver —

Otherwise known as; the largest gland in the human body. This particular organ is second only to the human brain in function. While the brain performs thousands of different functions daily, the liver performs at least five hundred complex functions on a daily basis. The liver is a large, highly - vascular organ with huge arteries that feed into it. And equally large veins that feed into the other organs of the body.

Now you may ask; Where is it located and how big is it?

Let's stop and do a little exercise here.

Hold your right hand out in front of you and cup it slightly. From your wrist to your fingertips is approximately the size and shape of one lobe of your liver. Anatomy tells us that we actually have five lobes, but three of those lobes are small. They are under the right lobe and are equal in size to one cupped hand. Cup your hands and layer one on top of the other (three lobes), right hand on top and then again on the bottom. With that third hand under the right side, this is equal to the size and shape of **your liver**.

Your hands, and your liver – this means that each individual can use his or her hands as an approximate measuring tool for their own body organs. A newborn baby will have a liver equal to the size of three of its own cupped hands. A newborn's liver is quite large since its hands are large in comparison to the rest of its body. The average adult liver is six to seven inches thick and eight to nine inches long.

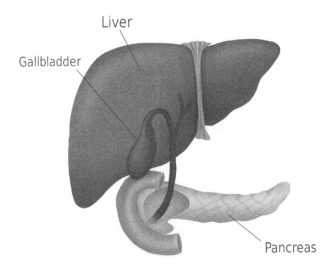

Make a fist with just one of your hands. That's the size of **your heart**—from the wrist out. It is not very big. People with bigger hands have bigger hearts. The hands are good measuring tools for organs.

While your hands are still cupped, stick out your right thumb at the bottom, from wrist to thumb tip. This is the approximate location, size and shape of your pancreas. That all-important organ produces insulin. It is not very big. The adult pancreas measures approximately five to six inches long and one to one and a half inches wide. Also in the same area, under the liver, is the gallbladder. The small sack is much like an inverted balloon and can inflate and deflate. It is about the size of your thumb (when deflated). Think of it as the storage container for toxic waste disposal from the liver. We will discuss this organ in more detail in later chapters.

The liver is, literally held in place by a large ligament that straps the organ to the back (posterior) abdominal wall. It sits under your right lower ribs with the diaphragm (muscle for breathing) and the right lung above, and the intestinal tract below.

The liver is an extremely - vascular organ. Large vessels run through it from the intestinal tract to and through the liver and exiting to the main circulation. **It is the first stop for all elements that are absorbed through the intestinal tract,** giving the liver a chance of filtering out and removing toxins and unwanted materials before they reach the rest of the body. Bondable fuels (bonded to insulin) have their 'get-out-of-jail-free' cards already punched so this nutrient goes straight to the cells. Unfortunately, the 'modern diet' has more chemicals and toxins than the liver can handle. Much of it slips past as the liver as it works hard to capture all non-bondable foods, unwanted proteins, and chemicals (including pharmaceuticals and direct toxins) for processing.

The liver is a great processing plant; that handles the breakdown of nutritional elements from proteins, fats, and sugars. It also manages the production and regulation of functional hormones, not just reproductive hormones, but those hormones necessary for tissue development, energy production, metabolism, brain stability and function, and so on, including all facets of body function, right down to regulating the volume, viscosity (thickness), and temperature of the blood.

The liver is also known as our toxic waste disposal plant. It attempts to break down chemical wastes and shuttles those waste products to the gallbladder, the kidneys, or the skin for excretion or disposal. Without this vital function, we could not dispose of toxins that manage to get past our intestinal tract and into the body. From a nutritional standpoint, we need to understand the how and why involved in the production of nutritional elements and toxic waste disposal.

Please remember; there is no 'magic bullet' that can improve your health.

No single supplement or pharmaceutical will ever return your body to

good health. It takes a community! The body must function as a whole—in conjunction with the type of nutrients you feed it. **Every element—vitamins, minerals, proteins, fats, and bondable fuels—must work together to create better health.**

So, let's connect the dots.

If the liver is the most important organ in the human body, then why do we abuse it? The American diet is literally toxic to the human liver. Some people say, "My liver is fine. I'm not sick, and my chemistries are normal. I'm okay, right?"

Wrong!

Think of the liver as a food processor that we overload on a daily basis with non-bondable fuels. The blade can only move at one speed, but we cram as much into it as possible. The blades continue to move even though the volume of fuels and toxins keeps increasing. When the blades begin to slow, the processed return becomes a thicker, unusable sludge, but that processor continues to function. The liver will continue to struggle to give the body the necessary raw materials, in proper balance, for continued function of the entire body—until the blades finally stop. In the meantime, other organs become affected, and the slow process of metabolic syndrome develops.

If you eat the modern American diet, you are causing unseen damage that will persist for years before you ever realize you are in trouble. If you are only slightly overweight, then the signs of trouble have just begun to show. Unfortunately, these signs are generally ignored until actual chemistries begin to change, usually just before those blades stop, or other organs begin to show damage.

So, what causes those blades to slow down?

If you have completed the chapter on bondable versus non-bondable fuels, then you understand that part of the problem is a lack of ghrelin production in the brain due to free insulin blocking leptin absorption. The result of this scenario is hunger, more food, and an increase in production of all the unwanted by-products, including more belly fat, which slowly increases the weight and pressure placed on the liver.

The liver sits in a fairly restricted area, it is confined by the diaphragm and the rib cage from above, and the twenty-six feet of intestine from below. It has a little bit of 'wiggle room', but increasing the volume of belly fat that surrounds and protects it, adds pressure that decreases the vascular flow through the liver and slows its overall function. Unprocessed toxins that can't be captured by the overburdened liver will continue to float throughout the body in the circulating blood, causing slow, untold damage (weakness, pain, functional damage, and even cancers) in other organs.

New exercise; what happens if you sit on your hand for a few minutes?

The compressive pressure to the tissues causes a loss of circulation, and the fingertips start to turn blue, due to loss of oxygen to the tissues. The signals from the nerves diminish (numbness), due to compressive pressure. The hand becomes blanched (little or no circulation), and movement and sensation are difficult and painful. If this pressure is allowed to continue, the tissues in the hand will begin to die, and sensation and movement will cease to exist. *You can stop sitting on your hand now.* This is the same problem that we see with increased 'belly fat' and increased compressive pressure to the liver. The processor blades slow—and you lose many of the five hundred vital, complex functions that keep you healthy, but you need every one of those functions to give the rest of the body good function.

Remember those five hundred different complex functions?

How many of them begin to fail long before we notice? Hormone imbalance, thyroid problems, depression, renal failure, loss of muscle strength, slow healing, failure to heal, infection, skin lesions and skin reactions, osteoporosis (mal-absorption syndrome), bone and muscle growth disturbances, and cancer are typical problems that we fail to associate with liver function. **The liver is of primary importance in the stable function of all other organs!**

We simply take a pill for the symptoms, and we never correct the real cause of the problem: **what we eat!**

Although the liver was designed to handle small amounts of non-bondable fuels, in the form of fruit sugars (fructose), it was never designed to handle the chemical breakdown of 80–95 percent non-bondable foods, which is what the American diet provides. The liver's main functions are toxic waste disposal and the formation of compounds used for organ and tissue function. When the liver is overwhelmed with excessive amounts of non-bondable foods, other functions within the liver will decrease to the point of destruction.

Added to this process is the increased production of toxic by-products (lactic acid, VSLDLs, and glycogen—a closed molecule) from processing those non-bondable fuels, which results in symptoms of metabolic syndrome. This is a long and slow degenerative process, that goes largely unseen for many years. The symptoms are sometimes not connected to liver function, but they are a distinct part of those five hundred other functions the liver performs. Do you really have a thyroid problem—or is it early stages of metabolic syndrome? Chemistries will **not** tell you the answer to that question, but **your weight and waist size can.**

Let's compare this to the reaction we see with large amounts of alcohol consumption.

We know that someone has a problem with controlling alcohol consumption since it also affects brain function with confusion, disorientation, and lack of motor function. We also see the slow and direct damage that becomes alcoholic liver failure. Large amounts of alcohol (a non-bondable sugar), ingested over a prolonged period of time will result in direct and distinctive liver failure, which can be seen in blood chemistries.

The prolonged use of non-bondable fuels will also result in metabolic syndrome or syndrome X, and liver failure, **but blood chemistries will not be elevated, until after diabetes, hypertension, and renal failure have already arrived.**

So, what does the liver need?

In short,   the liver needs a reduction in non-bondable fuels. For some people, this means consumption of only 5–10 percent non-bondable foods. For others who are very sensitive to these types of foods, it means no non-bondable fuels for at least six months, or until healthy liver function begins to return (usually after at least a twenty-pound weight loss).

We know how very important the liver truly is, but there is something marvelous about this organ as well. With as much damage we place upon it, once we reverse that damaging process, the liver will actually regenerate and heal. With a little help, it can return to near normal function—provided we haven't stopped the blades completely before we make those dietary changes.

One added note, for those who want to make significant health changes (reversing hypertension and type 2 diabetes, improving cholesterol balance, or improving cardiovascular function), **you will not succeed until your liver returns to near normal function.** This means weight loss with a BMI and waist measurement within acceptable range. Go to chapter 3 to set your goals. Give your liver a chance to do what it was designed to do. Use 80 percent bondable fuels (some people may need as much as 95 percent). Start with bondable versus non-bondable teaching, and change **what you eat.**

It's time to change the way you look at food and change your life!

Start the program, eliminate sugars (chapter 3), use bondable fuels only, and rebuild your liver's health by reducing compressive pressure on your vital organs. The liver is the only organ in the human body that will heal itself over time, and the end- result will be improved overall health, better tissue function (including the brain), no diabetes, no hypertension, and no metabolic syndrome. Once the compressive pressure is gone, the ability to rebuild with healthier foods will result in a longer, stronger, happier life.

Once your liver has improved, your body will respond to the changes **you want to make**, including the removal of pharmaceuticals and treatment for chronic disease or infections. Any further diet and exercise adjustments will become much easier.

CHAPTER 7

What Is Wrong with These Foods?

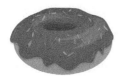 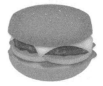

The knowledge you gain from this book will empower you to change your life and improve your health, but **your own actions truly give you that power.** When there are advised changes in the way you look at food, you need to know why. Why eat this and not that? Do I avoid or just eliminate—and how do I do that? And what is wrong with these foods?

Let's start with eliminating sugars from your diet.

Science has found that a persistent, elevated insulin level is one of the main causes of obesity, hypertension, and diabetes in this country. The use of fructose and sucrose in your diet will predispose you to metabolic syndrome (syndrome x), obesity, diabetes, heart disease (high blood pressure), and renal disease. **These sugars speed up disease by maintaining multiple insulin spikes long after your meal should have ended.**

Our bodies need glucose, which comes from vegetables and unrefined grains. Persistent insulin spikes come from excess fruit sugars and man-made or chemically derived sugars such as HFCS (high fructose corn syrup), sucrose, and artificial sugars. If we look at the glycemic index (charts and grafts), we notice that fructose, sucrose, and other fructose compounds have significant readings, which normally would indicate an insulin spike, but these sugars do not bond with insulin. **These forms of sugar (fructose compounds and artificial sugars), are only metabolized by the liver, and additional insulin spikes occur after the glycogen is produced by the liver (about one hour later).** These insulin spikes can be termed **secondary spikes** and they are the most damaging to your health since they block your ghrelin response from your brain that would normally stop hunger. As a result, your body believes you are starving—and you keep eating. The artificial sugars used today are synthetics or chemical foods that cause irreparable damage to the body directly.

If you look at the labels on the products in your pantry, you will find that 90 percent of them have one or more forms of toxic sugar in their ingredients. If your goal is to improve health, then eliminating these toxins must be your **first move.** Then start by removing sugars from your diet (chapter 3).

Other foods that cause persistent insulin spikes are refined grains, gluten, whey, and the heavy starches found in potatoes and white rice (non-bondable fuels). Let's take a look at each to see why the foods that used to be so good for us are not so good now.

Refined Grains

Fifty years ago, bread was baked with whole milled flower with no additives or preservatives. Today, bread and all forms of foods that contain grains are refined or processed. The grain is chemically separated with bleach and bromides, and the bran and germ are removed, which strips the grain of all its nutrients (most of, which are natural B vitamins and minerals). The vitamins are reintroduced by using synthetic or chemical forms. So; now we have added toxins, and to tip the scales, these products need to have a viable shelf life. Since breads fifty years ago only lasted two to four days, we now add chemical preservatives. Oh goody—more toxins! The bread found in fast-food hamburger buns lasts more than a year on the shelf. If they don't naturally deteriorate, how does your liver handle breaking it down?

Another problem with the use of wheat and barley flours.

These grains are now harvested under a method that has become popular in the past fifteen years. It's called **desiccation**. This is a process by, which the grain, just days before harvest, is literally soaked in an herbicide (the most popular is Roundup). This forces the grain to release more seed, thereby increasing the yield of the harvest. The problem lies in the herbicide that soaks into the grain and **cannot be removed.**

The main ingredient in Roundup is glyphosate, which is routinely found in wheat and barley products like breads and cereals. As a result, all products made from these grains contain an additional toxin: the herbicide glyphosate. Science tells us that herbicides in the intestinal tract of humans will alter the structure and function of beneficial gut bacteria (see chapter 20). This will destroy the bacteria's ability to break down proteins and release vitamins and minerals for absorption, causing malabsorption syndrome and a wide variety of health problems, including celiac disease. And as we eat ever-increasing quantities, this toxin can cause additional direct damage to the intestinal wall. Recently, glyphosate has been classified by the CDC (center fo disease control) as a possible carcinogen (stimulates cancer). Keep this in mind when eating grains. **With every bite of bread or cereal, you get a tiny dose or Roundup, and this will continue to accumulate. At present, there is no known way to counter the cumulative toxic effects.**

The goal is to improve total body function, which means the elimination of all toxic materials. Like a car engine, it will not run well if there is still sugar in the tank. Evidence shows that the use of refined grains results in far more negative effects on the body than those that may be positive. For this reason, the elimination of refined grains in the dietis advised. This goes for adults as well as children. Bread products, should be made at home with organic wheat or non-grain flours only.

Wheat, oats, barley, sugarcane, rice, seeds, dry beans, peas, sweet potatoes, and sugar beets are also processed with herbicide desiccation, which is another good reason to only use organic.

Gluten

Refined or unrefined wheat, rye, and barley grains produce a protein known as gluten, which further compromises the use of grains in foods. Gluten, has been found by researchers at the University of Maryland and Cornell University to be the trigger for the formation of allergenic reactions that appear to center in the gut. This allergic reaction is called **celiac disease.** These reactions have been further classified as autoimmune response because, an antibody is formed by the body to attack the gluten that clings to the intestinal wall. This causes damage to the intestinal wall and a cascade of resulting diseases: irritable bowel, impaired nutrient absorption (malabsorption syndrome), osteoporosis, multiple vitamin deficiencies, and a variety of neurological disorders (ADD, ASHD, Autism) occur, especially in children. Research at the University of Maryland has also found that untreated celiac disease is linked to an increased risk of certain types of cancers, particularly intestinal lymphoma.

New studies at these same institutes have found that sensitivity to gluten may be far more encompassing then we had imagined. **It appears that many people sensitive to gluten never show any of the classic gut symptoms, but they will test positive for celiac disease.** Classic gut symptoms include diarrhea, weight loss, constipation, abdominal pain, and bloating.

One out of every 133 Americans suffers from celiac disease. But since symptoms are not always present—and we do not routinely test for the disease in our children or ourselves—the number could be much higher.

If you want to improve your gut function and decrease or eliminate the development of such diseases, gluten should not be a part of your diet. If you wish to be tested, you can ask your doctor for a blood test for the presence of specific antibodies. Since gluten is found in products that already have been compromised with chemicals and artificial additives, the choice is simple. **No gluten!**

Whey? —— No Whey!

This is a destructive approach for the use of protein. Yes, the body needs protein, but the **twenty-five grams** of protein found in meat, fish, and vegetables is more than sufficient for any meal since that **is the maximum load the liver can handle at any one time.**

Whey products in the United States are produced (by law) from pasteurized, homogenized milk. Whole raw milk also produces whey to make cheese. These two products are diversely different. One is alive (raw) and healthy, and the other is dead (you can't make cheese from it).

So What is Whey?

Whey is what's left over after the pasteurization and homogenization of milk. Years ago, the farmer threw it out after processing the milk for the market or fed it to the pigs to make them fat. Blood serum from animals is used to precipitate caseins (whey) from milk to produce lactoserum. It consists of dead white blood cells, dead red blood cells, serum albumin (BSA is a nonspecific protein binder found in blood), dead bacteria, mucus, and residues of bovine hormones, including estrogen, progesterone, and growth hormones (IGF is insulin growth factor).

As the dairy industry grew, the problem of disposal of this waste product increased. Some of this whey was sold to cheese producers who inoculated the product with bacteria to make cheese (not a healthy product). Then someone suggested they could sell this product, since there's protein still found in this waste. So, a marketing program was developed to sell this 'protein-rich' product to the bodybuilding industry. The sales theory was to convince the industry that a high-protein intake (over thirty grams per meal) was a necessary part of a healthy diet. The fact that liver and kidney damage would result with doses over twenty-five grams, was never mentioned. This falsehood of 'high-protein intake' soon became truth, and as a result, a new and rapidly growing industry was developed.

At the same time, the waste material grew. Mass milk production involves the use of chemistry to stimulate larger quantities of milk from the cows. Steroids and growth hormones force increased production along with milking three to five times a day rather than the typical two times a day. The dairy cows developed udder infections, and the frequent machine milking caused traumatic tissue damage and pain. Some cows will actually bellow and even pass out from the pain, which requires antibiotics and large doses of pain medications.

The aggressive use of steroids and increased machine milking caused the formation of large amounts of mucus to form in the milk, as a defense mechanism against the continued traumatic injury (mechanical milking) to the udder of the cow. As an end- result of all this, we now have added to that toxic waste, pharmaceuticals, which include pain killers, steroids, and antibiotics, along with a large amount of mucus. Keep in mind there still has been **no development in science to safely remove the toxins from the whey.** Now, instead of feeding waste materials to pigs, we eat it, Oh, yummy! High-production dairy cows live only six to seven years out of a normal life span of twenty-one to twenty-three years. And pasteurized/homogenized milk fares no better. It has no nutritional value and poses the same health risks.

The consumption of organic, raw, unpasteurized milk and milk products, such as butter and cheese, especially for children is highly recommended. Raw milk contains all the essential nutrients, digestive enzymes, and bacteria needed for basic good health, but it must be organic and raw. Once milk is processed, it becomes pure toxins with no health benefits.

Now let's look at the health dangers of whey.

Unfortunately, whey is one of the main culprits in the formation of allergies, including lactose intolerance, respiratory diseases such as asthma, and multiple nasal allergies. Lactose intolerance can result in loss of energy, diarrhea, stomach pain, cramping, and excess gas.

The introduction of continuous small amounts of antibiotics into the human intestinal tract (found in whey) will weaken the immune system, killing off good as well as bad bacteria, thereby decreasing your ability to digest and utilize nutrients from your food.

It is believed that bovine protein is linked to the development of diabetes, particularly in children. If we ignore the protein, we can find other ingredients in this waste product that are also harmful to the body. Take insulin growth factor (IGF); which, has been indicated in several studies at the University of Illinois to show a significant link to the formation of cancers. Increased concentrations in the body are associated with an increased risk of lung, colon, and prostate cancer as well as premenopausal breast cancer.

Today we find whey protein in a growing number of products—from energy drinks to cereals—but the most disastrous use of this waste product is found in infant formula. Almost every formula on the market has whey protein as an ingredient. If you feed your baby formula with whey, you are giving him or her an overwhelming amount of hormones, antibiotics, and painkillers that could lead to diabetes, abrupt changes in growth and development patterns, slow neurological development, and create cancer. **Mom, please breastfeed your children for at least six months and move straight to raw organic milk (cow or goat) from there.**

What do we see when we look at Whey? **A toxic waste that should never be consumed by the human body.**

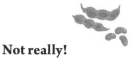

Is Soy the Miracle Cure?   **Not really!**

Let's look at soy (edamame) as a simple basic food. Twenty years ago, soy became a mass-produced commodity, but it had no market. Discovered in

China by an American, soy was a weed that could grow literally anywhere around the world in any soil. It was a bargain-basement bonanza for blockbuster sales by the US food industry. Again, the food industry devised a campaign that promoted the 'protein' found in soy as a miracle cure that fights cancer and reduces heart disease by lowering cholesterol.

Soy was promoted as a health food, was used as a protein additive, and put into 70 percent of all processed foods. It has been estimated, that more than thirty thousand grocery foods contain soy. It seems like soy popped up out of nowhere onto the market, but the industry promoted soy as a 'food staple' that had been used for centuries around the world. The truth of the matter is that **none of the statements made by the industry are true**.

Soy is a weed, that was used by the Chinese in the seventeenth century as a fermented form of spice. It was not a 'food staple'. In fact, it has never been a food staple in any diet—anywhere in the world—until the United States mass-produced it twenty years ago.

As for the miracle cure, let's look at the science.

Soy contains high levels of phytic acid, these levels only decrease with long fermentation (one to two years). The acid prevents the proper use of calcium, magnesium, copper, iron, and zinc in the body. This leads to malabsorption syndrome, osteoporosis, and growth problems, especially in children.

Soy contains phytoestrogens that mimic estrogen hormones in the body and disrupt endocrine function, which leads to infertility, and increase the risk of breast cancer. Ingestion of multiple soy-containing products can cause female sexual traits in males. These phytoestrogens also act as anti-thyroid agents, disrupting the thyroid's function and leading to hypothyroidism (severely low thyroid; seen as weight gain, low metabolism, and insulin spikes) and thyroid cancer.

The vitamin B12 found in soy cannot be absorbed by the human body and it actually increases the need for vitamin B12. Trypsin found in soy interferes with the digestion of proteins, and in animal studies, it causes stunted growth (see chapter 19).

The processing of soy actually destroys most of the protein that is promoted as so valuable. This processing also creates lyssomanine (a highly carcinogenic nitrate) and glutamic acid or MSG, which is a potent neurotoxin and appetite stimulant. Together they create multiple neurological diseases, including ADD, ASHD, autism, Alzheimer's, and a variety of cancers involving the nervous and reproductive systems.

And finally, soy contains high levels of **aluminum, which is a known toxin to the nervous system and the kidneys.**

In conclusion, soy is not a food staple. In fact, soy is a **pure toxin**

that should never have been introduced into the American diet. Unfortunately, it is spreading around the world.**There is no intrinsic value to the use of soy in any diet, including animal diets.** The saddest part of the soy story lies in the fact that we feed enormous amounts of this toxin to our children, starting from the day they are born.

Mothers, if you feed your baby soy formula, you are giving him or her a dose of female hormones—equal to four to six birth control pills a day. You will change their sexual and neurological development and start them on their journey toward autism, multiple neurological dysfunctions, and even cancer. **Please breastfeed your babies for the first six months and move straight to raw organic cow's or goat's milk from there.**

This story has become a nightmare (see Chapter 19).

White Potatoes and White Rice

These foods cause an insulin spike, and are classified as non-bondable since the breakdown of these foods in the liver causes the formation of glycogen (the closed molecule). For years, these types of foods have been classified by nutritionists; as empty calories, because they provide little or no nutrition to the diet—and almost no usable poly-glucose for cellular energy. They spike insulin levels, which results in a free flow of insulin in the body and blocks the reception of leptin in the brain, so ghrelin cannot be produced. And we have learned, that wthout ghrelin to shut down the stomach, we continue to feel hunger and eat.

These foods are now genetically modified (GMO's). So, white rice and potatoes are out.

The target is keeping your insulin levels low. All of the foods previously mentioned in this chapter, cause unnecessary and uncontrolled spikes in the body's insulin levels, which is the primary cause of metabolic syndrome or syndrome X. **If the goal here is weight loss, weight control, and lower blood pressure, then these foods should not be a part of your diet.**

In conclusion, a healthy diet consists of simple, straightforward foods, meat, and vegetables. Mediterranean people have known this for centuries; they are some of the healthiest people in the world. A healthy diet is designed to keep insulin levels low, eliminate toxic substances (no sugars, refined grains, gluten, soy, white rice, or potatoes), improve your overall health, eliminate obesity, lower blood pressure, eliminate pre-diabetes and diabetes diagnosis, and ultimately put you in control for a longer, healthier life.

CHAPTER 8
Bits and Pieces

In previous chapters, we have discussed the role that diet has on our body responses, including the liver and brain. There are also automatic responses in the nervous system that we cannot control directly.

Previously, we noted that the hormone leptin accumulates in the brain, causing uptake or absorption into the hypothalamus and the automatic formation of the hormone ghrelin, which is a direct stimulant to the vagus nerve to shut down the stomach.

The Vagus Nerve

This is actually a bundle of nerves; **that do not exit the brain through the spinal cord.** This bundle involves ten cranial nerves, which branch out and enter the face and neck. The tenth nerve (the vagus nerve) travels down the core of the body, touching or connecting to the throat, the lungs, the heart, the esophagus and stomach, the diaphragm, the spleen, the kidneys, and the digestive tract. Often referred to as the longest nerve in the human body; in Latin, **vagus** refers to wandering, hence the wandering nerve. It's true that this branch of nerves serves as sensory (sensation or feeling) as well as motor (motion or action) in function, but pressure stimulation from either end of the tenth cranial nerve (the vagus nerve) will automatically slow down whatever organ it branches to. So we can also call it the slow-down nerve.

For instance; we go out for a night on the town, eat and drink a little too much, we may find ourselves praying to the porcelain god. Nausea and vomiting cause pressure stimulation to the vagus nerve, which attaches to the stomach wall. This stimulus travels to the heart, slowing it down and causing a distinctive drop in pulse (slower heart rate) and blood pressure (decreased blood flow). With decreased blood flow to the brain, we pass out. Once the stimulus is gone (and we stop vomiting), the body recovers without difficulty. In other words, **this is a normal response. Problems arise when you hit your head on the way down after passing out.**

We already know that ghrelin stimulates the vagus nerve to slow the stomach down.

This is a **chemical response.** The inner lining of the stomach wall consists of cells containing ghrelin, which has a similar, but not identical structure to the ghrelin formed in the hypothalamus. Science has shown that these two elements **are attracted to each other, but they do not stimulate each other.** Ghrelin from the hypothalamus only stimulates the vagus nerve. This stimulus is specific to the stomach and slows it down since there is an attraction to the ghrelin in the stomach, but it does not stimulate the ghrelin in the stomach directly. That is the job of the salivary glands, which results in the production of hydrochloric acid. That is why we call ghrelin the hunger hormone. **Vagus nerve stimulation is chemical in nature, and each chemical stimulus appears to be specific to special organs.** The stimulus from ghrelin will slow down the stomach, but it will not slow down the heart.

When pressure is applied to the vagus nerve.

That pressure will cause the same stimulus to travel along the nerve root from either end of the nerve. Severe constipation, an extremely full bladder, or bearing down or rapidly emptying either organ (bladder or bowel) will also cause the same result: a decrease in pulse and blood pressure from a slow heart and a loss of consciousness.

We can take advantage of this automatic stimulus in cases that involve rapid heart rate, which is seen in atrial fibrillation. In the emergency room, the doctor can apply carotid massage with direct manual pressure to the vagus nerve in the neck. Again, this causes the heart to slow and—hopefully—the return of a normal rhythm.

Now you ask; Why should you know this?

First of all, everyone needs to know that **there are some instances where loss of consciousness is not a life-threatening condition.** If you get lightheaded, dizzy, or pass out in the middle of the night after emptying a full bladder or passing excessive constipation, as long as you have no adverse cardiac history, you are not overtly dehydrated (your pulse is not rapid), and you have sustained no injuries, just remain on the floor and slowly recover. If you don't improve over fifteen to twenty minutes, then call 911.

Second, we are reviewing basic body function—not just in relation to food but as a way for you to understand and follow what your body is telling you.

The vagus nerve (tenth cranial nerve) belongs in a bundle of nerves that has no connection to the spinal cord and the nerves that run from the spinal cord to the body. This bundle of nerves or branch starts midbrain, just below one of the ventricles (a vessel that manages fluid pressure in the brain). The vagus nerve (tenth cranial nerve) runs down the core of the body, connecting to all the vital organs.

We can control the nerves that transcend the spinal cord, that manage musculoskeletal or muscle and bone response throughout the body, including the respiratory tract and breathing. But the tenth cranial nerve (vagus nerve) **is part of a separate branch of nerves that is not under the brain's direct control (you cannot control its functions).** This is why people who suffer from neck fractures and spinal damage can eat, move facial muscles, digest food, and maintain organ function, but they are unable to maintain muscle control of some organs, including breathing, speaking, or emptying the bowel or bladder. This is good to know when your doctor tells you that your compressed vertebral disc in your spine is the cause of your gastric reflux or heartburn. Now you know that they are not connected.

One final point to keep in mind when listening to your body is that chemical messaging between the nerves for digestive function is **totally independent of brain function.** The salivary glands stimulate the stomach directly, the stomach stimulates the pancreas directly, the gallbladder is stimulated by the intestinal tract directly, and other internal organs can stimulate the liver directly, and so on. **None of these chemical messages needs to originate or go through the brain to maintain function of the body.** None of this is under your control (you can't think yourself thin), **but you can control these automatic functions by controlling what you eat, thereby controlling the stimulus.** When your doctor tells you that losing weight is a matter of willpower, you will know better. It is about what you put in your mouth, and it is not connected to drive or willpower. It's an automatic body function and you control it with food.

Caffeine is a neuro-stimulant as well as a vasodilator, so small amounts of coffee can help clear up your headache and give your brain a wide-awake feeling. It also makes the vagus nerve **hyperactive,** increasing the heart rate, raising blood pressure, which increases kidney function, and stimulating peristalsis or increased rhythmic contractions in the colon. You can pass stool more frequently, your kidneys filter more urine, and you feel invigorated. Once you have created this stimulus, **the vagus nerve will remain hyperactive until the stimulus is completely gone.** And there is such a thing as too much of a good thing.

Neuro-stimulants and neuro-blockers that affect the vagus nerve include;

Caffeine, ginseng, and electrolyte imbalances, including dehydration (including alcohol effect). Included in this category is sugar (non-bondables) because it causes brain stimulation much like an addition, and uncontrolled cravings for food (more sugar) due to a lack of ghrelin via the vagus nerve resulting in hunger. In other words, sugar is a neuro-stimulant in the brain, but not a vagus nerve stimulant. Some street drugs, pain medications and antidepressants will suppress (decrease function) the vagus nerve response. Vitamin B-12 is not a part of this list. B-12 actually stimulates the formation of hormones to maintain a balance in brain function, but it is not a neuro-stimulant.

Now drink four or five cups of coffee, or two double lattes, or heavy green tea, or a few energy drinks, and you will have put your vagus nerve into overdrive.

Your kidneys will continue to function at a high rate, and you will dehydrate. This will cause your already fast heart rate to increase even more in response to dehydration. Now we have a tumbleweed effect going, and even if you are drinking water, your heart will remain accelerated until that stimulus is completely gone. Some people call this 'increased metabolism', but we have already learned that metabolism must have fuel involved. The rapid release of large numbers of ketone bodies without exercise can be dangerous. Remember the body still is burning glucose, this can result in a distinctive increase in the PH levels of the blood (ketoacidosis), which is life-threatening and can only be countered by the presence of glucose.

Adding exercise doubles the risk of a cardiac event.

The heart is still in overdrive when you start exercising, and that exercise rapidly pushes that overdrive to super-overdrive. When you stop exercising, everything should slow and cool down. Instead, the heart is still in 'overdrive'. It's like hitting the brakes in a car and decelerating from ninety miles an hour, to zero, without a seatbelt. You have now entered 'Newton's law', as you continue to travel through the windshield. The same goes for your heart. It's still operating in overdrive, which results in damage. This includes increased frequency of arrhythmias (irregular heartbeats), that can lead to heart attacks and death. Whatever you do, never use neuro-stimulants and exercise, that's just asking for a heart attack. Better yet, **never use neuro-stimulants.** We are learning how to listen to our bodies and create better health, and **neuro-stimulants are uncontrollable and destructive.**

Keep in mind that the sensitivity of the vagus nerve increases with frequent irritation by stimulants.

So after using neuro-stimulants over a long period of time, once you have stopped their use, the **hypersensitive response will remain in that nerve for weeks or even months.** Any trigger—including a cardiac arrhythmia (one out-of-sync beat)—will trigger that hyperactive response. This response may only last a few seconds or a few minutes, but it can also cause that same heart attack.

Now you say; I'm healthy, I have no heart problems, I won't have a heart attack when using neuro-stimulants, right? —

Wrong!

Everyone has the occasional irregular heartbeat, and even the healthiest person can have a heart attack caused by one heartbeat at the wrong moment during a rapid heart rate. Yes! Healthy people have heart attacks! So, don't be lulled into a false sense of security just because your doctor says your heart is healthy.

So now we can see that what we eat or drink can not only control our responses to disease, but our level of fitness internally (healthy organ function). If we follow the bondable versus non-bondable teaching, **we can create the desired responses that will occur automatically.**

The Vagus Nerve

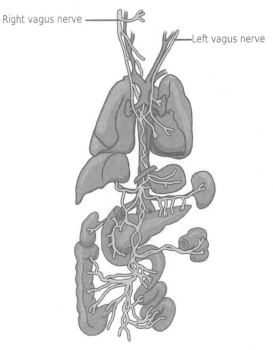

Right vagus nerve — | Left vagus nerve

(Single nerve that connects to every organ in the human body)

The knowledge and research surrounding the vagus nerve and its value are ongoing.

New York University's Langone Medical Center has been running a study on implanted small stimulators of the vagus nerve (in the neck). The stimulator, can be activated and slow or even stop epileptic seizures with minimal effects on other organs.

The School of Behavioral Brain Sciences at the University of Texas in Dallas is using a novel approach to treating tinnitus (ringing in the ears) and its associated hearing loss by stimulating the vagus nerve with sound.

There are clinical trials underway in three countries that are testing the use vagus nerve stimulation to slow the stomach, by bypassing the leptin-to-ghrelin signal and producing satiety in the patient without dietary changes. **This may be helpful, but if the diet does not change, then the metabolic syndrome will remain.**

CHAPTER 9

Tissue Regeneration: How Long Is This Going to Take?

Let's step back and look, we have changed the diet; now with bondable fuels only, healthy fats, minimal healthy proteins and no GMO's, and now you ask; how long will it take for the body to respond and begin to show improvement?

The answer to that question will vary with each person. It really depends on how far down the road you have already traveled to know how much time it will take to get back to where you started. How much damage has occurred? And what needs to recuperate besides the liver? This is precisely where we look. The liver needs to recover first. Until it is back to proper normal function, nothing else will happen.

That brings us to the question of <u>regeneration</u>, what does this term mean?

Throughout our lives, we continually replace cells throughout our bodies that are worn or too old to function properly. These cells die and simply dissolve into the extracellular fluids and are transported out of our system through the skin, kidneys, lymphocytic system, or gallbladder. This includes all cells; in blood, bone, soft tissues, and the brain. **Literally every cell in the body (all one trillion of them) will be replaced, and every organ, including the brain will be renewed every seven to ten years. So, you are not the person you were ten years ago.**

Now for a quick course in Embryology

Embriology;

The study and development of the human embryo; in other words, how our body develops. This is an extremely simplified version of how human embryos develop. It will give you a better understanding of how recovery or regeneration is an integral part of improving your health.

In school, we learned that we all start from one egg and one sperm.

These are both single-cell entities that come together, blend their DNA, and begin to divide. **This is the beginning of your basic cellular structure, and it stays with you for the rest of your life.**

As these cells rapidly divide, they continue to carry the exact same blueprint of the original egg and sperm. These cells form a hollow ball with a single layer of cells on the outside. This ball begins to elongate and fold upon itself, over and over again, forming cavities, organs, and bone structure. Each of these structures has a base layer of **stem cells** that are a part of that original single layer of cells.

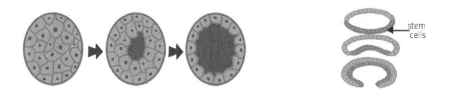

For example; The brain folds into five different cavities. The center of each contains a ventricle (fluid-filled cavity). The spinal fluid, flowing through the ventricle, feeds the base cells (stem cells) the essential nutrients they need to continue to divide and grow. The layer of stem cells is where your new brain cells come from to replace the damaged and dead cells that dissolve back into the fluid bed. **This repetitive process continues for the rest of your life in all of your tissues;** every cell in your body is eventually replaced within that seven to ten year span.

Stem cells in each organ divide and add new layers of cells to the organ at different rates.

The brain reproduces cells every thirty to fifty hours, laying down a new layer of cells every three to four days. The liver grows cells much slower, approximately every five months. Depending on the thickness (layers) of the organ, total cellular replacement of this organ takes three to six years. Most muscles replace cells within four to six months—with total tissue replacement in three to five years.

Keep in mind that bodybuilders develop large amounts of muscle tissue by creating tissue damage that requires structural repair. The elements of this repair come from our food—in the form of cholesterol sulfate and not base stem cells.

Our red blood cells, which are made in our bone marrow (the soft center of long bones), are replaced every three to four months. And the most important to the diabetic is the pancreas, which is the slowest growing of them all. Pancreatic stem cells (beta cells, which produce insulin) reproduce at a rate of every nine to twelve months. This may be the reason why cancer in this organ is so hard to detect. By the time it is detected, this small organ has already lost half of its total cells—or more. There is a new train of thought in the scientific community, with studies showing healthy stem cell regeneration at a higher rate with exercise and fasting, which forces the body to burn fat for fuel.

You now have enough base information in embryology to continue And since we are looking at the recovery of the liver as the first step in total body recovery, it will take a minimum of three months to see functional results. Since each person has a different level of liver damage to deal with, the time can vary, usually from three months to two years. In some cases, it could take up to ten years, depending on the level of illness or disease already present.

When considering illness, the 'cancer' factor must also be utilized.

Ketosis and the ketogenic diet have been found to be effective in the treatment of cancers. When looking at hundreds of cases of full ketosis as a treatment for cancer, most of the cases cited were cancer-free in approximately four to six months. Remember, these are sick cells that die and need to be replaced with healthy growth from stem cells. But at present, not enough studies exist to show a comparison for health when stem cell cancer is involved. There is no definitive science in this particular area since it has yet to be thoroughly researched. But we can assume that the organs involved require even more time for full regeneration, depending on the extent of the damage and the number of stem cells that need to take up the workload or replace, those stem cells that were damaged or lost due to cancer.

Again, considering time factors and illness, we as humans are poorly adaptable when it comes to changes in our environment.

It takes two to three generations for the human body to adapt or evolve (changing DNA structure) to minute changes in our environment (air, water, and food). If the oxygen in our environment drastically increases or decreases, our bodies will either, adapt or die. Fortunately, most natural environmental changes are small and gradual, taking thousands of years, and giving humans a chance to change their DNA and slowly adapt.

As an example; When the earth was formed, thousands of years ago, the oxygen content was much lower. Animal body structure, size, function, and lung capacity were all radically different. As the oxygen content increased slowly, these adaptations also adjusted. When humans came onto the scene, the oxygen content in the air was not much lower than it is now. Today the oxygen in our air is 28 percent. We have slowly adjusted to changes in DNA structure in order to adapt to changes in weather and the presence or absence of food over multiple generations.

Our bodies cannot adapt to environmental changes in any less than three to four generations (about one hundred years), but our biologics (gut bacteria) don't have that problem. The bacteria in our intestinal tracts grow and reproduce at a very rapid rate, with new generations in days instead of years. This gives our bodies a little advantage.

Science has determined, that our biologics are divided into **enterotypes** by the types of foods they utilize or ferment. There are two enterotypes;

prevotella-type bacteria, which ferment (break down and consume) the sugars in food, and **bacteroides,** which ferment (break down and consume) protein and fats found in food.

Our gut bacteria will automatically produce larger colonies of each enterotype, depending on the types of foods consumed.

When we eat only bondable foods, balanced protein, and fats, the majority of enterotypes will be bacteroides, which will produce higher quantities of vitamins and elevated quantities of healthy proteins and fats, which are available for improved body function. This is exactly the enterotype we all need, especially the type 2 diabetic —with less sugar absorption and better sugar control.

Science has shown that this **major shift in gut enterotypes occurs in ten days.** Any dietary changes will take ten days to show active results. A consistent, stable dietary regime will prevent a continuous shift in gut enterotype colonies and prevent digestive problems. The fewer monkey wrenches (non-bondables or sugars) thrown into the machinery, the better the machinery will operate. It makes sense to follow bondable versus non-bondable teaching.

If our bodies are exposed to extreme changes, the effects can be devastating (see chapter 19).

Over the past twenty years, the presence of ever-increasing toxins in our food through chemical additives, preservatives, pesticides, herbicides, and GMOs (genetically altered organisms) has caused structural changes in our DNA. It has resulted in multiple diseases and cancers, **and we can plainly see that we are not adapting!**

These changes are too abundant, aggressive, and fast for the human body to adapt and make the adjustments to maintain health and survival. Some of these toxins (especially GMOs) are causing **direct DNA changes that cannot be undone.** Some GMOs create **horizontal gene transfer** (the alteration of genetic structure of our bacteria – chapter19). When we change the structural DNA of our enterotypes (bacteria), they lose the ability to ferment some forms of foods, resulting in severe vitamin deficiencies and loss of vital fats, proteins, and minerals. These changes in structure will result in disease and cancers. **This is not improved health, and it is not natural human adaptation.**

So now you ask, what does this mean for me?

It only takes ten days for our biologics to form healthy colonies in response to the types of foods we eat, and this is a direct and efficient form of health improvement. However, it still takes three to four generations (about one hundred years) for the human body to adapt to genetic changes. **The changes that are rapidly occurring today are creating disease rather than health.**

We need to step back and look at what supplies our bodies are using.

We need to maintain a toxin-free environment for our bodies and for the biologics that help feed and maintain our health. We need to **reduce or eliminate non-bondable and unhealthy foods**, allowing the bacteria to adjust from excess sugar fermentation to protein and fat fermentation. This includes herbicides, pesticides, chemicals, pharmaceuticals, and GMOs. It will prevent direct DNA damage from these toxins. We need to stop this experiment in toxic evolution; **we are not adapting.**

Keep in mind that the more significant the health problems, the longer it will take to regenerate healthy tissue for overall healthy function. Now we can see that in order to grow and repair tissues, we need a healthy base of stem cells that is nourished by the proper nutrients that are supplied by healthy biologics. If we want healthy structure, we need to pay attention to **what we eat.** Since we depend on our biologics to provide sufficient quantities of healthy nutrients, we must provide them with toxic-free foods as well.

CHAPTERS 10 AND 11
Protein and Fats

(Healthy versus Unhealthy)

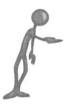 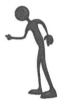

This would be a good time to discuss the last two elements of a balanced diet. We included those normally used for fuel, but tissue formation and maintenance to this point have largely been ignored. Proteins and fats are those elements necessary for this task.

When we discuss bondable versus non-bondable, we are looking at insulin stimulation and its bonds with foods. Most proteins and all fats do not cause direct increase in insulin production, depending on the food (most protein foods contain sugars), so generally, no bonding is present. Both fats and proteins, must be processed through the liver, to become usable by the body. Since these elements do not generally stimulate insulin, we can place them in a new category: **healthy versus unhealthy**. Some vegetables fall into both categories if they contain small amounts of fats, bondable sugars, and protein (healthy). Others contain sugars as well as proteins but are genetically or chemically altered (unhealthy).

Protein by definition; is any class of high-molecular-weight polymer compound composed of a variety of amino acids joined by a peptide linkage (usually sulfur).

Protein comprises 50 percent by dry weight of a cell, remember there are about one trillion cells in the human body (give or take a few hundred). Hundreds of proteins have been identified, and **all contain; carbon, hydrogen, and oxygen**, and nearly all contain **sulfur**. All of these structures are based on twenty amino acids, **eight of which are essential or must come from food.** Without these eight, we cannot form the remaining twelve in the body. These proteins form linkages or polypeptide chains. Formation of each of these chains results in more than one hundred thousand different molecular structures in the human body. These structures involve almost every aspect of human growth, development, and function—from basic tissue formation and repair to the regulatory hormones that maintain that function.

Protein; **'the building blocks of healthy tissue'**, that provides not only structure, but peptides, enzymes, and hormones for the control of growth and cell division, which is necessary for every cell throughout the body. This source of protein is listed in most nutrition manuals as; **histidine, isoleucine, leucine, lysine, methionine and cysteine, phenylalanine and tyrosine, threonine, tryptophan, and valine (valine is necessary for infants and children)**. Methionine converts to cysteine, and phenylalanine converts to tyrosine in the body. These amino acids are available in both animal- and plant-based proteins and cannot be synthesized by the body. They must be found in foods.

The most complete form of protein (containing all the needed amino acids) is found in human milk and eggs.

Healthy proteins are found in organic sources of meat (including fish and poultry), raw milk, whole raw cheese, eggs, beans, peas, raw nuts, organic oats, and brown or wild rice. **Protein can also be used as a fuel—but only when all other fuels are completely gone.**

If the body has burned its available poly-glucose and all available fats, the only remaining fuel is protein. This is seen only in two circumstances.

The first is starvation, when the body literally cannibalizes its own muscles for fuel in order to survive, **and this is <u>extremely</u> rare.**

The second is when the body is forced to use protein as fuel in extreme bodybuilding, which rapidly depletes all available fuels. Please understand that extreme bodybuilding involves aggressive exercise and forced tissue damage for two to five hours every day. This group includes a few professional sports, and these types of bodybuilders are rare. They are not your usual gym enthusiast who pushes weights. Most of the people who use a gym and exercise regularly do not need to increase their protein intake beyond the maximum recommendations of seventy-five grams per day. According to the United States and Canadian Dietary reference intake guidelines; to avoid deficiency, **adult women need to consume a minimum of forty-six grams of protein a day, and adult males need fifty-six grams per day.** These guidelines will vary according to age and activity as well as pregnancy. For instance, a pregnant woman (150 pounds) will need approximately sixty-seven grams per day. A pregnant teen (110 pounds) will need at least sixty-two grams per day, which boils down to **25 percent more protein during pregnancy.**

The easy way to find a balance between the two is to use a simple guideline.

If you are relatively inactive, consume no more than eighteen grams of protein per meal (three ounces of meat, including eggs or fish, each meal, over three meals a day). If you are physically active with mild daily exercise, then you need no more than twenty grams (three to four ounces) per meal. If you exercise heavily, you need no more than twenty-five grams (5 to 6 ounces) per meal. Healthy proteins are found in plants, including legumes (a wide variety of beans, nuts, and seeds). **Whey, corn (a GMO), soybeans (a toxic GMO), and roasted peanuts are all non-bondable foods and** unhealthy forms of protein. These forms of food should not be included in any diet.

Healthy proteins consist of ;

Organic (preferably grass-fed) beef, organic whole raw milk and cheeses, organic free-range chicken (including eggs) or turkey, wild game, and wild-caught cold-water fish and seafood. The goal is to eliminate the toxins that flow through the liver, giving it a chance to recover and become healthier. For this reason, any meat consumed should have no chemical additives (including hormones and antibiotics) and should be free of toxic GMOs (found in most animal feed). At the very least, opt for no added steroids, hormones, or antibiotics in your meats. Be careful when choosing fish. The packaging should read "wild-caught" and not just wild. That is the only way you will know that your fish is not farmed. Also, if it comes from the state of Alaska then it is wild-caught since it does not allow commercial fish farming. **All commercially farmed fish is either genetically engineered or grown with large amounts of GMO feed and antibiotics.**

When we consume protein, the body expects to receive simple amino acid chains with no chemical bonds. The protein found in corn, whey, gluten, soy, and casein are chemically bonded or genetically altered. **These so-called forms of protein should never be ingested by the human body.** Even if you are an aggressive athlete or power bodybuilder, never use these forms of protein to supplement your diet. For extreme bodybuilders, the maximum protein intake (in healthy meat and plant sources only) needs to be calculated according to your type of exercise, and general diet, but an intake of more than eighty grams a day could be dangerous.

Our bodies do not store protein.

Studies have found that our bodies actually break down or use up our daily intake of protein in thirty-six hours because the **nitrogen content** is no longer available for building tissue. So, what you ate on Monday will no longer be useable on Wednesday. Also, proteins act as cholesterol carriers and form enzymes and hormones in the liver. Any excess is funneled through the liver for complete breakdown and disposal through the kidneys.

Let's look at how this takes place.

When we consume **just three ounces of protein,** the hydrochloric acid and enzyme pepsin in the stomach break down the fibers into long chain molecules attached to fats. In the small intestine (duodenum, first ten inches of the small intestine), these molecules are further broken down by digestive enzymes and bile that come from the gallbladder, separating the fat molecules and reducing both chains for further consumption by bacteria. Beneficial bacteria completes this breakdown to a single molecule and very short chain molecules of fatty acids and amino acids (proteins). These molecules pass through the intestinal wall and are sent to the liver. These amino acids (*hundreds of them, remember this came from just three ounces*) **reformulate to form thousands of different structural molecules,** each with a different purpose such as forming sex hormones, new digestive enzymes, and new tissue. These structural molecules are **used by every organ, bone, and tissue in the body—right down the very structure of each and every single cell in the body.**

Now you ask; If we don't store protein, can we just flush out the excess?

Yes, but at the expense of our kidneys, blood pressure, and brains.

We have learned that one of the by-products of non-bondable fuels (sugars) is uric acid (chapter 2). This is the same by-product, that is formulated with the breakdown of **excess proteins,** since protein breakdown uses the same pathway in the liver. The result is damage to the small blood vessels in the periphery (hands and feet) and in the renal tubules of the kidneys (renal failure) and blocked formation of nitric oxide, resulting in elevated blood pressure. Once protein has been used, after thirty-six hours, the nitrogen content is gone. At this point the kidneys can dispose of this form without damage. **So it's the excess protein that still contains nitrogen, which is the element we need to concern ourselves with.**

Recent studies have found that the **loss of nitric oxide** in the circulation will also result in increased platelet activation. Since nitric oxide; is derived or pulled from the circulating platelets in the blood (pulled from the platelets and deposited in the endothelial beds of artery walls and the skin), the body is trying to replenish its supply of nitric oxide. This produces a loss of control of clot formation in the blood (increased formation of blood clots from too many platelets). **In an effort to provide increased nitric oxide for blood pressure control, the body inadvertently increases the platelet count and the formation of clots. This may be the reason why those who take blood pressure medication also need to take aspirin or anticoagulants.**

For this same reason, protein should never be used as a form of energy. <u>Protein is not fuel!</u>

During the disposal of excess protein, this process requires the kidneys to break down the nitrogen in the protein, called **deamonization**, which increases tissue stress and kidney damage since nitrogen is **destructive to the fine renal tubules of the kidneys.**

Free amino acid fragments or Glutamine.

The accumulation of excess free amino acid fragments (unhealthy proteins or excess proteins not yet filtered out by the liver) is seen as glycol-proteins (also known as **glutamine**) from non-bondable foods. Foods that contain sugars and protein (whey, soy, corn, gluten, wheat, rye, and processed milk) will accumulate outside the brain. These proteins are a direct irritant to the arterial walls surrounding the brain (blood-brain barrier), resulting in inflammatory response.

As glutamine creates the **inflammatory response** (irritation to the tissues causes swelling and a separation of the bonds between the cells that form a defensive wall); it can then diffuse across the blood-brain barrier by slipping

 between the cell wall gaps to create a cascade of inflammatory reactions. These reactions, within the brain, will result in multiple neurological problems; seizures (epilepsy), stroke, Alzheimer's, autism, multiple sclerosis, and ALS. **These proteins cause the same response in the intestinal tract, which is known as 'leaky gut syndrome'.**

The result of too much protein is;

Renal failure (kidney failure), multiple forms of neurological damage, hypertension, and coagulation disturbances. This failure can cascade into a litany of other health problems that most physicians never associate with excess protein intake. Such problems include mineral imbalances (especially magnesium), which can cascade into dehydration and muscle cramping, arthritis and joint pain, hypothyroidism, decreased immune response, and even increased inflammatory response.

Since the liver can only handle the primary processing of a maximum of twenty-five grams of healthy protein in any given six-to-eight-hour period, anything over this range is going to increase the liver's workload and result in tissue damage. Even extreme sports enthusiasts and bodybuilders should space their intake of protein (in healthy meat sources only) to not exceed that twenty-five-gram marker (every six to eight hours).

Studies have also shown that the excess protein excreted through the kidneys as uric acid-bonded proteins causes a direct and equal loss of sulfur and vitamin D, which are critical elements in health maintenance. These two elements will be discussed in more detail later.

Fats

Misinformation, and the poor use of healthy fats has led this country in the wrong direction.

When the government decided that this country had to reduce its fat consumption by 20 percent, the unfortunate story of metabolic syndrome started. The food industry took out the fat and replaced it with sugar, and a new nation of obesity, diabetes, heart disease, and renal disease began.

Up until recently, it was believed that the body was composed of fat molecules that came from our food. In other words 'fat makes you fat'. Science has completely turned this theory on its ear. It has proven that the base layers of fat that form your body, line and protect your organs, cushion muscle tissue, and protect and support your very structure has been in place since the day you were born. And these fat cells only increase in size with the excessive consumption of non-bondable fuels (sugars).

Your base number of fat cells never changes.

It can only grow or shrink in size. It's interesting to note that you can surgically remove fat cells from a given area in your body, but those fat cells that are left behind will grow larger with the excess consumption of non-bondable fuels. You will end up with fewer fat cells, but they can grow large enough to replace those that are lost.

The point here is;

The fat in your food, has nothing to do with the actual fat cells in your body, or how you got your spare tire.

Dietary Fats: The Fat in Your Food

The nutrition industry will break fats down into several categories: essential fatty acids, those that must be obtained from foods, and nonessential fatty acids, those fats the body can produce or synthesize from chemical bonds to essential fats. In other words, we need fatty acids.

For a better understanding of fats we use, look to the 'types of fats' as a more concise description of the necessary elements for good health.

Animal Fats

Alpha-linolenic acid (ALA) and saturated fatty acids are also known as omega-3 fats. These fats turn solid at room temperature and consist of animal fats, butter fat, beef fat, and chicken fat. In this category, fish fat, eggs, coconut oil, nuts, and some seeds are included since they have the same physical structure. Generally, fish fat is a combination of saturated and unsaturated fats.

Plant Fats

Linolenic acid (LA) and monounsaturated and polyunsaturated fatty acids are also known as omega-6 fats (plant sources). These fats remain liquid at room temperature and include olive oil (75 percent oleic acid), cocoa and real chocolate, nuts, seeds, sunflower, safflower, sesame oils, avocados, and olives (unrefined and cold-pressed). **Not included are corn, cottonseed, canola (also known as rapeseed oil), vegetable oils, or soy in any form. These are all toxic GMOs and are no longer a healthy form of fat.**

For some strange reason, the health food industry and the medical industry have convinced the general public that omega-3 fatty acids are somehow different. All fats can become a part of cholesterol formation, and healthy fats and sterols (fat cofactors found in vegetables are also known as dietary cholesterol) provide the lipids that become the body's form of cholesterol, which is otherwise known as lipoprotein (chapter 13).

For years, saturated fats (animal fats) have been classified as the 'bad guys' in our diets, but the opposite is true.

We need a variety of fats, including saturated and unsaturated fats, to maintain the essential functions involved in cell structure and transport of nutrients and vitamins throughout the body.

Let's make things even simpler.

Our bodies have a way of simplifying this fat conundrum. Linolenic acid will convert to arachidic acid (unsaturated to saturated). These are unrefined, cold-pressed fats or oils.

ALA (alpha-liolenic acid) converts to EPA (eicosapentaenoic acid), which converts to DHA (docosahexaenoic acid). Each time this conversion is made in the body, the end- product becomes smaller. Only 9 percent of EPA becomes DHA . **As the result of all these conversions, we end up with usable omega-3 fats and saturated fats.**

Think of fats as two sources: **plant and animal.** Since animal meats naturally have a lower fat content—and we generally need to limit protein intake— the use of fats found in plants must also be a healthy part of the diet. This includes organic olive oil, coconut oil, sesame and sunflower oils, olives, nuts, and seeds. Again, use unrefined and cold-pressed oils.

So what does a healthy body really need?

When it comes to fats, we need a balance of **animal source fats to plant- source fats; one to one.**

Now it's time for a little biology; Cell Wall Structure

To understand the function of lipids or fatty acids, we need to look at the actual structure of each of the trillion cells that comprise our bodies.

If we look closely at cell wall structure, we find the lipid bi-layer.

The wall seals out the outside fluids and protects the **cell's contents** where multiple chemical reactions occur and energy is produced. Also where we store our precious **DNA (diribonucleic acid) and RNA (ribonucleic acid),** which contains our genetic code. This particular structure looks a little like an 'Oreo cookie' —two layers of LDL cholesterol (low-density lipoprotein containing fatty acids) separated by a layer of sulfa-bonded protein. The protein binds and holds the layers in place and gives structure to its shape.

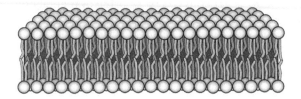

The 'Oreo cookie structure' (cell wall) or the **lipid bi-layer** has two layers of fat held together by a layer of sulfated protein. This cell wall is highly resistant to damage, but it is not completely impervious. The cell wall can be

damaged by **free radicals** . These are elements that float around in the system in an unbounded state. Their outer shell of electrons is out of balance and needs electrons from other elements to become complete, but instead of bonding to other elements (like insulin to glucose), they simply steal electrons to balance their own structure. In doing so, they cause damage to the structures from which they steal, this is called **oxidation**. **Most of the elements in our body must remain bonded to prevent damage to structures by oxidation.**

Remember, in earlier chapters we discussed the formation of type-two diabetes? When bondable glucose is allowed to float free in the system (unbounded means there is no available insulin to bond to it), it becomes a **free radical** and is extremely damaging (**oxidation**) to our cell walls, resulting in symptoms seen in diabetes: peripheral neuropathy (pain and numbness in hands and feet), renal failure (kidney damage), and retinal damage (blindness). **There are multiple elements in the body, that are vital to good health, but if allowed to become free radicals (unbounded), they will cause untold damage.**

If we only look at the individual cells and their needs, we find that each cell needs cholesterol or fatty acids found in LDLs (low-density lipoproteins) to replenish and fortify the cell wall. The inside and outside layers of this cell wall, need to be supported with fresh cholesterol on a regular basis. When an injury occurs, be it inside of the body or out, a large quantity of cholesterol is necessary to heal the area. Think of LDLs or cholesterol as your **internal Band-Aids**. This explains why cholesterol levels rise after an illness or injury. **It is a direct result of the inflammatory response.** It is also **the reason why people with chronic disease always have elevated cholesterol readings. That elevated reading is not a bad thing.**

If we multiply the needs of one cell by one trillion, tack on the need for vitamin transport, and the transport of other nutrients such as CoQ-10, we now have a significant need for **healthy fats** in the diet. Strangely enough, most of those fats are saturated (coming from animal fat) the same place we get our healthy proteins.

When we use the word fats, we must include plant sources.

In our efforts to make foods more convenient, the food industry developed hydrogenated and partially hydrogenated fats. This turns a liquid form of oil (from vegetable sources) into a solid form of oil that lasts longer on the shelf. This hydrogenated oil became known as trans fats (not a healthy form of fat). Initially, it was believed that this form of fat was the same as the trans fats found in butter fat, which found naturally in nature and is a healthy form of fat. Science has shown that these **trans fats** (hydrogenated oils) **form molecules that are not found in nature at all. They are the culprits in the formation of heart disease rather than cholesterol.** It's the type of fat used in the formation of our cholesterol that makes all the difference in our health.

When these hydrogenated and partially hydrogenated oils were first made, they were made from soy oil—and then corn oil was added. Today, a wide variety of oils, classed as vegetable oils, are used to make these solid forms of fat (margarine and soft spreads), and hydrogenated fats replaced lard in baking.

The change in structure of these trans fats actually blocks or prevents the body from forming a balance between **prostacyclin and thromboxane** in the blood. **These two elements have opposing but balancing effects.** Prostacyclin maintains blood flow (think of it as blood thinning), and thromboxane maintains effective blood clotting. With the consumption of healthy fats, these two elements maintain a delicate balance. One thickens, and one thins—maintaining healthy blood flow. When trans fats are present, this balance is lost and clotting occurs—along with heart disease. Today, the use of trans fats as hydrogenated oils is banned in the United States. Caution must still be applied since many oils are still **partially** hydrogenated, including some forms of healthy fats (coconut or avocado oils). Read your labels. **Vegetable oils at high heat (as in frying) can also become trans fats.**

When we use the word **healthy** in reference to fats and proteins, this means organic, especially when it comes to products like butter. All mammals store toxins in the same tissues (fat cells). When we eat butter that is not organic, we are basically eating pure toxic material since butter is concentrated fat. If that butter is homogenized, then the fat cells are broken, releasing all the toxins inside. Oh, goody! Instant toxins for rapid absorption, we don't even have to break down the fat cell. The same goes for animal fat in the form of DHA.

DHA is animal fat, which can be found in its pure form, in fish oils.

If you use supplemental fish oils, this oil should come from healthy wild-caught fish or Alaskan fish. Farmed fish is either genetically altered, or fed toxic materials, and these toxins are stored in the fats. Since some DHA supplements are pure toxic material, **read your labels and be cautious.**

As for healthy, foods that are not included are any hydrogenated oils (trans fats), corn or corn oil products, soy oil, palm oil, cottonseed, rapeseed, or canola oil products. At one time, these were thought to be good sources of fats, but since the advent of food processing and genetically altered foods, these are now classified as pure toxins.

Avoid processed oils or fats of any kind, including margarines and spreads.

Look for the words **cold-pressed** and **unrefined.** When looking at fats, we must consider their structure. Using chemicals, heat, and hydrogenation with processed fats changes their structures just as heat and chemicals change the structures of sugars with an unusable, non-bondable outer shell. The same goes for fats. Once the structure has changed, the ability of the body to use them has also changed. The changes create severe damage since they become free radical elements.

So now you ask; how Much Fat?

Multiple groups advocate a wide variety of numerical ranges for fat consumption. Keep in mind, in the United States, the government still believes that "fat makes you fat." They advocate little or no fat in diets. If we look at the enormous need, for fat in every cell in the body, we can plainly see that this country is suffering from severe fat deficiency. This will be seen more clearly in future chapters.

The only fats that should be put into the body, are those that are classified as **healthy fats**. Only consume USDA organic fats, including, animal fats found in taro, organic butter, cheeses, meat, fish, poultry, eggs, nuts, seeds, olive, coconut, avocado, sunflower, safflower, and flaxseed oils. All oils should be organic, cold-pressed and unrefined.

If you want a complete balance of all healthy fats in one economic package, use free-range organic eggs or raw milk.

When it comes to eggs, there is healthy fat in both the yolk and the white of the egg. The yolk has a higher nutritional value with the presence of vitamins and minerals, but the balance of healthy fats and proteins is found in both white and yolk, together. The whole egg is the perfect nutritional package. Egg whites only contain partial nutrition, and if eggs are powdered, they can cause oxidation of your healthy cholesterol, which is not good. Milk is a complete source of balanced fats and proteins. Newborns and infants get the best of all balanced foods: mother's milk, it's perfect. If you wish to consume dairy with your children, be sure it is unprocessed whole raw milk—either goat or cow, which is another perfect package. Raw goat's milk is almost identical to mother's milk and can be an alternative for mothers who are unable to nurse.

For a minimum requirement to maintain a healthy function and find a balance that improves overall health; look to the Japan Society of Lipid Nutrition.

Their recommendations include omega-6 fatty acids at fourteen grams daily intake, which calculates to approximately one tablespoon of fat derived from olive oil, coconut oil, nuts, chocolate, sunflower, safflower, and sesame seeds, avocados, and olives. Remember that this is approximately fourteen grams, which converts to one tablespoon of plant-source fats.

And 2.6 grams of omega-3 fatty acids, animal source fats, converts to one teaspoon of fat derived from animal fat (beef, poultry, butter, and eggs), fish (at least twice a week), and whole raw milk for children.

There is a slight difference in concentration of solid and liquid forms of fats. One tablespoon of solid fat equal to 9.3 grams, and one tablespoon of liquid fat is approximately fourteen grams. This gives us one tablespoon of liquid to one teaspoon of solid (2.6 grams). This is just an approximation, but it is a way to remember basic ratios for fat use in any diet. With the liquid in a higher concentration, think of solid fats in teaspoon increments. And those liquid fats should be cold-pressed or cold-processed since heat will convert the fatty acid to a trans-fatty acid (see chapter 13). This comes back to our one tablespoon to one teaspoon requirement for plant- and animal-derived fats.

If I'm eating a high-fat diet, does it all go into making cholesterol?

No! When we consume animal fats or plant-sourced fats, our bodies make cholesterol from the abundant supply (see chapter 13). The remaining fats become free fatty acids, which are converted to ketone bodies in the circulation and are used at the cellular level as necessary fuel for energy production by every cell, especially after all forms of poly-glucose have been burned. Remember, our bodies do not store fat, so these extra free fatty acids become ketone bodies. Ketone bodies that are not used by the cells for energy will be flushed from the body by the kidneys (Ketonuria— ketones in the urine) and the lungs.

Caution needs to be taken by type 1 diabetics since excessive levels of fat appear to interfere with base insulin adjustments (injectable insulin) to maintain the basal blood sugars. Instead, raise your fat levels slowly while monitoring your blood sugars. A full ketogenic diet (75–90 percent fat) in most individuals will usually maintain a basal blood sugar of sixty.

What is the maximum amount of necessary healthy fats?

No one has ever established a figure.

Nutritional training tells us that each person has a different total calorie intake requirement to maintain body weight. If we use this figure as a guide, we could replace some of the non-bondable food calories with those in healthy fats. Although calorie counting is not recommended, this could be used as a guide to increase fat intake above that 1:1 ratio without increasing the need for more required exercise to burn or utilize aggressive deposits of ketone bodies (see chapter 4).

When we force large amounts of ketone bodies to be rapidly produced, this production can overwhelm the body. If the body has not converted completely to ketosis and, is still burning glucose, then the presence of high numbers of ketone bodies in the circulation can become too much for the tissues to consume and the kidneys to filter out in a short period of time. This causes the pH of the blood to rise too high and too fast, creating acidosis, which can be dangerous. The solution is slowly increasing the fat levels in the diet, after eliminating the sugars, while staying within the bounds of the body's caloric needs for that weight. When the percentage of fat consumed goes over the 60 percent marker, blood and urine testing for acidity is necessary.

An increase in fat above the minimum needed of 40 percent in your diet will stop you from losing weight.

If you want to raise your fat intake, do so **only after** you have arrived at your desired BMI and waist size. Once you start adding healthy fats, what is already stored in fat cells will remain in storage. It has also been noted that those who are on a high fat diet (healthy fats) may consume glucose, which also goes to storage. Once the fat is trapped in the fat cells, **the only way to remove it is by fasting and exercise,** which returns the body to an elevated ketone state. **This is the reason why ketogenic diets recommend intermittent fasting.**

If you wish to measure the general caloric need of your body at your present or future weight, use this calculation

- women (desired weight) x 3.95 + 825 = caloric limit for that weight
- men (desired weight) x 5.3 + 879 = caloric limit for that weight

A relatively high-fat diet (30 to 60 percent of the total caloric intake daily), remaining within the body's approximate caloric needs, along with intermittent fasting is highly recommended. The need for fats is vital in maintenance of health of every organ in the body. Once you have reached your BMI and waist measurement goals, you can begin to increase your fat intake. Start with animal fats in teaspoon increments, and you will see a noticeable difference in energy and health levels. And animal- and plant-sourced fats should come from healthy sources. For those who want to learn more about fat metabolism and its role in cancer, please refer to the chapter on ketosis (chapter 5) and ketogenesis.com.

So are we deficient in healthy fats?

Scientific research indicates, yes!

It has been noted that people on low-to-no-fat diets appear to have a higher incidence of illness and disease, and this may be a good indication to increase the intake of healthy fats.

Improvement; has been seen in people who are recovering from illness or who have chronic illness when they increase their intake of healthy fats to as high as two tablespoons each of animal- and plant-based fats, which could include omega-3 supplementation (DHA) of up to two grams daily. This increase should remain generally within your total body caloric requirement, adjusting for increase or decrease in exercise to burn higher levels of rapidly occurring ketones. This also means sacrificing all non-bondable and some bondable fuels (vegetables) for healthy fats.

Keep in mind that in the ketogenic diet, the intake of healthy fats is 75–90 percent of the total diet (total caloric intake for that specific weight). The rapid or aggressive introduction of this diet (ketogenesis – as seen in cancer treatment) is not recommended, without counseling and assistance from an experienced expert or physician well versed in this field since the changes require close monitoring of blood sugars and urine when starting this type of diet and intermittent fasting for diet maintenance.

Plant-Sourced Fats (Sterols and Sterolins)

Sterols and sterolins; are found in plant fats that act as immune modulators. They support the function of the immune system and aid in disease resistance as vitamin and mineral adjuncts like vitamin D2. They can also aid in balance of hormones during periods of stress. Think of them as **fat cofactors**.

Sterols are also found in **animal fats**. They are commonly seen as cholesterol and are classed as **zoosterols**. **Plant** sterols are classed as **phytosterols**, and both can become a part of human cholesterol formation.

All raw vegetables contain between five and forty milligrams of plant sterols.

This concentration can easily increase with drying since plants contain 80 percent water. Fruit contains two to thirty milligrams of sterols, and all seeds are rich in sterols at maturity, including nuts, beans, seeds, and spices. Kelp and other seaweeds are rich in sterols, which may be one of the reasons why people in Asian countries have less incidence of degenerative disease. Sterols are also found in fungi or mushrooms.

There is something to be said for the paleo diet, the Mediterranean diet, and vegan and vegetarian diets.

They all consume substantial amounts of raw foods. They follow the recommendation that 50–80 percent of the food in any diet, should be consumed raw(uncooked). As we progress you will see why a substantial amount of all diets should be raw in form.

Slicing, grating, macerating, or juicing fresh plants does not affect plant fats (sterols), but heat (above eighty-two degrees fahrenheit) and extreme cold (freezing) does.

If you cook or freeze your vegetables, you will destroy their sterols. Also, most chemicals used in food processing, oil extraction, and preservation, including esterification, will destroy vital sterols found in plant fats.

Grains and wheat and crude plant oils (canola or rapeseed, cottonseed, and corn) are all high in plant fats and sterols commonly seen as vegetable oils, but most—if not all—the sterols are destroyed with refining and are basically nonfunctional or dead sterols, having no functional effect on the body (you can't make healthy cholesterol out of it). These are also hydrogenated oils (as seen in artificial spreads) that become trans fats, and cold-processed vegetable oils that are heated also become trans fats and are not recommended.

Plant sterols have no antioxidant properties.

But natural plant sterols in the diet will enhance the absorption and utilization of 'B' vitamins, vitamin D, and many minerals. Plant sterols appear to enhance the production of DHEA (dehydroepiandrosterone), a steroid hormone that reduces stress in the body, which is seen in blood tests as elevated cortisol levels (our stress hormone). DHEA actually forces down cortisol, creating a balance in stress levels. DHEA will also enhance all other hormone production. So, estrogen, progesterone, and testosterone will remain active. This stimulates the thyroid hormone and human growth hormone function. And last but not least, plant fats are one of the lipids used by the body to produce cholesterol, a necessary component of the 'Oreo cookie' structure for every cell in the body.

Two hundred and fifty individual different sterols (both plant and animal source) have been identified to date. A wide action of these sterols has been recorded, including precursors to hormones and vitamins, mechanical strength, as well as behavior of cell membranes, synthesis of progesterone and vitamin D, the formation of Walzen factor (a potential anti-inflammatory compound), which inhibits the inflammatory matrix involved in arthritis and cartilage formation.

In recent studies on plant sterols, all the previous benefits just mentioned have been ignored, and much concentration has been placed on sterols as an LDL cholesterol-reducing agent in the human body. The supplemental industry now promotes artificial and processed forms of sterols for cholesterol reduction. And we now know that true natural sterols are destroyed by these processes. This research is inappropriate and misguided since the important benefits in sterols, found in plant sources, lies in whole food consumption (raw). When the overall diet improves, the body's cholesterol will normalize naturally.

There is still much debate as to the quantity of raw vegetables required for a healthy diet.

We are just discussing the fats and sterols found in those vegetables, and given the fact that plant food comprises 70 to 80 percent of what should be a healthy diet. Then a diet consisting of at least 60 percent raw organic vegetables (including juicing or a big salad every day) and 20 percent lightly cooked organic vegetables would form a minimum base for a 'healthy diet'. **This gives you 80 percent plant-sourced foods, and 20 percent animal-sourced foods. And fats come from both sources.**

Essential Fatty Acids (Animal-Source Fats)

Any nutritional supplementation would not be complete without a thorough review of essential fatty acids. The most important of the essential fatty acids are called omega-3 and omega-6 fatty acids. Omega-3 fatty acids are found in fish oils. These are eicosapentaenoic acids (EPA) and docosahexaenoic acid (DHA). Omega-6 fatty acids and linoleic acids (LA) are found in healthy oils (safflower and sunflower oils), nuts and flaxseeds that are raw and cold-processed and without chemicals.

Typical Western diets are much higher in omega-6 fatty acids than omega-3s. These are typically processed oils with no sterols. Damaged fatty acids that cannot be used by the body. Omega-6 fatty acids can overpower and destroy the functional value of omega-3 fatty acids. The increased use or supplementation of omega-6 in the diet is not recommended. The use of DHA and EPA has been studied extensively in such areas as heart disease, diabetes, depression, and schizophrenia. **Omega-3 fatty acids, by classification, cannot be synthesized (made) by the human body.**

Some Food Sources of EPA (20:5n-3) and DHA (22:6n-3) (3)				
Food	Serving	EPA (g)	DHA (g)	Amount providing 1 g of EPA + DHA
Herring, Pacific	3 oz*	1.06	0.75	1.5 oz
Salmon, chinook	3 oz	0.86	0.62	2 oz
Sardines, Pacific	3 oz	0.45	0.74	2.5 oz
Salmon, Atlantic	3 oz	0.28	0.95	2.5 oz
Oysters, Pacific	3 oz	0.75	0.43	2.5 oz
Salmon, sockeye	3 oz	0.45	0.60	3 oz
Trout, rainbow	3 oz	0.40	0.44	3.5 oz
Tuna, canned, white	3 oz	0.20	0.54	4 oz
Crab, Dungeness	3 oz	0.24	0.10	9 oz
Tuna, canned, light	3 oz	0.04	0.19	12 oz

*A 3-oz serving of fish is about the size of a deck of cards.

3-oz serving of fish about the size of a deck of cards
USDA Food Database

Research provided over the past twenty years has shown us that saturated fatty acids, are found in **all cell membranes** (the membranes formed by active cholesterol sulfate) and are a vital part of cell structure, and function throughout the entire body. (chapter13) Its presence has a marked effect on vision, reduces the inflammatory response that is seen in vascular disease (various forms of heart disease), and is a vital component of the gray matter of the brain (a major portion of the central nervous system containing layers of neurons). It is a major component of the sheaths or protective coating of all neurons (nerve cells). Its presence is essential in the chain formation of DNA and RNA (our genetic structure). Multiple studies from 2003 to 2008 (see references) have shown that omega-3 supplementation during pregnancy can significantly reduce the risk of premature births. During lactation, it appears to improve the neurological formation and growth of the brain in babies of nursing mothers.

Supplementation with omega-3 fatty acids decreases the risk of cardiovascular disease and stroke, lowers blood pressure, decreases inflammatory response, and helps control Crohn's disease (inflammatory bowel disease) and arthritis. In clinical trials, it has shown to have a direct effect on depression and the treatment of schizophrenia. **Some drugs (pharmaceuticals) used to treat depression and schizophrenia will actually block the absorption and use of omega-3 fatty acids.**

Vitamin E prevents the oxidation of omega-3 fatty acids within the body. For this reason, the use of low-dose (400 milligrams) vitamin E (non-esterified) is advised while supplementing with omega-3 fatty acids (EPA, DHA). **Be aware that many vitamin E supplements are derived from genetically altered corn or soy.**

Adult Daily	RDA	Over 50	Integrative use	Pregnancy	Maximum
Omega 3 total DHA	1.6 Gm (1600mg)	1.6 Gm	2 to 4 Gm	1.4 Gm	None
Vit. E	400 mg	400 mg	400 mg	400 mg	1 Gm

1000 milligrams = 1 Gram

If you are confused about the dosage you need, simply follow DHA content as a guide (one thousand milligrams equals one gram). According to the FDA, the minimum daily DHA for the healthy adult is five hundred milligrams. The RDA (recommended daily allowance) for the adult is 1.6 Grams (1600 milligrams) For illness, prevention of heart disease, treatment of neurological disorders, treatment of arthritis, and good health during pregnancy, the minimum DHA dose should start at 1,600 milligrams and may increase to as much as 4 Grams (4000 milligrams). Most commercial preparations contain more EPA than DHA. **The goal should be to get higher levels of DHA without the blood-thinning increase provided by EPA.** Too much EPA can actually prevent DHA from crossing the blood-brain barrier and getting into your brain where it is needed, **so any product you use should be 50 percent DHA and 10 percent EPA.** Keep in mind that these two elements balance each other, so they both need to be a part of any supplement you may use. Never use either DHA or EPA alone (as 100%), such products do not create balance, and may cause damage.

A four-ounce serving of wild-caught salmon or tuna will give you approximately two thousand milligrams of EPA/DHA (1,200 milligrams of EPA and 800 milligrams of DHA).

Since omega-6 is so plentiful in normal diets, it is recommended that—if you choose to supplement—use products that contain only *omega-3 oils at a 5:1 ratio.* If you are using fish oil capsules, keep in mind that most commercial formulas of fish oil contain only 10–20 percent of the needed EPA/DHA. In order to get the needed one thousand milligrams of DHA, you would have to take five to ten capsules of fish oil daily. It is also worthy to note that many fish oil products today are manufactured from fish farming operations. Along with those oils, you also get pesticides and GMOs stored in the fish fats. Please read labels and be cautious.

Commercially available omega-3 supplements have been tested, by several independent laboratories, and have been found to be free of methylmercury, polychlorinated biphenyls, and other environmental contaminants. Infant formula is not recommended, but DHA enrichment in infant formula was found to be safe.

Caution should be taken by people using borage oil supplements (a plant-based ALA that yields only 2–5 percent omega-3 fatty acids) to certify that the product is free of pyrrolizidine alkaloids (a common environmental contaminant). High doses of primrose oil and borage oil may cause seizures in people taking phenothiazines such as chlorpromazine (a seizure medication). **Although cod liver oil is rich in EPA and DHA,** some preparations **may contain preformed vitamin A (not recommended – chapter 18), which blocks absorption of vitamin D and other essential vitamins.**

A new trend has begun in the integrative medicine field, which involves the encouragement of the use of high-quality krill oil in place of omega-3 or fish oil supplements. Research has found that krill oil is a pure form of uncontaminated omega-3 oils in high concentration. The evidence so far has only shown that this form of omega-3 fatty acids is pure and free of mercury contamination. The dose of DHA present in most preparations may require an increase in the number of tablets taken daily.

There has also been interest in the use of green-lipped mussel products. Claims have been made that this product actually replaces the need for DHA/EPA in the diet. Studies are limited, but they have shown that this product may be effective in the treatment of the inflammatory response seen in arthritis. However, there is no evidence that it can actually replace the use of EPA/DHA found in omega-3 oils.

If you choose not to use supplementation, then follow United States Department of Health and Human Services in the recommendation that all people eat up to twelve ounces (two to three average meals) per week of a variety of fish that are low in mercury. Fish that are high in mercury are shark, swordfish, king mackerel, or tile fish (also known as golden bass or golden snapper). High-mercury fish should be consumed no more than once a month. For those of you who already use omega-3 supplementation, the addition of wild-caught fresh fish and shellfish at least two times a week is still recommended. And remember, 'wild caught' only.

To date, an increase of healthy fats has not scientifically shown any detrimental effects on total body function, and all indications of improved health at the cellular level has been verified scientifically. And the use of pharmaceuticals is never the answer to any cholesterol problem.

So, throw out that breakfast cereal full of processed grains and sugars, eat your eggs, and give the kids a glass of raw milk to follow their eggs. Soon, we will be able to say, "An egg a day keeps the doctor away."

CHAPTER 12
The Overlooked Elements of Good Health

There are three elements, that we continually ignore when we want to improve our health. And most physicians never discuss them since they assume that these are routine needs of everyday life. For our purposes we cannot ignore the basics. **Water, sleep, and exercise** are the basic elements that receive little if any attention and are **of crucial importance** when it comes to achieving your goals and becoming healthy for many, many years.

Water

Even though 72 percent of the body's weight is water, most people don't drink enough of it.

A large percentage of our population spends all day in a state of mild dehydration. They are never aware of its presence, and the symptoms are minimal (usually just an elevated heart rate). However, **continuous dehydration can aggravate and even accelerate the disease process.**

If we look closely at the chemical formations at the cellular level, we see that water becomes an important element. The fluid that surrounds our tissues and gives our blood and other body fluids their consistency is, basically, water. When chemical reactions occur, the elements in water (hydrogen and oxygen), can be utilized. The most important reaction that occurs naturally at the cellular level is with the antioxidant known as CoQ-10. As this element breaks down, it releases an oxygen molecule. When sufficient quantities

of water are present, the formation of **hydrogen peroxide** can occur. This is a vital protective element for cell wall health since hydrogen peroxide becomes an antioxidant that prevents damage from free radicals. Think of this antioxidant as **'our internal street sweeper'** that **cleans up the extra cellular tissues by removing bacteria, viruses, toxins, and heavy metals.** When dehydration is present, the formation of hydrogen peroxide becomes limited. Any disease present can get the upper hand.

As an example, in previous chapters we learned that the liver controls the body's temperature. This is accomplished by hormone signaling to the kidneys and heart to control fluid concentrations as well as sodium concentrations in the blood through dieresis (increased kidney flow). Without water, the liver cannot control the body's temperature efficiently with increasing or decreasing fluid levels, and this gives the disease process a foothold. By the same token, the lymphatic system (chapter sixteen) controls the flow of toxins and debris out of the body. It is dependent on fluid flow in the form of water. Without fluid flow, debris and toxins can become trapped in the lymph glands, which can lead to disease.

The consumption of coffee or alcohol and exercise will increase dehydration.

As a general rule, **adults and children should drink half of their body weight in ounces of water daily.** If you weigh 150 pounds, you would need to drink 75 ounces of water daily. At the very minimum, to keep the body hydrated, an adult must drink one eight-ounce glass of water four to eight times a day, depending on body weight—with an added glass of water for every cup of coffee, glass of alcohol, or hour of exercise.

The recommendation here is filtered water, preferably by **reverse osmosis,** which **removes toxins, heavy metals, fluorides, and chlorines,** unfortunately it also removes most of the minerals. For those who use reverse osmosis water, the use of an electrolyte solution, made with trace minerals or sea salts—without sugars or chemicals of any kind—added to filtered water, will maintain fluid and mineral balance.

Again remember, there can be 'too much of a good thing'.

The overconsumption of water can lead to severe electrolyte imbalances, specifically not enough sodium in the tissues.

If you remember our review of biochemistry 101, you remember that the movement of electrical charges in and out of the cell is dependent on a positive charge outside of the cell and a negative charge inside the cell. Even with the electron transport chain present (chapter 14), we cannot move that positive charge into the cell if it is not there. When there is not enough sodium ions inside and outside the cell – too much water – not enough minerals – this is known as dilution. As a result, the individual cells attempt to compensate for the loss of ions by absorbing (osmosis) the extracellular fluid in an attempt to concentrate the levels of sodium that may remain in that fluid. The cell is trying to create an electrical balance and replenish its own sodium concentrations. When this happens, all cells swell, including brain cells, which can result in progressive loss of neurological function and even death.

As stated before, the use of filtered water, preferably by reverse osmosis is recommended. This process removes the chemicals, clorine and fluorides, which in today's world is necessary. But it also removes the **mineral balance,** so this form of water needs mineral replacement, or the liberal use of sea salt.

To keep it simple, just follow the basic guidelines by consuming half your body weight (in pounds) in ounces of water daily. If you weigh one hundred pounds, drink fifty ounces of mineralized water daily. If you exercise vigorously, use an electrolyte solution (trace minerals) to rehydrate—one with no sugars or chemicals of any kind. Also remember that those who use sea salt in their daily foods will have fairly well-balanced minerals, which can be tilted in the wrong direction with the aggressive use of too much water.

Sleep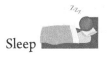

Along with a healthy diet and routine physical exercise, we must include sleep.

Without proper sleep, you are doomed to fail in your attempts to attain good health. One of the most important ingredients in a healthy life is sleep. **Not only is the length of sleep important but the quality of that sleep as well.** Below is a scale of the minimum sleep required for progressive age levels (developed by the National Sleep Foundation, National institute of Neurological Disorders and Stroke):

- children one to three years of age require twelve to fourteen hours of un-medicated sleep
- children three to five years of age require eleven to thirteen hours of un-medicated sleep
- children five to twelve years of age require ten to eleven hours of un-medicated sleep
- teenagers thirteen to nineteen years of age require minimum nine hours of un-medicated sleep
- adults and seniors require seven to eight hours of un-medicated sleep

Neurological studies done by the National Institute of Health on sleep and sleep deprivation found that **the brain reinforces and intensifies electrical patterns that maintain memory and learning, during REM (rapid eye movement) sleep, otherwise known as dreaming.** New cells are formed in the brain every four days and become imprinted with the special memory or body function that was originated by the brain since its formation (childhood) and with continual growth. This would include things like walking and talking.

Scientific research has found that people who awaken from long-term medicated or medically induced comas will require training to learn such things as walking again. Since medicated comas override REM sleep and dreaming, this needed electrical activity does not occur. **Without this electrical activity in the brain during sleep, memory and learning patterns are lost.**

Sleep is composed of two cycles:

REM (rapid eye movement) and NREM (non-rapid eye movement). During **NREM sleep, all body systems decrease activity—and even breathing slows.** This is the closest the body ever comes to total body rest, which may account for sleep apnea (the temporary cessation of breathing during sleep).

The healthy brain loses surface cells and re-grows new cells every four days. **During NREM sleep, science has shown a mild form of shrinkage in all brain cells.** This allows the free flow of spinal fluid throughout the brain and the flushing of dead cells and debris to the ventricles for continued disposal out of the body. These cycles of REM and NREM sleep alternate throughout the night every one to two hours. **The continuous reinforcement of those established electrical patterns and disposal of dead cells and debris is necessary in <u>all ages</u>,** with sleep deprivation, these vital functions are curtailed.

Psychiatric studies have shown that increasing levels of sleep deprivation cause increasing levels of depression (negative mood and emotions) as well as a progressive increase in the degenerative process, affecting cognitive function (perception and memory). Most institutionalized psychiatric patients suffer from varying degrees of sleep deprivation. Severe chronic sleep deprivation can result in psychosis, acute depression, hallucinations, and even suicide. In this country, there are 750,000 attempted suicides each year—and 30,000 of those attempts succeed. On the other hand, mild sleep deprivation causes an imbalance in leptin and ghrelin (your appetite regulators), resulting in decreased leptin absorption, decreased ghrelin formation, and loss of satiety. This trickle-down effect results in weight gain (the midnight refrigerator raid), decreased athletic performance, and increased anxiety. Sleep deprivation and their disturbances (loss of REM sleep) are common in children with ADD (attention deficit disorder). Loss of REM sleep is common in sleep-medicated adults and those with Alzheimer's disease.

Sleep deprivation in childhood begins at the age of five or six years.

If left unchecked, it will result in depression during the teen years. It appears that this scenario begins with the introduction of foods containing high glycemic index, non-bondable fuels found in sugar and processed grains, particularly high-fructose corn syrup, into the child's diet. Along with the lack of structured sleeping habits, the presence of these non-bondable fuels delays the onset of sleep and appears to counteract both NREM and REM sleep. This slow, accumulative progression decreases total sleep time and disturbs sleep quality. This may be a part of the explanation as to the increase in psychiatric disorders and even suicide in teens and young adults.

Most people suffering from lack of sleep don't consider seeking help or view a lack of sleep as a medical problem.

Instead, they choose simply to live with it, which could be a life-threatening mistake.

The mind provides a form of defense to sleep deprivation. The brain will actually cause momentary lapses in consciousness (the brain is trying to sleep) that last only seconds. Over a prolonged period of sleep deprivation, the seconds can progress into minutes. This is completely uncontrolled by the body (**it's an off switch you cannot control**). If you are driving a car or operating machinery, those seconds could become hazardous to your health. **An extra cup of coffee will not make a difference since caffeine has no effect on this particular off switch.**

Snoring and sleep apnea (the temporary cessation of breathing while sleeping) are health problems that need to be addressed. These problems increase in severity with the loss of REM sleep. They appear to be exaggerated in patients with existing respiratory problems (asthma, COPD) and those suffering from excessive weight gain.

Most doctors do not recognize lack of sleep as a medical problem— hence the 'sleeping pill'.

The routine use of prescription medications for improved sleep **is not advised** since these medications diminish electrical activity in the brain, **resulting in loss of REM sleep.**

Remedies for improved sleep include the removal stimulants for four hours prior to sleep, no caffeine, no alcohol, and no products containing sugars (this means no food for three to four hours prior to sleep) for children as well as some adults. Adhere to bondable foods only, decreased stimulation during sleep (no lights or music) and, if needed, use natural supplements to aid in the initiation of sleeping: 5–HTP (slows frontal neuro-excitability), melatonin, or L-tryptophan (enhances the brain's distinction of day to night or the brain's 'sleep clock').

Exercise

Even if you are at a healthy body weight, you still need to exercise—no matter what your age.

An inactive body functions very poorly. In fact, most disease processes diminish with the advent of exercise. A simple example of this is the combination of weight training and the increased consumption of vitamin D, resulting in increased bone density. It has been clearly shown that a proper diet (80 percent bondable fuels) and daily exercise can prevent and even reverse type 2 diabetes. It has also been found that even those diagnosed with diseases such as cancer, profit from an exercise program (ketosis or ketogenesis).

In short, exercise is **a precise tool for strengthening the body and fighting off many devastating illnesses,** including obesity, diabetes, heart disease, arthritis, and even cancer. If you already have an exercise program, keep moving. If not, set your goals and start now.

If we use common logic, we can see why our bodies improve with exercise. The advent of exercise causes many changes in the body. Just think of the process as 'shake and bake'. First, it increases the circulation with an increase in the heart rate (speed of the heart). This is followed by increased chemical reactions throughout the body due to increased ion exchanges (positive to negative flow, provided by 80 percent bondable fuels), which all come from that increased circulation. An increase in oxygen content in the blood as well as the tissues at the cellular level will increase the transfer of elements into the cells with the creation of ATP. Adenosine triphosphate (ATP) is metabolism inside the cell or energy. With exercise, the formation of cell by-products such as hormones increases, which improves organ function. This improved function goes for all organs throughout the entire body.

Our bodies are actually aggressive, defensive fighting machines bent on survival. The body knows what to do—even if you don't. It will actually sacrifice a portion of its necessary function for the purpose of survival.

In times of disease or illness; when nutrition levels are low, and the vital organs (heart, brain, and liver) have used up all available glucose and fats. And even if you do not exercise at all, the body can actually cannibalize your muscle tissue for the necessary fuel (protein metabolism) that it needs to maintain all the bodies other functions in order to survive. This is normally, seen in starvation and is the body's form of survival. This can also happen with improper dieting (non-bondable fuels and little or no fats—the junk food diet) along with aggressive exercise as seen in overtraining (often seen as rhabdomyolysis - see chapter 20).

Always start with mild exercise, and slowly progress to more aggressive forms of physical activity, eventually using all methods that involve total body response. Not everyone needs aggressive training to keep the body in proper function, but all ages should use a form of exercise that utilizes every muscle in the body. **"If you don't use it, you lose it"**. In Japan, people of all ages employ a form of exercise that is progressive and slow. It involves every muscle in controlled movement. Exercise does not have to be gym-style aggressive activity. It can be as simple as walking, riding a bike, or swimming. The goal is improvement of total body function—not 'six-pack abs'. If your goal is to lose weight, use bondable fuels only in your diet along with basic fat and protein requirements and exercise before breakfast (ketosis). Use your physical tolerance as a way to monitor your progress. You want to create better health—not injury.

The end-result will be the improvement of total body muscle fiber response. This response throughout your body will result in the increased production of human growth hormone and testosterone, thyroid stimulation, and the release of endorphins into the brain (the feel-good hormone). This cascade results in stronger muscle tissue with decreased fat stores (ketosis), improved metabolic rate with increased energy, increased mental function, including memory and cognitive abilities, and a decrease in depression. **Remarkably, you will see an increase in cognitive function with a distinctive improvement in sleep (both REM and NREM). This is true for all ages, including the very young and the elderly.**

When we consider exercise and sleep, we must consider the effects beyond just general functional improvement, involving improved circulation and nutrient transport (chemical changes throughout the body, especially the brain). We discussed the leptin-to-ghrelin signaling in the hypothalamus in chapter 2. This organ (hypothalamus) appears to function much like a master control switch that can turn up or down those functional responses in the kidneys, intestines, skin, thyroid, spleen, heart, and liver. All of these functional responses, are activated via brain neurotransmitters or hormones that travel to each of the necessary organs via the vagus nerve and the bloodstream. This particular organ has the ability to synthesize or formulate several different hormones, each of which is, released into the body in response to—and as a regulator for—improved function.

There are six major hormones.

The leptin-to-ghrelin response, is seen after meals, and **ghrelin** controls hunger. **Corticotrophins** are the steroid hormones that heighten or raise stress response. **Dopamine** increases the positive forms of brain or neurological function (the feel-good hormone). **Human growth hormone** (a major controller of all other hormones) will increase production by the liver for fats and amino acids and provide the growth stimulus to all tissues, including bones and muscles. **Thyrotropin hormone** for regulation of the thyroid gland stimulates tissue growth and function in all cells, especially skin nails and hair. Via the pituitary gland (attached to and located just below the hypothalamus), we get the **hypothalamic-pituitary hormones,** which include the male and female sex hormones that regulate reproductive behavior.

By definition, the hypothalamus means "chamber under the brain."

This walnut-sized gland is located under the brain (midbrain), behind the eyes, and above the pituitary gland.

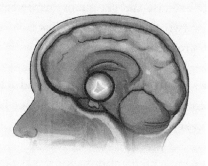

It provides most of the hormones that regulate the body's and brain's growth and function. **And yes, the liver is still the most important organ; without it, we cannot get the proteins needed for formation of these hormones.**

Now you ask; what does this have to do with exercise and sleep?

During REM sleep, we produce the highest levels of human growth hormones.

At that same time, we have the highest productive rate from the liver. Researchers at Washington University School of Medicine have found that human growth hormone generally increases during the first two to three hours of initial REM sleep and then slowly decreases. This increase does not appear to be influenced or affected by insulin the presence of glucose, but it is affected by the presence of cortisol (our stress hormone). When cortisol increases, human growth hormone decreases. **When your stress level is high, you have difficulty losing weight and difficulty sleeping.** A helpful counterpoint for this problem is the supportive levels of B vitamins and DHEA (dehydroepiandrosterone, a minor hormone in the human growth hormone complex). Both of B vitamins and DHEA appear to counterbalance or depress cortisol. See chapter 18.

Researchers at the Washington University School of Medicine also found that human growth hormone is stimulated within thirty minutes of vigorous exercise and is highest during periods of fasting prior to exercise. Now we can see that we can get a dose of human growth hormones in two ways. It is very important to exercise and get quality as well as a good quantity of sleep. Without these two elements, our bodies have a very difficult time maintaining proper growth and function.

So, get up and move—walk, run, or swim—spend at least thirty minutes to an hour in the sun every day, and get eight to ten hours of restful (un-medicated) sleep every night.

Most commercial sleeping preparations suppress the production of human growth hormone and REM sleep. And when it comes to children and their need for proper growth as well as function, they need to go outside and play for at least one hour and sleep (un-medicated, which means no sugars in the diet) for ten to twelve hours every night.

This is also an effective counterpoint for depression, behavioral problems, and stress-induced weight-loss prevention. Active, vigorous exercise will promote restful sleep, which promotes improved hormone production.

Thus, one aids and improves the other. Good exercise promotes better growth, better health, and better sleep, which promotes better growth and health.

If you want to stay fit, improve your body function, fight off disease, sleep better, improve your brain function, rid yourself of depression, or lose weight, you can't do it sitting in that chair. Get up and start moving!

Water, sleep, and exercise work well for the average Joe, but what if you are Joe plus one or Joe plus three.

The high-volume, fast-paced, overworked, and stressed out-human has trouble losing weight, sleeping, or relaxing. This Joe can also have other problems that tend to follow him and linger, like persistent colds, digestive problems, intermittent infections, allergic flare-ups, and episodes of depression. One of the biggest problems that hampers health recovery and/ or maintenance is excessive stress.

Stress Reduction

The human immune system will function at its peak if we function at our peak. If we push the envelope and make ourselves work past the point of healthy endurance, we risk significant damage to that very system that keeps illness at bay.

Our bodies must take rest periods and recuperate so that our peak performance can continue.

For the average adult, seven to eight hours of un-medicated, restful sleep is required. For children, ten to twelve hours is necessary. The key is un-medicated or restful sleep, and for some people, this is extremely difficult to do. Research shows that restful sleep or REM and NREM sleep occur when the mind and body are at complete rest simultaneously. The mind and body must be without stimulation for seven to eight hours, and there are several steps to take for this to occur.

Avoid caffeine and caffeine-containing products for six to eight hours prior to sleep.

Avoid that cup of caffeinated coffee or tea after dinner. Decaf or herbal is the answer—and eat that chocolate desert after lunch.

Noise and sounds stimulate the brain during sleep, decreasing the body's total rest time.

Keep televisions, radios, and computers out of the bedroom, and that includes the trusty iPod.

Light is also a brain stimulant, even during sleep.

Use nothing bigger than a nightlight in the bedroom. Since relaxation is the key to total body rest, it is recommended that we relax or become calm for one full hour prior to attempting sleep. This means no business calls or stressful activities for at least one hour. Attempting to sleep when you are anxious, angry, or still problem-solving will be futile.

Stress reduction plays a key role in the total performance of the immune system.

It can make or break us. A small amount of stress in our daily lives gives our immune system that extra boost to maintain peak function, but there can be too much of a good thing. When this occurs, the immune system can break down like a burned-out car on the freeway. And keeping a healthy balance, for some, is easier said than done.

Many researchers believe that excessive stress and its negative effects on the body are more common in this country than the common cold. Excessive stress, lack of effective sleep, and poor nutrition are a recipe for severe debilitating illness. Although we may not be aware, there are many stressors that affect our daily lives: noise, environmental pollutants, lack of exposure to the sun, freeway driving, racism, crime, work or school, negative emotions, over-exercising, chronic allergies, intense exposure to heat or cold, angry emotions, depression, loneliness, and much more.

When we are exposed to stressors, our bodies secrete the stress hormone cortisol, which causes a corresponding drop in our aging and immune-enhancing hormone DHEA (dehydroepiandrosterone). **This will return and rebalance with proper exercise and un-medicated sleep, but what about Joe plus one, two, or three?**

We can measure DHEA levels, and low levels are prominent in severely depressed or excessively stressed people. These same people often suffer from a variety of other health problems, including immune deficiency, arteriosclerosis (hardening of the arteries—early heart disease), diabetes, and other chronic illnesses. **If Joe still has stress-related elevated cortisol and low DHEA after exercise and restful sleep, a dose of DHEA supplement might be in order along with stress reduction.**

Where does the healthy immune-stimulating stress end and the damaging cortisol-increasing stress begin? Can we tell without a blood test?

This can vary from person to person and depends on physical and emotional tolerances developed from childhood, and it is usually not noticed or tested for, until disease has arrived.

Below, you will find a series of questions that were designed as a form of stress test to help you determine your own personal stress status. For each action or feeling that describes you, give yourself the appropriate points.

Stress Test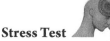

Frequent episodes of insomnia or difficulty sleeping: 1
Frequent feelings of loneliness: 1
Changes in appetite, excessive appetite/loss of appetite: 1

Fidgeting or restlessness, feeling loss of control: 1
Anxiety with inability to relax: 1
Feelings of aggression or suppressed anger: 1
Social fears, not wanting to socialize with friends: 1
Unconscious fears, using antibacterial soaps: 1
Conscious fears, fear of getting a disease like cancer: 2
Mood swings, feelings of inadequacy: 2
Mood swings, lack of confidence, or being self-critical: 2
Mood swings, inability to can't cope, or feeling trapped: 2
Mood swings, feelings of guilt: 2
Mood swings, frequent feelings of anxiety or depression: 2
Poor nutrition or emotional eating: 2
Will not take vitamin or mineral supplements: 2
A drive or need for over-exercising (more than four times a week) or not exercising at all: 3
Frequent bouts of nausea, irritable bowel, or digestive problems: 3
Frequent episodes of lack of desire for sex: 3
Frequent headaches, muscle tension, or joint pain: 3
Need for appetite stimulation with excessive sugar consumption or use of sugar substitutes: 3
Dependent on the use of alcohol, cigarettes, caffeine, or taking more than one prescription medication: 3
Frequent, unexplained irregular heartbeat and/or shortness of breath: 3
Unexplained episodes of unusual tiredness or dizziness: 3

How Did You Score?

If you scored twelve or more, you are putting yourself at risk for stress overload and eventual health problems. Improve your diet with bondable versus non-bondable, immediately adopt the recommendations below, and focus on stress reduction.

If you scored between six and twelve, you are still coping with stress. You need to slow down, learn to say no, improve your diet with bondable versus non-bondable teaching, and join a meditation group.

If you are between one and five, you are in peak range. Keep up the pace. Your hormones will remain balanced—and you will stay healthy. Keep on trucking.

Stress-Busting Tips

- **Stop, take ten, and breathe**. Deep breathing is a powerful stress-reducing tool. Several times a day, fill your lungs to their full capacity with air (deep breath), then slowly exhale through your mouth until your lungs are completely empty. Repeat this exercise five times in a row, slowly.
- **Get a minimum of eight hours of restful, un-medicated sleep every night**.
- **Just say no, limit tasks** when you have too much to accomplish in one day.
- **Share the household workload** with other members of the family—and make it fun.
- **Eat eight servings of healthy vegetables every day.**
- **Smile, laugh, and purge yourself of negative emotions** such as anger and hatred. Find something funny in life every day. Laughing long and hard is the ultimate cure.
- **Get help in dealing with grief**. Loss of a loved one, a divorce, or the loss of a job can all create a form of grief. Stress is the result of grief, that is never dealt with.
- **Carpe diem; seize the day**, and live it to its fullest. Stop worrying about tomorrow.
- **Believe in yourself**. Negative self-talk and continually doubting your abilities, hampers your hormone balance and your body's ability to heal.
- **Notice the beauty around you**, stop and smell the flowers, watch sunsets, listen to the wind, relax, and enjoy nature.
- **Love your family and your friends**—and be forgiving. Love is a strong emotion that can reverse mood swings.
- **Be good to yourself**. Most of us are our own worst enemies. We tend to focus on our weaknesses and minimize our strengths. Wake

up each day and tell yourself that you are a good and useful human being. This is a powerful force to reverse mood swings.

- **Do the things that you have always wanted to do**—learn to ice skate, sing in a choir, write a book, or tell stories to children—and create whatever makes you happy. Happiness is also a strong emotion that drives hormone balance.

- **Seek your spiritual side.** This does not have to be religious, although those with strong beliefs in God generally live at peace and feel protected. Most of us believe in something greater than ourselves—a spiritual power that offers solace and helps us find that quiet place within. This quiet response relieves anxiety, improves appetite, and aids in DHEA response within the body.

Researchers in China, Korea, and the United States found that yoga or controlled breathing exercises like swimming are excellent mood swing breakers. Those who suffer from anger problems or have difficulty with emotional control can also break this cycle with the use of aggression therapy, which involves emotional release with a punching bag or pillow—or boxing or kickboxing classes. **These therapies help you return to the quiet side of your emotions so that stressors can be eliminated, and your DHEA levels will once again rise.**

Your moods and emotions, are directly affected by your levels of neurological hormones.

A person who has difficulty with stress control tends to develop symptoms of depression. In today's medical community, the treatment for stress-related depression tends to rely on pharmaceuticals. These forms of treatment appear to have the opposite desired effect. Instead of 'getting up off of the sofa' to an improved mood and life, with the use of pharmaceuticals, you 'become the sofa'. Statistical evidence shows us that the incidence of homicide and suicide rises in parallel with the use of pharmaceuticals. As a result, this strategy for depression or stress reduction cannot be recommended. Stick to using the natural stress-buster methods and counseling (conversation) to improve your neurological hormone levels.

CHAPTER 13
The Missing Elements

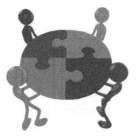

Human Cholesterol

Healthy Cholesterol versus Unhealthy Cholesterol
(The element necessary for every cell and is made by the human body)

In chapter 11, we discussed the need for fatty acids in the diet. The combination of plant- and animal-source fatty acids creates an end- product of DHA. It combines with methionine or cysteine (animal and plant source, sulfur-bonded proteins) in the liver. We get LDLs (low-density lipoproteins or triglycerides); otherwise known as cholesterol.

This element, has been given a 'bad reputation' by the pharmaceutical industry.

Why?

The theory put forth by the pharmaceutical industry is that cholesterol (in the form of LDLs) is the direct contributor to heart attacks in this country.

Scientific research in this area refutes this theory. Findings show a connection between the formation of plaque from LDLs (low-density lipoproteins), but plaque **does not have** any direct connection to the cause of heart attacks. While increased plaque formation is stimulated by increased consumption of non-bondable foods (Chapter 2), some of that same plaque may be beneficial. We have also seen that unhealthy LDLs in large quantities does cause a condition known as peripheral artery disease or hardening of the arteries, which again, has no direct connection to heart attacks. We will also see how the use of pharmaceuticals in this area is unnecessary when we understand the formation and action of healthy cholesterol.

So, where to start?

Cholesterol comes from the Greek word *chole*, meaning *bile*, and *stereos*, meaning solid. The chemical suffix *ol* means *alcohol*. This hydrocarbon organic molecule (found in nature) is a lipid or fat molecule that is **biosynthesized (or made) by all animal cells**. This is an essential structural component of all animal cell membranes (including human cells).

When we look at the word **cholesterol**, all sorts of images come to mind—from the list of ingredients on that food product you bought at the store to the doctor who tells you that you must control your cholesterol. And much of what you have learned to this point, from basic education, commercial advertising, and even your doctor, is either misleading or outright false.

So, what is cholesterol anyway?

Cholesterol is a specific molecule in a broad class that encompasses all forms of sterols (plant and animal fats) in the body. Fatty acids and sterols enter the liver and are broken down to the basic lipid droplet. During a process called the Krebs cycle, this droplet becomes coated in proteins, which is the beginning of what we call cholesterol.

Cholesterol is one of the most important elements your body produces, and it is used by every cell in the body.

The laundry list of its applications include; repair of cell wall structure, providing strength and structure, and the ability of the cell to allow or prevent permeability through its membranes and its bonds between cells. Cholesterol is the precursor to vitamin D and the sex hormones: estrogen, progesterone, and testosterone. Some cholesterol particles can even help fight infections.

Confused? Just think; stronger, longer-lasting, healthier cells throughout the entire body.

Now let's look at the total body's needs for healthy cholesterol.

Our bodies are composed of about one trillion cells. If we multiply this by the number of days each organ produces replacement cells, we can see that maintaining cell structure and preventing premature cell death is vitally necessary and takes a large quantity of cholesterol.

If we look at brain structure alone, we find that the dry weight of the brain is about 35–40 percent cholesterol. Depending on which area of the brain you are looking, the total lipids (all forms of fatty acids or fats) by dry weight are 40–80 percent of the brain. Dr. Fred A. Kummerow, head of research at the University of Illinois, said, "If someone calls you a fat head, thank him. It's really a compliment."

If we replace cells several hundred layers thick with a new layer every four days, then all of those layers must be maintained as long as possible. The new cells that are provided by stem cell growth must have healthy active cholesterol sulfate, as well as those already produced, to maintain integrity and prevent early cell death. This prevents brain structural loss (shrinking) and damage to vital functions. This makes the constant and continuous production of healthy cholesterol (active cholesterol sulfate) a monumental job that requires large levels of healthy fats in the diet.

Add to this the fact that hormones in the brain are carried and transferred (end coated) through healthy levels of fatty acids. So, direct brain health (mood, emotion, and function) increases the need for healthy fats in the diet.

Again, add to this the fact that cholesterol sulfate is the mending material required to repair injuries inside and outside the body as a response to injury, or the inflammatory process (your internal Band-Aids), and all scar tissue in the body is composed of cholesterol, which increases that total need.

And for people who have chronic disease (arthritis, sinusitis, tendonitis, and so on), the continuous inflammatory response created by that disease forces a demand for even higher quantities of cholesterol. And for those who have suffered traumatic injuries, the need for cholesterol may very well be astronomic.

Before all the interest in lowering fats in the diet, the general population was stable, cardiac problems remained low, and cholesterol was not an issue. **The body knows what it needs, and it will provide for it to survive—even if that cholesterol is made from unhealthy materials**.

No one knows what the level of cholesterol should be—

No one number fits all—and science has shown that the use of pharmaceuticals has increased our deficiency in healthy cholesterol. Since a healthy body can actually utilize ketone bodies (fatty acids) as fuel, the premise that fat makes you fat, can now be dismissed.

Cholesterol is the element;

That transports the raw materials in a neat little package to all cells, remember the 'Oreo cookie' structure? The **fat** and **protein** along with **phosphorous** and **sulfur** are the basic contents of that package, which will **form the lipid raft**. This includes nerve cells and their intricate coating or myelin sheaths and Schwann cells (found in the brain), which are both rich in cholesterol.

Cholesterol also acts as a transporter of fat-soluble vitamins A, D, E, and K. It has been found to be a necessary component for the formation of vitamin D, and hormones formed in the adrenal gland (on the kidneys), specifically steroid hormones and sex hormones. **Without cholesterol, we cannot formulate vitamin D or any of our vital hormones. Ouch!**

The medical industry will discuss triglycerides, LDLs, and HDLs. They look at what's good, what's bad, and how they believe cholesterol should be controlled.

So what is the point here, and what do we need to know?

First of all, **we must get rid of this idea of control**. All cholesterol, in every un-oxidized form, is good for you, and all forms of cholesterol, are controlled by the liver. We don't need to use any controls other than supplying the healthy forms of fats, proteins, and minerals that contribute to their formation. This is **what we eat**! Remember; **the only harmful LDL is a damaged LDL and the most useful LDL is a sulfated one.** The body knows how to control cholesterol. All we need to know is what to feed it, so that the healthy forms of cholesterol are made.

When we look at cholesterol in food, we must remember that this too does not need to be controlled.

Dietary cholesterol (cholesterol found in food) is a part of the total cholesterol that our bodies use. Typically, the body absorbs 30–60 percent of the cholesterol found in food. In an average diet, this is approximately four hundred milligrams. The liver uses this and makes more. The use of dietary cholesterol by the body is highly dependent on the quality and abundance of probiotics or beneficial bacteria in the intestinal tract. **Without beneficial bacteria, we cannot break down or absorb dietary cholesterol**, which is highly - valued by the body, and used in the formation of sex hormones and human growth hormones. So the cholesterol from foods is not something to avoid, but the increase in healthy bacteria is important for the body's production of high-quality, healthy cholesterol.

Dr. Kummerow Ph.D., (head of research at the University of Illinois) found that studies vary, but the total cholesterol made by the body is 360–1,400 milligrams in a twenty-four-hour period, with the average daily production of cholesterol at approximately 900 milligrams. This means the liver is left with the job of formulating or synthesizing approximately 300–400 milligrams of cholesterol daily. The liver also has the ability to stop that production when proper or needed levels have been achieved. This means your liver makes sure you have enough—even in times of illness and injury—but not too much.

Are you starting to realize how important the health of your liver is?

The liver makes that cholesterol from the supplies provided whether they are healthy sources or not. Again, we return to the original premise: healthy versus unhealthy. **This is what we eat.**

Remember the term, un-oxidized cholesterol?

The damage to our cholesterol (oxidation) and the diseases that result (from heart disease to cancers) boils down to the **types of foods that change cellular structure.** These changes result in damage to the cholesterol directly and damage to those defenses our bodies have to prevent this damage. This disables the cholesterol and its protective defenses. We need to learn how to use the change in those types of foods and how to enhance natural defenses to prevent disease.

To understand the process of damage, we need to look at free radicals and oxidation.

Healthy cholesterol is that form of cholesterol that is un-oxidized. It comes from your food, is made by your liver, and is utilized by all cells throughout the body. Unhealthy cholesterol is oxidized, contains extra oxygen, or has been changed or transformed into a new compound, and is used improperly by the body, and there are two ways this damage can occur.

Keep in mind that healthy or un-oxidized cholesterol is used by our cells, and during that process, some oxidation will occur, producing what is called

oxysterols, which can be beneficial. These oxysterols help regulate liver production and the liver's control of cholesterol. They are also the basic foundation or precursor on which steroid hormones, testosterone, estrogen, progesterone, and cortisol are produced within the adrenal glands (glands located on the kidneys).

To date, there have been 40 different derivatives or types of oxysterols that have been identified, and are produced in the human body. Most of these derivatives are beneficial and can be recycled as bile or new cholesterol once utilized by other tissues and organs.

Dr. Kummerow, PhD has been working in this field for sixty years. **He has found seven of those oxysterols to be what he titles "lethal" oxysterols.**

These are the forms of damaged cholesterol that will lead to heart disease and other diseases as a result of **direct tissue damage**. Two of these "lethal" oxysterols come from your diet and can be avoided.

One comes from fried foods.

Polyunsaturated fats, which are commonly seen as vegetable fats (usually made from a combination of corn, soy, cottonseed, or rapeseed oils) that are used for frying at high heat. Which converts the fats in fried foods to **trans fats, which become free radicals** in the body, causing direct damage to

cholesterol and resulting in lethal oxysterols.

Remember, free radicals create lots of damage to cholesterol, and they destroy vitamins A, D, C, and E in the body.

Research at the University of Illinois found that foods cooked in butter, for a shorter period of time, at lower temperatures, does not form trans fats that cause this damage. It was also found that frying fish in either saturated or unsaturated oils causes a dramatic increase in free radical trans fats since fish is high in unsaturated fatty acid content. Again, the end- result is lethal oxysterols.

So, heating fats changes their structure.

The fats found in roasted peanuts have an altered composition that will rapidly deteriorate and become rancid (more oxidation). This means that vegetable oils cooked at high heat will become trans fats. Thus, **rancid oils and heated vegetable oils become trans fats and free radicals**, resulting

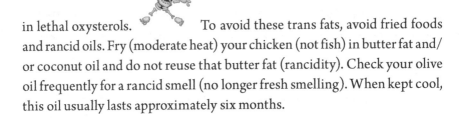

in lethal oxysterols. To avoid these trans fats, avoid fried foods and rancid oils. Fry (moderate heat) your chicken (not fish) in butter fat and/or coconut oil and do not reuse that butter fat (rancidity). Check your olive oil frequently for a rancid smell (no longer fresh smelling). When kept cool, this oil usually lasts approximately six months.

The second form of "lethal" oxysterols comes from powdered egg yolks.

The processing of egg yolks into a powdered form causes the fat in the yolk

to become trans-fat. So, to avoid; **don't eat powdered eggs.**

The other five forms of "lethal" oxysterols can be avoided by altering your diet.

These are forms of **trans fats created by hydrogenation or partial hydrogenation** (the conversion of liquid oils to solid oils by processing) of vegetable fats. This means 'read your labels' an extremely large percentage of processed foods on the market today contain hydrogenated or partially hydrogenated oils in various amounts. This also means that all spreads and margarines should also, be avoided, since these contain hydrogenated or partially hydrogenated fats. This also means "read your healthy fat labels", healthy oils such as coconut or avocado must remain in a liquid state at room temperature. Today many companies feel a solid fat is more convenient, as a result hydrogenation is used and this changes your healthy fat to an trans fat 'without labeling'. So if that healthy fat is not a liquid at room temperature avoid it, or find a product that states no hydrogenation or trans fats.

If we look closely we will notice that there are two types of trans fats.

These are trans fats from saturated fats of animals, and trans fats produced by excessive (high) heat and hydrogenation (also known as artificial trans-fat) found in food processing.

Saturated fats, from animals contain trans fats (produced by animals) that are found naturally in nature. These fats, are easily recognized and used by the body. But artificially produced trans fats are not found in nature, and are not recognized by the body, causing multiple forms of damage, including multiple forms of heart disease and cancers. **In other words, it's 'artificial' and not the real deal.**

As a small side note:

Known carcinogens (agents in foods that are known to stimulate or cause cancer) when cooked at high temperatures as in frying, has been found to cause cancer. Think about that while you're eating your chicken 'nuggets' or 'wings' that are coated in a soy based batter and fried at high heat. **That's a triple whammy: 'lethal' oxysterols, soy (which is food for cancer), and GMOs (see chapter 3 and 19). OOuch!**

Now let's look at how the body controls those other thirty-three oxysterols, the nonlethal ones.

Our bodies have several mechanisms that effectively neutralize oxidation, some act as precursors to or even direct antioxidants. These agents are found in vitamins C, E, B6, along with enzymes (like CoQ-10), and protein bonded elements such as fibrinogen, and albumin (elements found in human blood). **These elements form a defense against oxidative stress, and oxidative stress is now seen as inflammatory response,** and is directly related to such diseases as heart disease. All of these protective elements are formed, with the help of probiotics and the liver, from healthy source whole vitamins and proteins.

If you stick to healthy source foods (fats and proteins) and ferment your own foods.

These foods contain a healthy source of whole vitamins and probiotics, then your liver will have its own arsenal for fighting disease and maintaining healthy cholesterol, which is so vital for your entire body.

When we use the word cholesterol:

We are actually looking at multiple functions throughout the body. This element, in all its various forms, whether it is an LDL, or HDL particle, is the main supplier of critical molecules that influence the function of every organ in the body, from the liver to the brain and even to the blood that flows in between. **So, damage to this element we call cholesterol, is something we simply cannot afford if we want to stay healthy.**

How do trans fats affect blood flow;

Dr. Kummerow found that trans fats in the bloodstream will inhibit the production of prostacyclin, an enzyme that maintains blood flow by preventing excessive clot formation, this keeps blood flowing. When trans fats are consumed, prostacyclin is blocked with a resulting increase in thromboxane, an enzyme that increases blood clotting and allows an increase in calcium deposits in the arterial walls (hardening of the arteries and heart disease). There is a delicate balance between these two enzymes, and **the balance is broken by trans fats.**

In chapter one we discussed the need for nitric oxide.

Our bodies store nitric oxide in the endothelial (reticular) layers of the skin, a bed of connective tissues that supports skin structure, which is high in protein. Nitric oxide is produced by endothelial cells that line the inner walls of the arteries in the body. Like a battery, the skin absorbs sunlight, and the electrons in that sunlight cause a reaction with that nitric oxide. It produces a sulfate anion, this process is called *ENOS* **(endothelial nitric oxide synthase).** This sulfated ion binds to the cholesterol molecule, making it water-soluble and fat-soluble. **When sulfated (bonded), this molecule can travel anywhere throughout the body, making this form of cholesterol more valuable since it can now be used in the brain, bones, muscles,**

and so on. This form of cholesterol is an efficient form of rapid repair of our bodies, including the heart and brain during times of injury.

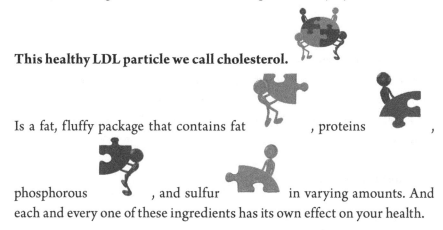

This healthy LDL particle we call cholesterol.

Is a fat, fluffy package that contains fat   , proteins   ,

phosphorous   , and sulfur   in varying amounts. And each and every one of these ingredients has its own effect on your health.

Cholesterol particles (LDL and HDL) are fat droplets coated in various forms of proteins, and the proteins are the main difference in their structures.

Remember when we learned that just three ounces of healthy protein will produce thousands of protein molecules. These protein molecules can form thousands of different combinations for different structures throughout the body. Some will be specific for formation of brain hormones, some for thyroid hormones, and some for tissue formation like muscle or tendons, and so on. There are literally thousands of combinations of protein molecules, that form strength and structure throughout the body, **and they are all utilized in cholesterol formation so the cholesterol can be specific to a given area.**

Cholesterol traveling throughout the body, is guided by the type of protein that it is coated in.

That **protein becomes the carrier of the cholesterol** it is bonded to. And this bonding process is controlled by the liver. If you consume less than the minimum required amount of healthy protein in your diet, you will be unable to carry the needed cholesterol through the bloodstream to its needed destination (the cells). The liver will attempt to compensate and raise the cholesterol level by using incomplete forms of amino acids (unhealthy source proteins) to provide the proper supplies. This results in

unstable, poorly formed cholesterol that oxidizes easily (oxysterols) . The end – result is seen in illness and disease. We need a minimum amount of healthy source proteins to maintain the healthy building blocks called cholesterol (see chapter 10) and healthy proteins from animal and plant sources.

The highest source of healthy protein:

This is found in eggs and whole milk (organic and unpasteurized), beef, chicken, and fish (free range and wild caught). For healthy plant-sourced proteins, look to legumes (organically grown) including green peas, beans, raw nuts, and brown rice.

The highest and healthiest forms of proteins and fats can be found in mother's milk.

The nursing infant gets the best, but it has also been found that trans fats, these "lethal" oxysterols, consumed by the mother, will also be found in

her milk — —and newborns will actually develop early stages of heart disease. Mom, think about what you are eating while feeding that baby. Do you really need that burger and fries? Did you use canola oil to fry that chicken? And what's in those chicken nuggets? Do you really need them?

In the United States, the unhealthy sources of proteins in foods are numerous and can be dangerous.

Most unhealthy source proteins are found in processed foods, and some can even become free radicals as soon as they arrive in the intestinal tract. Glutamine is found in wheat, rye, soy, corn, whey, and processed milk. The consumption of healthy foods rather than unhealthy foods is a primary factor here (see chapter 7). The proteins found in wheat, rye, whey, corn, soy, and pasteurized milk are not healthy forms of protein.

Cholesterol, in all of its forms, also contains phosphorous.

Phosphorous is the pilot light that lights up ATP for energy, and the mineral that bonds with calcium for the bone matrix. The level of phosphorous increases with the level of protein. The phosphorous found in cholesterol comes from foods that contain healthy proteins. **If your consumption of healthy protein is sufficient (minimum needed), then the phosphorous will be sufficient as well.**

Each cholesterol particle also contains sulfur.

We still need more research to find its limits, but science shows us that we are all deficient in this mineral. We can only assume that those lipids formed in the skin have a higher level of sulfur since that is where UV rays and ENOS occurs (see chapter 15).

When we look to cholesterol, we look for that **fat, fluffy valuable LDL with sulfur-bonded to it.** It is now healthy because it is supported by cholesterol sulfate. Since this protein is bonded to sulfur that has been activated by skin exposure to UV light (using the process of ENOS), it will also contain vitamin D sulfate, which we will learn more about later.

Cholesterol levels rise in response to inflammation or injury.

The lipids (cholesterol sulfate) enter the damaged cells in an attempt to salvage the cell and pass through the lipid membrane of the cell easily since they are sulfated and fat- and liquid-soluble. Like little ghosts, they move freely through any tissue. There are protective membranes, found throughout the body, that selectively prevent elements from passing. **Tissues from the brain (blood-brain barrier), the intestinal wall, bone, and fetal membranes require sulfated cholesterol.** Once sulfated, this cholesterol passes into the area to prevent cell damage and early cell death and heal those tissues.

Once the cholesterol sulfate is inside the cell.

The neet little package opens, some of the sulfur breaks away. The protein and remaining sulfur are pulled into the inner lining of the cell wall (cell wall thickening),—followed by the cholesterol. **And the cell wall has just been reinforced or rebuilt, with new inner layers of the 'Oreo cookie' structure**

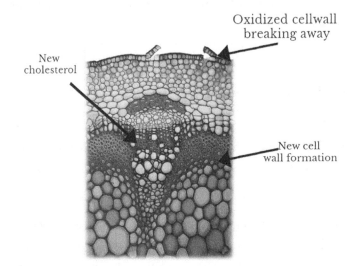

The CoQ-10 and the phosphorous enter the mitochondria (the cell's energy factory) to aid in production of ATP (adenosine triphosphate, otherwise known as energy). The extra sulfur also enters the mitochondria and is utilized for the formation of multiple substances, including glutathione, an enzyme used to control the aggressive nature of powerful antioxidants such as hydrogen peroxide.

Scientists in China have found that the formation of HDLs is dependent on the presence of LDLs or cholesterol inside the cell before the cell wall ruptures.

If the cholesterol sulfate is in the endoplasmic reticulum (inside the cell), then the cell wall thickens and the outer cell wall (old or damaged cell wall) breaks away. This process protects the delicate structures inside the cell, preventing damage to DNA and RNA. The cholesterol sulfate (LDL) needs to be inside the cell before the rupture of the cell wall. This affords a longer and stronger life to that cell. When the cholesterol is not present inside the cell—and if the cell is becoming oxidized or damaged—when the cell ruptures, the entire cell is lost. **This is a form of early cell death (necrosis), and when early cell death occurs, it shortens the human life span.**

The newly formed HDL:

Formed from cell wall fragments from ruptured cells, which clump together (nonlethal oxysterols) and are carried by the bloodstream back to the liver for recycling. The percentage of HDL's returning to the liver appears to be the stimulous for the liver to make more or less cholesterol. More HDL's and the liver makes more cholesterol (increased loss of cellular structure). Less HDL's and the liver reduces its production (cellular structure remains healthy).

Once filtered by the liver, the HDLs are broken down to form bile, which aids in the breakdown and absorption of free fatty acids in the intestinal tract, or reformulated to form new triglycerides.

The end- result of unhealthy foods (fats or proteins) is basically the formation of small, poor-performing lipids that are unstable and can

become oxidized easily (oxysterols) **along with the formation**

of "lethal" oxysterols **that cause direct damage to the body and our natural defense systems.**

What about deficiency?

The government mandated the 20 percent reduction in the use of fats in this country about thirty years ago, and those fats were replaced by sugars. This scenario created less healthy cholesterol and more unhealthy cholesterol, which started the roller coaster toward our slow and eventual destruction of the use of healthy fatty acids in the diet.

When our healthy cholesterol is low, body functions diminish—and illness takes hold.

This encompasses all forms of illness since cholesterol sulfate is necessary for every cell in the body. Without it, our cells die.

Now you ask, What is the maximum amount of necessary healthy fats?

No one has ever established a figure.

Nutritional training tells us that each person has a different total calorie intake requirement to maintain proper body weight. If we use this figure as a guide, then we could replace some of those non-bondable food calories with those in healthy fats. Without counting calories the total calorie need could be used as a guide to increase fat intake calories above that 1:1 marker—without increasing the need for ketosis (see chapter 4 and chapter 11).

When we force large amounts of ketone bodies to be rapidly produced, this production can overwhelm the body. If the body has not converted completely to a ketogenic diet, then the presence of high numbers of ketone bodies in the circulation can become literally too much for the tissues to consume and the kidneys to filter out in a short period of time. This causes the pH of the blood to rise too high and too fast, creating acidosis, which can be dangerous.

The solution here -

is slowly increasing the fat levels in the diet above that minimum 40 percent marker. When the percentage of fat consumed goes over the 60 percent marker (remaining within your caloric limit for your weight), blood and urine testing for acidity is necessary. Avoid elevated fats in the diet, until healthy BMI and waist measurements have been achieved. In other words, lose your spare tire before increasing the fats above the 40 percent marker in your diet.

When you raise your intake of healthy fats, you provide the body with ketone bodies. As a result, fatty acids trapped in your fat cells and will not be released to become ketone bodies. Instead, you will burn those ketones in your diet—and your spare tire will remain in place. Use bondable fuels only with minimum fats (40 percent) in your diet if you want to burn off that spare tire.

If you wish to measure the general caloric need of your body at your present or future weight use this calculation

Women: desired weight x 3.95 + 825 = caloric limit for that weight

Men: desired weight x 5.3 + 879 = caloric limit for that weight

Are We Deficient in Healthy Fats?

Everyone's need for fat in the diet will vary.

Our production of healthy cholesterol (cholesterol sulfate) is dependent on a minimum intake of animal- and plant-sourced healthy fats at 1:1 (one tablespoon plant to one teaspoon animal each) daily. A minimum intake of healthy proteins, particularly those that are sulfur-bonded (methionine, cysteine, and sulfotyrosine), and exposure to sunlight (preferably sunbathing) at least twenty minutes, three times a week will provide the synthesis of vitamins and activation of sulfur (vitamin D sulfate).

Every person needs cholesterol at a different level.

People on low-to-no-fat diets appear to have a higher incidence of illness and disease, and this may be a good indication to increase the intake of healthy fats.

Improvement has been seen, in studies, in people who are recovering from illness or who have chronic illness when they increase their intake of healthy fats, which could include omega-3 supplementation (DHA) up to two grams daily. This increase should remain generally within your total body caloric requirement, adjusting for increase or decrease in exercise to burn those higher levels of rapidly occurring ketone bodies. This will also mean sacrificing all non-bondable and some bondable fuels (vegetables) for healthy fats.

In the ketogenic diet, the intake of healthy fats is 75–90 percent of the total diet (total caloric intake for that specific weight). The aggressive or rapid change to this diet (ketogenesis) is not recommended, without counseling and assistance from an experienced expert or physician well versed in this field since the changes require close monitoring of blood and urine when starting the diet.

To date, an increase of healthy fats has not scientifically shown any detrimental effects on total body function, and all indications of improved health at the cellular level have been verified scientifically. And the use of pharmaceuticals is never the answer to any cholesterol problem.

Cholesterol sulfate also contains protein, but how much do we need?

Protein molecules are compact and abundant, and we only need the minimum recommended level: 45–55 grams for females, with 25 percent increase for pregnancy, and 55–65 grams for males (see chapter 10). Extreme athletes and bodybuilders may need more, but this should to be adjusted according to activity and not exceed 75 grams in a twenty-four-hour period—and it should only be from healthy animal- and plant-sourced proteins with no exceptions. **Added protein will only cause damage to the body. The double-down theory—if one is good, then two is better—does not work here.**

Blood Testing

Cholesterol control is unnecessary.

138

It appears that the medical field leans too heavily in this area and not enough credit is given to the human body and its capability when it comes to producing that fat- fluffy- healthy cholesterol, which increases during times of need. Yet this controversy exists, and we all end up with those incriminating blood tests, it might be worth your while to learn how to read this test so you can adjust your diet for improvements if needed.

This NMR LipoProfile test appears to be much more reliable than the old studies. It will tell you the number of LDLs floating in your bloodstream and measure the size of the particles. The test uses the words particles when describing each product or form of cholesterol that the body produces. There appears to be a lot of misconceptions in regard to how this test should be read. Some physicians still look at the number of particles and not the **size**, which is actually the main determining factor in reading this test. Let's look at each of these forms and their numbers and sizes so you can interpret the test yourself.

Cholesterol control in any form other than food is not recommended. That said, this test can be a guide for you to help improve the necessary foods (ingredients) that make up healthy cholesterol. You can improve your cholesterol yourself—and you will know when your doctor doesn't understand how to interpret a cholesterol reading.

- LDL-P (LDL particle number) range <1000nmol/L
- Lipids   LDL-C (calculated) range <100 milligrams/dL
- HDL-C (calculated) range >40 milligrams/dL
- Triglycerides range <150 milligrams/dL
- Total cholesterol range 200 to 330 milligrams/dL
- Particles HDL-P (total) range >30.5 umol/L
- Small LDL-P range <530 nmol/L
- LDL Size >20.5 nm

Lipids

The normal total cholesterol level was set by the pharmaceutical industry twenty years ago at 240 milligrams/dL, and has been reduced intermittently as the sales of cholesterol-lowering drugs (statin drugs) decreased over the years. Today, the suggested range is set below 200 milligrams/dL, but cholesterol, is controlled by the liver, to maintain and repair all cellular structures, especially during illness or injury.

No one number fits any one person, but this number will vary with types of foods consumed and episodes of illness, injury, infection, or disease, especially chronic disease.

Triglycerides

Modern medicine places the measurement of triglycerides to HDL as the most important factor. You can divide your triglyceride level by your HDL level, and the end- result should be two percent or less. Total triglycerides should be below 150 milligrams/dL. **The lower this number, the smaller the number of by-products you are producing (see chapter 2). The use of non-bondable fuels at 20 percent or less will produce a triglyceride count of around 50–100 mg/dL.** And healthy triglycerides are produced when healthy protein and fats are consumed.

Total HDL-C (Calculated)

The total HDL (calculated) should be above 40 milligrams/dL. **Remember that these are the cell wall fragments that clump and return to the liver, so the higher the number, the better, especially during times of injury.**

Early destruction of cell walls (cell death) can be caused, by traumatic injury, oxidative damage (free radicals), or the use of pharmaceuticals (statins). **In this scenario, we need to eliminate the cause (free radicals or pharmaceuticals)**, consider supplementation with CoQ-10, and avoid the formation of "lethal" oxysterols, trans fats, and foods that create oxidation (fried foods, powdered eggs, rancid oils, and hydrogenated and partially hydrogenated oils). Increase the use of healthy fats and minimum amounts of healthy proteins to form active cholesterol sulfate for mending of tissues, preventing further early cell destruction, and eliminating drugs that control cholesterol.

LDL-P (LDL Particle Number) Minus Small LDL-P

As for LDL particle number, this will vary with several important factors that need to be accounted for. As referenced by the National Cholesterol Education Program and Shafer EJ, in the results from the Framingham Offspring Study, the LDL particle number and size and subspecies must be assessed. **The total LDL particle number—be it high or low—needs to have the small particle number subtracted from it.** Small particles are basically poor quality or damaged (oxidized) cholesterol (nonlethal oxysterols) and will eventually either be recycled by the liver or be consumed by macrophages (our internal trash compactors). So, subtract this number.

LDL Size

The remaining number (LDL-P minus small LDL-P) now needs one more comparison: size. **If the LDL size is above 20.5 nm, then it is fat, fluffy, and healthy.** These forms of cholesterol can cause no damage to your circulating system or heart. **When the size drops below the 20.5 nm marker, we need to look at just what we are eating. Are we using healthy fats and proteins?**

When we use unhealthy fats and proteins, our triglycerides can become nonfunctional or poorly functional—with early cell death. If we are consuming trans fats, then we will be dealing with oxidation and altered blood flow.

LDL-P (total LDL particle number)

If the LDL particle number, is1000 nmol/L or less (minus the small particles), then the body is functioning at a healthy level. **If the number is high—be it healthy or unhealthy LDLs (size)—then we need to look for signs of injury, illness, or disease.** Since inflammatory response causes an increase in cholesterol production, we may see a much higher particle number after an injury or during illness or disease. Which may return to lower levels after the illness, injury, or disease has resolved. This is an area that needs more research and may be a good way to pinpoint early disease that has yet to develop outward symptoms.

The calculated LDL (LDL-C) number is not included here. It is not significant, if the HDL and triglycerides are within appropriate range and the LDL particle number and size are within acceptable ranges for each individual. **Always take into account the foods consumed and the presence of illness or injury.**

To sum it up:

These numbers can help you adjust your dietary regime to improve your body's production of healthy cholesterol. That neat little package of elements, that gives every cell in the body renewed strength and structure for improved overall health and growth. And our need for statins or cholesterol-lowering drugs is completely unnecessary.

If we know, where the damage comes from, follow bondable versus non-bondable teaching, and provide the body with healthy foods (fats and proteins). **Then we can prevent unhealthy cholesterol, simply by changing what we eat!** Remember, the only bad cholesterol is a damaged or oxidized one, and the best cholesterol is a sulfated one.

What have we learned — Dorothy?

Cholesterol, in all its various forms—whether it be LDL or HDL particle—forms a neat little package that contains various levels of fat, proteins, phosphorous, and sulfur. When healthy, it is fat and fluffy and can cause no damage to the body. When damaged or oxidized, it can cause multiple forms of damage—from heart disease to cancers. Damage to cholesterol (oxidation) comes from two sources: trans fats and free radical oxidation.

There are two types of trans fats:

Trans fats from saturated fats from animals that are made by animals and found in nature (healthy form) and trans fats from artificial hydrogenation of vegetable oil, which are not found in nature (unhealthy).

To prevent damage from trans fats:

"Lethal" oxysterols, found in fried foods, margarines, soft spreads, partially hydrogenated and hydrogenated vegetable oils, heated vegetable oils, rancid oils, and powdered eggs need to be removed from the diet. The basic cooking oils in any house should be organic, cold-processed olive oil, coconut oil, and butter (and tallow and lard for baking). Margarines, corn oil, soy oil, palm oil, cottonseed oil, or rapeseed oil are not recommended since these are not healthy forms of oils.

To prevent oxidative damage to our natural body defenses:

Avoid trans fats (free radical damage) and incorporate the use of vitamins C, E, B6, and CoQ-10 as natural antioxidants to enhance the body's defenses. All of these elements, can be found in healthy-source whole vitamins and proteins.

The healthy forms of protein should always be used.

This includes eggs (organic), whole milk (unpasteurized), hard cheeses (unprocessed and not artificial), meat and poultry (organic and grass-fed), fish (wild-caught and not fried), legumes (including green peas), raw nuts, and brown rice (all organically grown). Unhealthy source proteins can also provide forms of oxidation seen as protein fragments (glutamine).

We do not need to avoid dietary cholesterol, but we need to read our labels.

A high percentage of the processed food in the United States contains varying amounts of hydrogenated as well as partially hydrogenated oils and unhealthy fats and proteins. You may find yourself with little to no processed food in your cupboard and refrigerator as a result of these chapters. That's okay! Simple, whole foods are precisely the direction to travel here.

It's not how you eat, when you eat, how much you eat, or how little you eat—it's what you eat that makes the difference.

CHAPTER 14

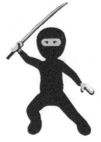

CoQ-10: The Soldiers That Protect Our Cells

This element has been mentioned before, but its importance requires a better understanding of its relationship with each and every cell—throughout the body.

We can use the health of one cell (cellular health) as the basis for almost all the information provided in these teachings. Think of the cell as a micro unit of yourself. All cells perform the same basic functions. In mass, they work together to support each other for survival. The important word here is **survival.** Multiply that one cellular unit by one trillion.

CoQ-10 is a vital element for every cell in the body.

Each and every cell makes CoQ-10 from proteins (amino acids) that are mostly found in beef, fish, chicken, eggs, and some vegetables.

In the body, this element can be found in three (redox or reducible) states.

- fully oxidized = **ubiquinone** (forms the electron transport chain)
- partially oxidized = **semiubiquinone** (antioxidant coats cell walls, produces hydrogen peroxide)
- fully reduced = **ubiqunol** (antioxidant cotes cell walls, attracts CoQ-10)

This molecule is unique;

It is the only molecule, produced by the cell, that can exist as fully oxidized as well as fully reduced state, and remain stable to perform their functions. Which include formation of the electron transport chain as well as formation of antioxidants (protecting the cell from oxidative damage). It is also a primary ingredient in the formation of ATP (adenosine triphosphate) otherwise known as energy, which every cell makes.

As the element ubiqunol coats the exterior of the cell wall, it tends to attract other CoQ-10 in the surrounding area. As it begins to break down or oxidize, it forms semiubiquinone and produces a by-product of hydrogen peroxide, which is actually a form of free radical that provides the antioxidant protection against other free radicals, including heavy metal ions and bacteria. **This antioxidant (hydrogen peroxide) literally cleans up the area by killing bacteria and viruses and neutralizing heavy metals. Our**

internal sweeper.

Once fully oxidized, semiubiquinone becomes ubiquinone, forming a chain of molecules (the electron transport chain) that actually pierces the cell wall.

CoQ-10 enters the cell by crossing the electron transport chain, created by ubiquinone, and it is a vital element in the formation of that energy (ATP) inside the mitochondria (the energy factory).

A by-product of that ATP is acetyl-CoA;

Which is the necessary element for the formation of more CoQ-10. This CoQ-10 also changes its redox state, becoming semiubiquinone **inside the cell,** forming hydrogen peroxide for protection **inside of the cell,** before it reduces again, becoming ubiquinone and creating that electron transport chain **to exit the cell.**

Outside the cell, ubiquinone picks up vitamin E.

And again becomes ubiqunol, supplying a new exterior coat to that newly created cell wall and protecting it from damage. This process repeats itself until the components are depleted. As long as the cells have a supply of healthy proteins, this process will repeat itself over and over, protecting each and every cell. Problems arise when the supply of healthy proteins or vitamins is diminished. We need to maintain that minimum supply of healthy proteins, and only the minimum, since excess only creates damage.

The hydrogen peroxide exists for a short time inside and outside the cell.

Since this free radical (hydrogen peroxide) can become damaging to the cell wall in large quantities, it is neutralized by an enzyme called glutathione (a sulfa-bonded antioxidant and oxidation regulator) created by the sulfur, brought into the cell by the cholesterol sulfate, and produced during the formation of ATP. The hydrogen peroxide is neutralized to become water, oxygen, and sometimes hydrogen sulfide. Hydrogen sulfide is a gas and can exit the cell, converting back to a solid, so this process repeats itself over and over again.

In areas of heavy connective tissue, we find strands of protein-coated cells.

These strands of protein appear to be more abundant in the skin. In these strands or beds, the protein present is high in sulfur as well as CoQ-10. It is interesting to note that the level of CoQ-10 is highest in these beds, where ENOS and higher levels of protein are present. So, the throry is, that cholesterol, with its protein coating, can pick up CoQ-10 as its hitchhiker in the skin during its travels through the bloodstream, and it can travel to its destination without being damaged by those free radicals that appear to be more plentiful in the bloodstream than in the extracellular fluids.

There are no set values for normal levels of CoQ-10 in the body—

Whether it is tested in the blood or tissues, no one knows how much your body needs, and to make it more difficult, levels of CoQ-10 vary throughout the body. Different levels are found in blood, bones, soft tissue, the liver, and the heart.

The need for increased cholesterol flow in the body, is triggered by the inflammatory response and is regulated by the liver. This response may also serve as a CoQ-10 regulator, increasing levels in areas of the body when needed since the two appear to work together.

There is no scale to measure deficiencies of CoQ-10.

But decreased levels of CoQ-10, have been noted in areas affected by illness. Cardiac studies have shown that, when increased cardiac disease is found—such as with congestive heart failure—significant decreases in levels of CoQ-10 have also been found. This indicates an increased demand for CoQ-10 during illness. **We can conclude that physical activity and overall health (amount of illness present) are directly related to CoQ-10 production.**

Let's take another look at those one trillion cells that make up our bodies.

If every cell makes its own CoQ-10 to remain in a protected state and there is still the need for CoQ-10 in transport and protection of lipids and proteins, where does that extra CoQ-10 come from?

The reticular layer or beds in the skin appear to have a much higher level of CoQ-10, and these beds consist predominantly of fat cells and interlinked protein fibers. Since fat cells don't make CoQ-10, the theory is that the extra CoQ-10 comes from the interlaced protein fibers. CoQ-10 comes from protein, and this bed is predominantly protein. These beds also appear to be the source of proteins that provide the needed base to maintain the sulfur created by ENOS from sunlight (the extra sulfur and oxygen molecules). These protein fibers, can be viewed as a form of protein storage bed, that continues to be replenished by amino acids provided by the minimum dietary supply.

Let's sum it up and look at what we know.

CoQ-10 is a primary source of energy for the cell. **It is made by every cell in the body using amino acids (protein) provided by the diet.** It is necessary for lipid (fat) and protein protection as an antioxidant. It produces hydrogen peroxide, which also acts as a free radical that neutralizes other more dangerous free radicals, including heavy metals, toxins, and bacteria. It is also a main ingredient in the formation of ATP, our cellular energy. Our cells continually recycle this element until it is no longer usable. At that time, the cells pull more CoQ-10 from proteins provided in the diet.

There are no set maximum or minimum levels of CoQ-10 for dietary needs.

But is has been noted that the average dietary intake of CoQ-10 is approximately ten milligrams daily. This number may be substantially lower than the body's actual needs for necessary concentrations. **Food sources** of CoQ-10 are beef, fish, chicken, nuts, vegetables, and eggs. Levels in food sources decrease with frying during preparation. Some strict vegetarian diets should consider supplementation at any age—but especially over the age of thirty.

Since CoQ-10 works in such a close relationship with other elements, this relationship is critical to overall health of the entire body.

Deficiency?

To see deficiency, we need to look at overall health status and the presence of illness. Overall health needs to be looked at in the form of that energy necessary to be active for a twelve-hour period. This includes the presence of weak or tired muscles and the inability to concentrate or perform functional tasks. **The presence of any illness or injury may be an indicator of**

CoQ-10 deficiency. When these signs occur, supplementation may be necessary.

The healthy human body absorbs, breaks down, and creates CO Q-10 by biosynthesis from healthy source proteins from birth to age twenty. At that point, natural biosynthesis begins to decrease. Healthy adults over the age of twenty and those people of any age (including children) who are ill should supplement, depending on the severity of the illness.

If we look at bondable versus non-bondable, we can see that the use of non-bondable foods over time will foster the production of metabolic syndrome, which will drive up the need for higher levels of CoQ-10 in the diet. As a result, people attempting health improvement and physical change should also supplement.

Today, it appears that almost all conventional medical therapy of patients with heart disease in any form, includes the use of statin or cholesterol-lowering drug therapy. Since statin drugs, including red yeast rice, block the formation of CoQ-10 within the body, and reduce the flow of healthy cholesterol in the blood, both of which are vital elements for maintaining good health. Then it can be assumed, that the tissue demand for energy frequently outweighs the supply, in the presence of these drugs. This can be termed a **drug-induced deficiency**, which results in the progressive formation and increase of disease in the heart and in all tissues of the body.

And last, when considering the quantity of protein, we must also consider the quality (healthy sources only). Since the highest quantities of CoQ-10

are seen in soy—and since soy is a toxin — —Any commercial supplements that contain soy in an unfermented state are not recommended. Avoid unfermented soy in your supplements. **If it contains soy, it must be fermented only.**

Healthy maintenance over 30	Adult age recovery from illness	Adult age during illness	Any age high dose Rx
100mg/day or 50mg absorbed	200mg/day or 100mg absorbed	200 -800mg/day ^200mg absorbed	200 - 1200mg/day
	Child by wt.	Child/physician	Adult /Child Per physician

A general guide for CoQ-10 supplementation.

CHAPTER 15

Sulfur

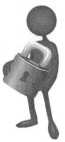

**The Mover, the Shaker, the Element Maker
The Key to Cell Strength and Mobility**

This particular element has been, for the most part, ignored by biochemistry studies.

And until recently, it was never considered an important element in our health. The evidence is starting to show us that sulfur is a vital element in the role of maintaining cell health and its integrity. It may very well be found to be the most important element in the body since it provides calls with a long and healthy life.

To date we have learned that a large portion of the sulfur in the body is synthesized in the skin by exposure to UV rays (sunlight) as vitamin D sulfate and cholesterol sulfate. **We can absorb sulfur four ways: eat it in food, drink it in the water, synthesize it in our skin, and absorb it directly through the skin as seen in swimming or soaking.**

Sulfur is a natural mineral that comes from soils formed by natural volcanic activity.

Elevated concentrations of sulfur in the soil and water appear to occur in and around areas formed from active volcanoes. The foods grown in these regions and the fish that thrive in these waters are high in sulfur. Comparative studies have shown us, that people who live in those areas, eat the plants from the soils and the fish from the waters, and swim in the waters have extremely good health and little or no heart disease.

Modern science, commercial food processing, and the use of herbicides and pesticides have severely depleted the availability of sulfur in our foods. Commercial food processing and the use of chemicals can limit the absorption and usability of sulfur by the body. Pesticides and herbicides block plants' absorption of this precious element, so it is not available in our foods.

Sulfur is the most abundant element in the human body after phosphorus and calcium. It is an essential component for all living cells. Under normal conditions, a human body weighing 154 pounds will contain approximately 140 grams of sulfur.

So, what is it about sulfur that makes it so important?

The Mover!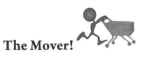

Fifty years ago, sulfur was looked at as just a binder of protein molecules.

Recently, it has been discovered that sulfur, when exposed to UV light, has the ability to move through any tissues (liquid and fat-soluble). This mobility gives sulfur the ability to cross the blood-brain barrier and the fetal barrier with ease. Along with its protein bonds, it can carry elements anywhere.

In bondable versus non-bondable, we see insulin and glucose bonding (poly-glucose with a sulfur bond). The sulfur gives the molecule mobility. The insulin—a polypeptide with a sulfur bond—can also move freely throughout the body, accumulate in the brain, and block leptin-to-ghrelin signaling.

The sulfur found in active cholesterol sulfate gives the entire element mobility. This is particularly important for transport of hormones (transported by active cholesterol sulfate), especially those in the brain that maintain emotion, mood, and cognitive function.

Sulfur will bond with almost all the elements in the human body.

But it has a particular affinity for proteins, which appear to be the strongest of all the bonds. It is a natural element found in methionine and cysteine (animal- and plant-sourced proteins), which are elements the body cannot synthesize. Those proteins must come from food.

The liver will form a sulfur bond between tyrosine (a non-sulfated plant- and animal-based amino acid) and sulfur (derived from the diet). This bond is called sulfotyrosine. This bond is so strong that the sulfur **cannot be removed**. This amino acid becomes a major component in brain hormones and neurotransmitters such as dopamine, epinephrine, and norepinephrine. It is also a major contributor to the formation of thyroid hormones.

Sulfur will bond with and carry oxygen through the circulating blood

It will carry oxygen to the tissues where it also aids in the chemical reactions involving oxygen. Oxygen by itself becomes a free radical and can damage other elements and tissues. Sulfur, by itself, will form a strong bond to other sulfur molecules, creating an unusable jell-like mass that can be dangerous in the circulation. **Sulfur is never left unbounded, and there is always another chemical reaction or combination that utilizes sulfur.** The most important of these reactions is found in the intracellular and extracellular regions. This involves the formation of an enzyme called **glutathione.**

Glutathione acts as the <u>master controller</u> of oxygen-oriented reactions.

It will neutralize hydrogen peroxide, keeping this free radical (hydrogen

peroxide 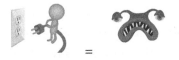) from getting out of control and destroying more than just the heavy metals and bacteria in the area. Glutathione can form almost anywhere in the body, but it cannot form without sulfur. **Think of hydrogen peroxide as the internal sweeper that cleans up the area and the glutathione as the robot that unplugs it, cutting off its power and limiting any damage.**

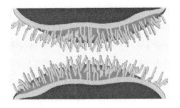

When we look at the average cell wall;

We see the lipid bi-layer (the 'Oreo cookie' structure). As the layers compress against the protein center, it forces fragments of the protein to extrude from the outer cell wall, giving the appearance of cilia or small hair-like projections of sulfur-bonded protein outside the cell wall.

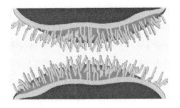

These projections or cilia will bond to the cilia extruding from the cells next to it,

And the sulfur in the extruded protein will bond tightly (sulfur–to–sulfur bond). Between epithelial cells in the intestinal lining, the skin and those found in the lining of the arteries—or even those that line and protect the unborn fetus—we find this **sulfur-to-sulfur bond.** We get sulfur bonding (**a double bond**) that pulls the cells closer together and bonds them tightly. Think of these bonds as the body's form of glue, and we need the highest-quality glue (sulfur to sulfur) to form the strongest bonds, giving our cellular structure the ability to lock out or prevent unwanted elements from getting into areas where they can cause damage and disease. **This bond can create a watertight seal between cells. This seal is so tight that it will even hold out bacteria.**

Science has found these bonds;

On the surface of the skin, in the lining of the arteries and veins, in the inner lining of the heart wall, and in the lining of the intestinal wall. Although it has not yet been scientifically proven, it is also believed to be an important element in the blood-brain barrier, the inner lining of the arteries that surround and feed the brain. This bond keeps destructive bacteria out of the skin, keeps bacteria and platelets out of arterial walls (as seen in peripheral artery disease), and seals out chemicals and free radical proteins and bacteria. It prevents intestinal absorption through the gut wall (leaky gut syndrome). It is believed that this bond provides the same protection for the brain.

When considering protein-to-protein bonds, we must remember that the critical element involved in this process is the sulfur (the glue). A majority of those bonds occur as a result of the presence of active cholesterol sulfate. The neat little package provides strength in the form of energy and structure in the form of reinforced or rebuilt cell walls.

With this in mind, consider a theory that has yet to be proven by science. A sulfur deficiency along with a lack of insulin control in the American diet may be one of the main causes of many of today's diseases. We need to look specifically at a deficiency of active cholesterol Sulfate in the body. **This sulfated element can pass through any tissue, and it can only be produced by exposure to UV rays (sunlight).**

If we look at bone cells, they appear much like tissue cells.

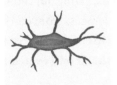

The protein extruding from the cell wall is long and interlaces with strands from other cells (the protein-to-protein bond). These cells are farther apart, not pushed up against each other like they are in the arterial wall lining. The sulfur from the active cholesterol sulfate that made that cell wall bonds with the strands of neighboring cells, leaving open spaces between the bonded strands where mineral deposits solidify and form crystals.

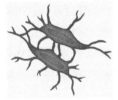

This creates a double bond with exceptional strength and flexibility (bone).

Bone cells are alive and just as functional as any other cell in the body. They need to be reinforced or restructured like all other cells, but the only way they can get the proper restructuring elements is through active cholesterol sulfate since it is the only element that can pass through the dense mineral formations (water and fat soluable) to actually get to the cell. Blood vessels pass through bone, but they do not diffuse into tiny arteries and veins like they do in soft tissue. The elements in the blood must pass or diffuse through the artery wall by osmosis –

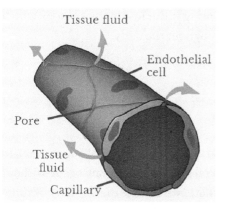

Tissue fluid

Endothelial cell

Pore

Tissue fluid

Capillary

- and get to the outermost densely packed cells of the bone to provide new cell wall structure and minerals to maintain density. **Without active cholesterol sulfate this osmosis cannot occur, the bone cell itself, remains locked in that densely packed structure and cannot maintain its strength and its own bonds (otherwise seen as osteoporosis).**

Cholesterol with no UV ray exposure (no ENOS);

Although it still contains sulfur, is a weaker molecule. It is not completely liquid- and fat- soluble and cannot pass into the bone cells or cross the blood-brain barrier or fetal barrier. This form of cholesterol may still be useful to other more easily assessable tissue cells, but it will not be useful to the brain, bone cells, or fetal growth.

It appears that the activation of cholesterol sulfate, is actually induced by the formation of vitamin D sulfate, which is also created, by UV ray exposure. These two elements look the same, and it actually seems like one blends into the other. Vitamin D sulfate activates the cholesterol sulfate, becoming a part of its molecular makeup and making it water- and fat-soluble. It becomes active cholesterol sulfate and moves freely through any tissue.

This may be the reason why most studies involving supplemental vitamin D3 have not significantly shown improvement at the cellular level because this form of vitamin D is not sulfated by exposure to sunlight. Although vitamin D3 as a supplement; has been shown to be a form of stabilizer of sulfur levels within the body by preventing sulfur loss in the kidneys, which could minimize sulfur deficiency throughout the body.

The Shaker and the Element Maker

There are many chemical bonds that are formed to assist in, or react to the formation of hormones and enzymes, and that cannot occur without sulfur. Without active cholesterol sulfate, we cannot make many of these compounds. We also cannot grow, maintain, or repair organ, bone, and even brain function. Whether cholesterol sulfate is active or inactive (with or without UV ray exposure), this element is the foundation on which the body is built. Some of the functional compounds the body makes using sulfur are listed below

- **Glycoaminoglycans**: glutamine sulfate and chondroitin sulfate = major components of synovial fluid (in joints), connective tissue and cartilage
- **Cerebroside Sulfate**: a major component of myelin membranes in the brain, essential in the formation of Schwann cells (protective coating on neurons)
- **Heparin Sulfate**: anticoagulant and the component that forms insulin
- **Sodium Sulfate**: cotransporter for oxygen
- **Keratin Sulfate**: a major component found in skin, hair, and nails
- **Poly-glucose with a Sulfa Bond**: bondable fuel for the cells

Digestive enzymes require the presence of sulfur to activate.

Sulfur is the primary component in the formation of **synovial fluid for joints.** The presence of sulfur compounds in the blood assists in the maintenance **mineral and PH balance** as well as **platelet aggregation (stickiness).** And sulfur is one of the main **transporters of oxygen to the tissues.** Without sulfur, oxygen would remain in your hemoglobin and never get to your cells. Sulfur is necessary for **the release of nitric oxide from platelets** that are formed in the marrow (core) of large bones. As platelets carrying nitric oxide flow through the circulating system and pass through the reticular beds, sulfur pulls the nitric oxide out of those platelets for deposit in the tissues.

Platelets also provide a secondary or backup system for cholesterol formation in times of need.

Scientists at MIT have found that cells circulating in the bloodstream (platelets and red blood cells) can actually produce cholesterol sulfate when needed in abundance, which is seen in acute trauma, heart failure, and severe brain damage. When large quantities of cholesterol sulfate are needed, the platelets can produce cholesterol sulfate from damaged triglycerides and LDLs, that the liver has difficulty filtering out, putting them back into the blood directly, by-passing the need for the liver's production. This process appears to be stimulated by the presence of elevated levels of LDLs.

The platelets receive the lipids as HDL-1 (in plaque) from macrophages and then use the ATP and sulfur from red blood cells to produce a healthy, undamaged LDL that is sulfated and can provide those healing measures to our damaged cells. Dr. Seneff, senior scientist at MIT, said, "This is a backup mechanism to keep the heart and brain as healthy as possible. It also reduces the circulating debris in the bloodstream and reduces the load on the liver."

Nitric oxide is used for maintenance of normal blood pressures and platelet activation (the formation of clots) and the formation of ENOS (oxygen and the sulfated ion). The presence of sulfur compounds in the circulating blood maintains a negative charge on most elements so they may move freely in the system without clumping. Sulfation (the addition of sulfur to other compounds) which creates, the binding and removal of toxins, heavy metals, and aluminum from the tissues, especially in the brain; this also requires sulfur.

We are beginning to see how important sulfur is to the body,

Yet there is **no clinical measurement of quantity or quality of sulfur in the blood or anywhere else in the body.** We can detect the presence of sulfur by measuring the presence or activity of sulfur-containing hormones and enzymes, which may give us an indication of a need for more sulfur in the body. In scientific studies, sulfur in the urine, is measured as a comparison to protein loss. The loss of excess protein from the kidneys will cause an equal loss of sulfur and vitamin D, but this measurement is not routinely used in medicine.

Are we sulfur deficient?

Yes!

Modern science, commercial food processing, and the use of herbicides and pesticides have severely depleted the availability of sulfur in our foods.

The lack of sulfur may also be a result of cascading losses created by stealing. Yes, the body will steal sulfur from one area of the body to supply another in order to maintain function and survival.

The first in line to steal is the liver.

This organ virtually cannot live without adequate supplies of sulfur. It is the first organ to receive nutrients from the digestive tract, including sulfur-bearing amino acids and sulfur compounds. When the liver is struggling to maintain all of its functions and produce sufficient quantities of elements for the rest of the body, then its own requirement for glutathione (which must have sulfur to form) will rise to maintain control of oxygen-oriented free radical production (free radicals containing oxygen). This increase in the need for sulfur will deplete the sulfur availability somewhere else down the line. Just as stealing from the minerals held by the bones for correcting or adjusting to a mineral imbalance (usually seen during pregnancy), the body will steal sulfur. The body suffers damage in the form of disease as a direct result of the theft or intake deficiency.

If we look at a variety of diseases that are not directly related to metabolic syndrome, we might get a gist of the pattern seen in direct relation to sulfur deficiency.

Let's start with osteoporosis and arthritis (osteoarthritis).

Mineral deficiency is a minor problem in this disease, which can easily be corrected by hair mineral analysis and adjustments in mineral consumption—rebalancing the body minerals (not just calcium).

If we look back on the section involving cholesterol, we can see that bone cells play a major role in bone density. These cells must remain healthy, functional, and alive to prevent structural loss and maintain its fragile bonds that give the bone its strength. Earlier we noted that bone cells receive their restructuring elements via active cholesterol sulfate. If the bone cells do not get sufficient nutrition and restructuring materials, the cells die, leaving a gap or hole in the bone (increased bone porosity) and eventual bone death.

If cholesterol is not sulfated or active, then it cannot reach that bone cell for nutrition and restructuring. The lack of activated sulfur is the basic cause of this disease, and the crucial ingredient missing in healthy bone formation is active colesterol sulfate. And since Chondroitin sulfate is the main component in the formation of synovial fluid in joints, provides protection of joint cartilage, and can only form with sulfur present. Then this is a directly related factor with another sulfur deficiency.

Science has found that people with osteoarthritis have extremely low or even nonexistent levels of **chondroitin sulfate** in the body (sulfur deficiency). Supplementation with synthetic derivatives has been poor to non-effective. This could be because we are not using the correct form of sulfur, which comes from sources of bondable fuels. Methionine and cysteine (sulfur-containing amino acids) can only be provided by food (healthy protein sources) and contain high levels of sulfur, along with the needed exposure to sunlight for activation of the sulfate in the cholesterol.

The brain is another area where barriers are involved.

The blood-brain barrier protects us from many forms of damage, much like the intestinal wall. It has been suggested that the increase in the sulfated bonds between the cells in this barrier (the inner lining of the arteries surrounding the brain) could improve its function and prevent diffusion of unwanted elements across the 'leaky' gap junctions (separations in cell-wall bonds due to inflammatory response) into the brain. **This is also seen in the intestinal wall and leaky gut syndrome.** With a loss of active cholesterol sulfate, it can also be seen as a form of sulfur deficiency.

The blood-brain barrier will selectively allow elements in and keep out most forms of bacteria and viruses. Even with this protection, sulfated ions can pass this barrier. The primary example of this would be insulin (two polypeptides with a sulfur bond), which can cross the blood- brain barrier and accumulate, blocking the absorption of leptin in the pituitary gland. This allows hunger to persist and also blocks the absorption of poly-glucose for healthy cell function, resulting in brain damage.

Some forms of non-sulfated free amino acids (glutamine), which are usually found in processed grains, milk, whey, soy, and corn, can accumulate outside the barrier. Accumulating heavy concentrations cause tissue irritation and inflammatory response (swelling in the cells). These amino acids (glutamine) cross into the brain as a result of accumulated numbers and squeeze between the leaky gap junctions during the inflammation of the barrier's structure.

In place of the normal neurotransmitters, this amino acid becomes a form of neuro-excito-toxin.

Creating a defensive response by nerve cells with the formation of ammonia (a free radical) in the brain that can cause early cell death of neurons. This can be seen in ALS (Lou Gehrig's disease) with high ammonia formations and neuron death. Along with the damage comes neuro-excitability seen in migraine headaches, seizures (epilepsy), strokes, Alzheimer's, and autism. These non-sulfated amino acids can block and prevent the proper use of healthy sulfated amino acids, which are the neurotransmitters that are needed to maintain brain balance and function.

This is a form of sulfur deficiency.

If we look back to bondable versus non-bondable, the main sources of glutamine are processed milk, gluten, grains, soy, corn, and whey, which are all non-bondable foods and unhealthy proteins.

Science has found that people with multiple sclerosis (a disease of the central nervous system) have extremely low levels of sulfa-bonded neurotransmitters in the brain and spinal cord, which may account for demyelination of nerves (loss of the myelin sheath that protects the nerve). This is another form of sulfur deficiency since the sheath can only form with sulfur present or active cholesterol sulfate.

Science tells us that people with psychiatric disorders or mood disorders (depression, anxiety, or loss of cognitive function) have increased levels of ammonia and decreased levels of sulfur-bonded neurotransmitters in the brain (sulfur deficiency). The most important source of neurotransmitters is found in active cholesterol sulfate and sulfur-bonded proteins (methionine, cysteine, and sulfotyrosine), which are found in a diet of healthy proteins. Active cholesterol sulfate is fat- and liquid-soluble, and as such, it can easily pass into the brain, improving the strength and structure of every cell in the brain, including the barrier itself. The result is normal function with a longer, healthier cell life.

Approximately 70 percent of the sulfur used by the liver comes from food.

These foods promote good health. This must include organically grown vegetables since the wide use of pesticides and herbicides in commercial farming actually destroys the absorption of sulfur from the soil. Animals that eat plants from organic soils also have healthier levels of sulfur.

When we eat foods that have healthy quantities of sulfur, the biologics in the intestinal tract get the first crack at them. When it comes to healthy proteins and their sulfur content, it appears that they are not readily separated. They cross into the bloodstream—across the intestinal lining (gut wall)—with the sulfur tightly bonded to the protein.

Other elements that contain sulfur have less stable bonds and tend to break down more easily.

The presence of **anaerobic (without oxygen) bacteria is also known as pathogenic (destructive) bacteria,** can colonize in the intestinal tract, and can convert our needed sulfate ($SO4(-2)$) to a sulfide ($S(2)$), which cannot be absorbed by the body. In other words, it breaks down the needed or absorbable form of sulfur (sulfate), essentially destroying its usability in the body. This creates another sulfur deficiency.

An increase in peptides -

Amino acid fragments that become glutamine in the body. Are created by bacterial breakdown of proteins from unhealthy sources (grains, processed milk, whey, soy, corn, and processed foods) will block and decrease the breakdown of sulfur-bonded proteins (healthy proteins— methionine and cysteine) and decrease sulfation (the bonding of sulfur to other molecules). This decreased sulfation results in the loss of amino acid (healthy protein) absorption. **The end – result of excess peptides is sulfur deficiency, and protein deficiency.**

If the sulfation is reduced, and a lack of healthy bacterial count in the digestive system persists, this process tumbleweeds upon itself.

Large amounts of peptides from excess casein, gluten, and whey (grains, corn, soy, processed milk, and whey, all non-bondable fuels and unhealthy proteins) accumulate and press against the intestinal wall, causing inflammation. This irritant to the intestinal lining results in an inflammatory response, and this resulting inflammatory response is seen **in irritable bowel, Crohn's disease, and GERD (gastro-esophageal reflux disease).**

The inflammation in the intestinal wall causes the cells to swell, and the bond between the cells (protein-to-protein bond) separates, allowing unwanted elements to squeeze between the cells crossing the wall. This process is called **leaky gut syndrome**. These excessive peptides can cross over into the bloodstream and travel back to the brain as excess glutamine.

The glutamine accumulates, causing another inflammatory-type response with separations in the cell junctions in the blood-brain barrier and allowing them to cross the blood-brain barrier again by squeezing between the cells or gaps in the junctions. They cause another inflammatory-type response within the brain cells, causing the cells to produce **ammonia**, which results in an opiate-like (morphine-like) effect on the brain (brain fog). With a continued trickle-down effect, the **excess ammonia blocks the absorption of sulfated proteins (cholesterol sulfate) into nerve cells.** This is seen in autism and Alzheimer's disease. This can progress to a resulting **loss of neurons by demyelination** (loss of the protective sheath on the nerves) and eventual cell death—ALS, Lou Gehrig's disease, and multiple sclerosis.

The digestive enzymes known as amylase and lipase must be sulfated in order to be active for digestion.

Science has noted a distinctive drop in amylase production when an increase in pathogenic bacteria is present. Two pathogens, H. pylori and candida, tend to increase and grow when sulfation is diminished in the meucin lining of the intestinal wall or gut. The health of our biologics or gut flora is directly related to the availability and usability of sulfur in the digestive tract, another sulfur deficiency (see chapter 3).

Gut permeability and leaky gut syndrome are a direct result of the loss of active cholesterol sulfate.

Since the cells in the intestinal wall cannot absorb sulfur directly from the intestine—and the sulfate bond that is required to bond cells tightly together preventing leaky gut is provided by active cholesterol sulfate—this form of sulfur needs to come from the inside of the body. Cholesterol sulfate is formed and controlled by the liver. This is a double-edged sword. If we cannot absorb the proper ingredients to make active cholesterol sulfate (methionine, cysteine, and sulfotyrosine), which is caused by leaky gut syndrome, we cannot prevent leaky gut syndrome. Ouch! More sulfur deficiency.

In each of the previous scenarios, the <u>solution</u> is the elimination of all unhealthy proteins and the increase of sulfur and healthy bacteria in the gut.

As an added note,

Several small, independent groups have found that the aggressive increase of biologics or probiotics in the intestinal tract contributes significantly to increased sulfation and utilization of sulfur throughout the body—with improved bonding in the body's defense walls. This has been accomplished with fermented foods, especially vegetables. References can be found in the back of the book on how to ferment your own vegetables.

In each of the previous instances, inflammation plays a key role.

The body responds to all insults in the body with aggressive inflammatory response. The difference in the effect lies in the quality of the cholesterol used by the body. **In other words, it's what you eat, and is it sulfated?**

When it comes to sulfur deficiency, there is one more area, that needs our attention: fetal development. We have already discussed the creation of stem cells in fetal development. These cells stay with you for life. Life begins with growth in the uterus, and that growth is influenced by the presence of multiple nutrients available in the maternal or mother's circulation. These nutrients must be able to pass across a barrier (decidua reflexa) that keeps the maternal circulation completely separate from the fetal circulation.

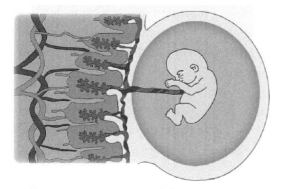

Note in the illustration that the two distinct circulations of the mother and the fetus are separated by a thick layer of epithelial cells;

This is the protective barrier, that is actually made up of epithelial cells in the uterine wall (not made by the fetus) that encase and protect the fetus along with its circulation from any outside sources, allowing only nutrients from the mother's circulation to pass. On either side of this barrier, two distinct and very separate arterial flows occur. For simplicity's sake, we call this the fetal barrier. **The blood of the mother never mixes with the blood of the fetus.**

Vitamins and minerals must pass across this barrier—along with fat and protein in the form of 'active cholesterol sulfate'. This wall must have a tightly bonded structure of epithelial cells. The bond must be a tight enough to prevent any unwanted elements from passing from the maternal circulation across to the fetal circulation, which can cause damage to fetal growth and development.

The same sulfur-to-sulfur bond is found in other barriers like the brain, the intestinal wall, the skin, and the inner lining of the arterial walls.

They are all made of tightly bonded epithelial cells. The main cause of separation of these tight bonds appears to be **inflammatory response,** which is the end - result of accumulation of unusable elements in the circulating system (in this instance, the maternal circulation). These elements can be chemical or pharmaceutical in nature or simply be the accumulation of too many elements like glutamine that remain in the circulation due to an overloaded liver, which cannot filter out these products in a timely manner. **Again we can see that the healthy function of the liver is of primary importance throughout our lives.**

This indicates the need for sulfur in the diet, along with the formation of active cholesterol sulfate in the mother to maintain proper structure (tight bond) and create healthier tissue growth of the fetus.

Sulfur is a major player in the maintenance of overall health throughout the body, but since there is little or no available independent research to indicate the quantities needed, it is impossible to tell how much sulfur our bodies are missing.

The deficiencies occur as evidenced by the formation of multiple diseases and physical dysfunctions that are prevented by the presence of sulfur. But where to draw the line defining deficiency has not yet been established. At present, we can only use those dysfunctions or diseases as an indication to change the diet and incorporate more sulfur.

On the other end of the scale,

There is little research on maximum dosage, but several private groups have been studying the individual uses of organic sulfur in the diet. They have found that the body only uses or absorbs what it needs. To date, an overdose of sulfur has not been noted; as a result, there is no maximum dosage.

We can take sulfur into the body in several different ways.

The simplest form is soaking. Epsom salts (magnesium/sulfate); both of these ions will soak through the skin easily. One half – to - one cup in a hot bath three times a week will improve skin function. Sun exposure three times a week for thirty minutes will produce ENOS (sulfur synthesis), and vitamin D sulfate will activate the cholesterol sulfate and maintain better sulfur bonds in the endothelial layers or protective barriers. **Or you could find a spa with hot mineral springs, usually located around volcanic activity, to jump into.**

The waters in and around volcanic activity (like Hawaii) are also high in sulfur content. It has been noted that people who use these forms of soaking actually acquire better utilization of the ultraviolet rays from the sun with improved tolerance to sun exposure. **Keep in mind, no chemicals on the skin, chemicals block ultraviolet absorption and cause skin cancer, and only spend thirty to forty minutes in the sun at one time.**

Pesticides and herbicides have severely depleted the soil of natural sulfur. For this reason, use only organic vegetables to improve sulfur content in the diet. Organic, rotational crop farming improves the soil mineral content and yields healthier plants that are rich in sulfur.

If we are discussing improvement to diets, the most important elements are those found in protein-bonded sulfur (meat and fish). The highest levels of sulfur-bonded proteins are found in wild-caught seafood and pastured organic eggs that are lightly cooked or raw.

Tap water contains sulfur,

But commercial water production (tap water) involves multiple damaging chemicals such as fluoride and chlorines. Even though tap water contains sulfur, because of the presence of other more damaging chemicals, reverse osmosis-filtered water can only be recommended, which also removes the sulfur. Those who use reverse osmosis filtering should also use trace minerals, to put balanced minerals, including sulfur, back in.

People who get their water from deep, natural wells or natural springs can be assured, that they are getting a natural and beneficial source of sulfur in their water, without toxins or the need for filtering.

How much is too much?

Unfortunately, no one has ever set a dosage for upper or lower limits. There are not enough studies to be able to set such values on the use of sulfur. We can only look at the health problems that involve sulfur and supplement via food, water, or application through the skin. The options available include soaking (three times a week), organic meats, fish, and vegetables, commercially produced supplements such as MSM (methysulfonylmethane), biotin (vitamin-like sulfur-bonded protein, also known as vitamin B7, vitamin H, or coenzyme R), or natural organic sulfur. For general use, follow label directions at one to two grams daily. If you choose a supplement, make sure it is non-GMO and contains no corn, wheat, or soy. And when attempting to conquer a long-standing health problem, the use of organic sulfur may be of more benefit since this form provides an increased bioavailability in the body. Independent, private studies appear to show a marked improvement in health response with organic sulfur.

In conclusion.

It can be said that, a majority of the American population is deficient in sulfur, but **the indiscriminate use of sulfur without improving overall health and the liver's function first may mask many problems.** Bondable versus non-bondable should be in place first. Once the foods that cause many of the inflammatory response problems have been eliminated, the improvement of healthy cholesterol sulfate with the addition of sulfur to the diet will result in noticeable improvement in all areas. We can conquer those diseases that have become so predominant in this country. **Remember, the body functions with all the proper elements in place, and sulfur, however important it may be, is still only one of those community members.**

CHAPTER 16
Detoxification

Over the years, the American diet has been continually changed, by the commercial food industry.

Today, processed food generally contains more chemicals than food. Our fruits and vegetables are grown with ever-increasing amounts of herbicides and pesticides. And genetic engineering has completely changed the structure of a large number of our staple crops. **It is now impossible to verify the safety of genetically engineered foods for human consumption.** As a result, these foods can no longer be considered part of a 'healthy diet'.

In the beginning of this book, we learned about extracellular environments.

We learned that all mammals store toxic or unusable elements, (excess polyglucose, metal ions, and toxins, particles from pharmaceuticals that are not filtered out buy the liver) in fat cells. The changes in our dietary supply have been ongoing for fifty years, so we have all accumulated varying amounts of toxins in our fat cells.

If changing our diets will eliminate a majority of the toxins we take into our bodies, than how do we get rid of what's already there?

Toxins pose a problem for the body, but the body has its own mechanisms for dealing with toxic or waste materials. There are **four ways** the body disposes of toxic or waste materials, this includes dead cellular material, and debris; via the **colon**, the **kidneys**, the **skin,** and the **gallbladder.**

But before we approach these end – points we need to start at the extracellular level where the fat cells are located.

When fat cells empty, the material inside becomes ketone bodies, along with waste products mixed with toxins. The cells burn the ketone bodies as fuel, and the waste materials and toxins are shuttled back into the circulating blood or out of the skin via a system called the lymphatic system.

Think of your lymphatic system as your solid and toxic waste disposal plant.

This is where dead bacteria, viruses, and cancer cells are shuttled. These materials are neutralized (becoming fat- and water-soluble) and are basically made 'safe' for disposal by this system. They are carried by white blood cells, glutathione, and macrophages (our trash compactors) mixed in with dead red and white blood cells, toxins, and heavy metals, shuttled from the tissues through the lymphatic system, back into the circulating blood, out of the skin via the sweat glands, or into the digestive system via the tonsils (lymphatic drainage from the head) or the gallbladder. This is a fluid system, so hydration (the maintenance of sufficient body fluids), and body temperature is very important. Without fluids, these lymphatic glands can become engorged and blocked, and health problems can result.

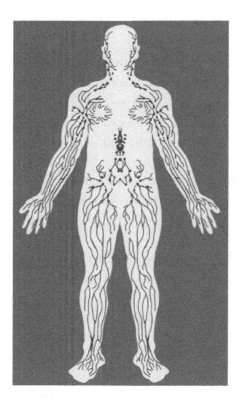

Elevated body temperature softens and facilitates the movement of lymphatic fluid.

This is why the body creates a fever when the immune system is fighting an infection or a virus. This helps the lymphatic system move the dead viruses or bacteria out of the body. This same theory is used in detoxification, as seen in hydrotherapies and the use of saunas.

Once returned to the circulating bloodstream, these products travel through the liver. The liver will filter out materials that are too large for other organs to handle. **Again we see the liver receiving a major portion of the burden in our health maintenance.** When we free up the pressure on the liver (decreased belly fat) and improve overall function by using organic bondable fuels, the filtering of the resulting smaller amount of waste products becomes highly efficient and very effective.

The liver shuttles these wastes to three areas.

- **The kidneys,** excess salts in the form of heavy metals, and ammonia, along with some chemicals are filtered through the kidneys.
- **The Skin,** the remaining salts, heavy metals, dilute ammonia and some chemicals can be excreted through the skin. The use of chemicals, especially antiperspirants and sun-block will prevent this function.
- **The gallbladder,** disposes of all complex chemicals and solid matter (dead cell fragments), via the intestinal tract, that the kidneys and skin cannot handle.

There are several acceptable forms of detoxification, that we can utilize to enhance these disposal routes or areas of body function.

People who do not need to lose any more than fifteen pounds will automatically improve their overall function and should not require aggressive forms of detoxification. For these people, one or two simple dietary forms of detoxification are usually sufficient. These forms of detoxification enhance the function of the intestinal tract and colon, preventing the ingestion of many toxins past the intestinal wall into the circulating bloodstream.

The colon should be at a fairly - normal functional level before detoxification should be attempted. A slow or poorly functioning colon can prevent the release of toxins and can even increase the re-absorption of those toxins into the body via inflammatory response. Those health problems seen in inflammatory response—irritable bowel, Crohn's disease, leaky gut syndrome, colitis, celiac disease, and even simple constipation—need to be addressed before using any oral forms of detoxification. This means the use of bondable versus non-bondable teaching, along with the removal of irritants that cause inflammatory response, processed milk, grains, gluten, whey, soy, corn, and GMOs. **The use of products beyond those mentioned in chapter 3 (adequate hydration and probiotics or fermented foods) for 'bowel cleansing' and improved function are discussed later in this chapter.**

Dietary Forms of Detoxification

- **Organic vitamin C** supplementation (organic whole food form), at one to three grams daily, will bind with toxins and prevent absorption.
- **Spirulina**, at one to three grams daily, will bind to heavy metals in the digestive tract, preventing absorption. They will also decrease toxic response from mercury-laced dental fillings, (silver fillings).
- **Chlorella**, at one to three grams a day, will bind to heavy metals in the digestive tract, preventing absorption. They will also decrease toxic response from mercury fillings.
- **Garlic, L-methionine, and selenium** also bind to heavy metals. Since doses will vary by manufacturer, follow the label instructions. Garlic is also a potent blood thinner.
- **Herbal teas aid in colon cleansing**, which assists in the disposal of accumulated waste materials in the colon and any toxic materials that may be present. This also enhances the overall function of the colon. Use caution since many over-the-counter products can cause dehydration and electrolyte (mineral) imbalances.
- **Chlorophyll-rich vegetables**, including parsley, can be added to a morning blend. They bind with heavy metals and decrease absorption via the digestive tract.

When looking to improve the skin's ability to dispose of toxic waste materials, hydrotherapy (water therapy) is the area of choice.

There are three forms that are well researched and safe to use.

- **Magnesium Sulfate (Epsom Salt) Baths** (Twenty-Minute Soaks): One half – to one cup in warm water to improve mineral absorption and increase the skin function for natural detoxification.
- **Baking Soda Baths or Soaks** (Minimum Twenty Minutes): Half to one pound in warm water for soaking, pulls toxins through the skin by osmosis. Particularly useful on insect bites and stings.
- **Hyperthermia.** The most efficient form of detoxification used for centuries, this therapy was even used by the ancient Greeks.

When the body temperature rises, the muscles increase their demand for fuel.

As a result, the fat cells deposit their contents in the extracellular tissues. Along with those ketones, the toxins become a problem in large quantities. The lymphatic system and muscles literally force many of these toxins to the skin's surface in the form of sweat via the sweat glands. Active mobilization of toxins can be accomplished with twenty to thirty minutes of exercise—preferably in the morning before eating—to provide the release of ketones from fat. Follow it with twenty to thirty minutes in a low heat (140–180 degrees) sauna. High heat can produce adverse mineral imbalances and can be dangerous. This sauna followed by a bath or shower in warm (75–85 degrees) water and then towel dry to prevent re-absorption of the toxins back into the skin. This process can be repeated over three to four days with heat exposure (sauna) at no more than thirty minutes each time. **So, find a local spa with a sauna.** Other more aggressive forms of hyperthermia should only be attempted with the assistance of a professional spa or clinic or alternative medicine physician who is well versed in this practice.

The goal of detoxification is the removal of toxins from the body after the fat cells have released their contents.

To improve the overall function of the lymphatic system, stretching, deep breathing, and lymphatic massage can be done each morning, after exercise. This is simple, safe, and effective. The combination of heat, fluids, and massage will improve the flow of lymphatic fluid and keep the vessels and nodes from becoming blocked. Lymphatic massage can also be performed by a trained therapist or physician. **This can also be found at your local spa.**

For those who want to lose more than fifteen pounds, a slightly more aggressive form of detoxification may be necessary.

That is over and above those already mentioned. As your weight loss increases, so does the level of toxins released into your system, **and when the body loses large amounts of weight, the risk of illness and cancer rises,** which is why detoxification is so important. More aggressive forms of detoxification can be safe, and others require the assistance of a physician.

A safe and effective method of removing larger amounts of accumulated toxins is by increased stimulation of the gallbladder.

The gallbladder is a sack that looks like an inverted balloon, located under the liver, which connects and empties into the duodenum (the first ten inches of the small intestine).

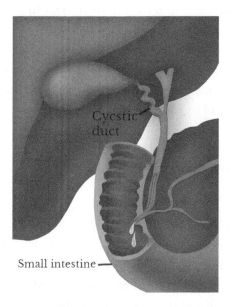

This sack fills with digestive enzymes, waste materials (dead cells), and toxins, but it will not contract and empty until it is triggered by sufficient amounts of fats in the diet. People on low-fat or no-fat diets cannot empty their gallbladders. This can lead to problems involving crystal formations in the sack (gallstones), which can block the channel or bile duct that flows to the duodenum.

A healthy diet consists of a minimum of 40 percent fat—40 percent of the total caloric intake daily should be healthy forms of fat. For some people, this can produce contractions of the gallbladder. But with large weight loss, frequent gallbladder contraction is necessary.

The use of coffee (caffeine) instilled into the colon (enema) causes dilation of the blood vessels and relaxation of the smooth muscle tissue found in the intestinal tract. This stimulation and relaxation effect travels the entire length of the intestine, dilates the common bile duct in the gallbladder, and causes contraction of the gallbladder itself.

Coffee enemas (instillations) have been used successfully for years by physicians in the treatment of cancer. This method of detoxification actually flushes dead cancer cells into the intestinal tract to pass out of the body. For cancer patients, this form of detoxification is routine and used two to three times a day without side effects. When coffee is consumed orally (by mouth), the acid in the stomach, neutralizes its positive effects, and it will actually cause adverse stimulation of the vagus nerve. **So, for those losing moderate to large amounts of weight, the use of coffee enemas is recommended.**

The colon is an organ of direct absorption to the circulating bloodstream.

Any chemical substances placed directly into the colon will be absorbed directly into the blood. The body provides some protection when toxins are swallowed, with the presence of hydrochloric acid in the stomach, digestive enzymes, and biologics. When any element is placed directly into the colon, these protections are no longer available. As a result, care must be taken to prevent, the introduction of direct toxins in this procedure. So, this form of detoxification requires organic, unflavored, natural coffee (one to one and a half cups), warm (not hot), processed with brown filters (white filters are processed with chorine), filtered water and avoiding the use of plastics that contain toxins that may leach into the coffee. The coffee is slowly instilled and held for as long as possible (around ten minutes). It is recommended in the morning after emptying the colon, the caffeine soaks readily into the tissues and does the rest.

If weight loss is already combined with illness or disease, such as heart disease, caution is recommended.

All the previous treatments mentioned can be used, but more aggressive forms of detoxification may be necessary after hair analysis for toxic levels.

For independent hair analysis, Dr. Thompson at aurorahealthandnutrition. com can also provide a phone consultation on the results.

When high levels of lead, mercury, cadmium, aluminum, calcium, and other heavy metals are detected, intravenous chelation therapy and hyperbaric oxygen therapy can be recommended Both of these forms of therapy, are administered by alternative medicine physicians who are well versed, trained, and certified in these areas.

Intravenous chelation;

Can involve the infusion of high doses of vitamin C or oxygen-treated hemoglobin in the circulating blood. Vitamin C will break down at the cellular level to become hydrogen peroxide (H_2O_2), also high-oxygen hemoglobin will result in elevated production of hydrogen peroxide. The end- result is an increase in free radical destruction of bacteria, viruses, and the binding of heavy metals, which are then captured by glutathione, and absorbed by the lymphatic system. The practice of stretching and lymphatic massage is helpful after these treatments.

Caution during these therapies is needed, as sufficient quantities of sulfur are necessary to carry the extra oxygen from the hemoglobin to the extracellular bed and to form glutathione (the master controller of oxygen radicals), controlling hydrogen peroxide and preventing the destruction of healthy cellular tissues during treatment. **This is also a recommended treatment combined with the ketogenic diet for the elimination of cancer.**

Intravenous chelation therapy

Can also be done using ethylenediaminetetraacetic acid (EDTA), which bonds to various heavy metals in the blood. This bond becomes water-soluble and is flushed through the kidneys. Again, sulfur levels should remain adequate since all heavy metals can bond to sulfur, and EDTA will lower the sulfur levels along with the heavy metals.

These therapies are only necessary when heavy metal toxicity is present or its resulting cellular damage (excessive cellular destruction and death) is present. It can be seen in such diseases as lead, mercury, or iron poisoning, osteoarthritis, hypercalcemia with acute hypothyroid function, many aggressive diseases, including cancers, and excessive weight loss (be it wanted or unwanted) with the release of elevated levels of toxins.

If someone loses a large amount of weight (more than thirty pounds) over a fairly - short period of time (less than one year), then hair analysis would be a good precautionary measure, making sure that toxins are not elevated to a point that would require these therapies.

Hyperbaric oxygen treatments;

Involve placing the body in a chamber filled with pure oxygen under pressure. The same principle applies here: the high oxygen content in the tissues will cause the formation of hydrogen peroxide (H_2O_2) and the subsequent destruction of bacteria, viruses, heavy metals, and cancer in the tissues. Again, a recommended treatment in conjunction with ketosis for eliminating cancer, keeping in mind that cancer cannot survive in an elevated-oxygen environment. This form of treatment, appears to induce rapid healing of tissues and has seen success in the treatment of stroke patients and those suffering from severe trauma. **The need for sufficient quantities of sulfur is again present.**

This particular therapy has become widely used in Europe, and is now being used with success, on serious injuries and illness in the United States. But obtaining this type of treatment in this country is difficult and expensive. **It has been noted, that there are approximately three or four hundred hyperbaric chambers in the United States, while there are more than two thousand in Russia alone.**

When we discuss detoxification of the body, it is important to understand that healthy colon function is necessary.

Without it, those toxins may become reabsorbed into the circulating system. Over the years, a slow or poorly functioning intestinal tract will result in gradual buildup of products of digestion that actually line the walls of the colon and harden. These products prevent absorption of nutrients and healthy function.

Healthy function involves the movement of foods through the intestinal tract in a timely manner, preventing buildup in the colon. So, what goes in should pass out of the colon in approximately twenty-four hours. If three meals a day are consumed, at least two stools a day should be passed. These stools should be soft and easy to pass, which indicates sufficient fluids (water) in the diet, and the color should be brown (presence of bile), which indicates sufficient fat consumption for gallbladder function.

When constipation is present in any form (frequent or intermittent), colon cleansing may be the first step in detoxification.

Once the colon is clear and functioning properly, other forms of detoxification, can be used with better effect. The absorption of vital nutrients will improve.

There are several, over-the-counter herbal mixes that work well for people who tend to have problems with constipation that is not resolved with the use of balanced, high-quality probiotics and adequate hydration (water intake). These remedies soften stool and gently cleanse the bowel, removing the accumulated residue that coats the walls of the colon. These herbal products contain cascara, senna leaf, fennel seed, kelp, black seed, rhubarb root, and corn silk or stigmas. **Bulk or fiber laxatives of any kind are not recommended. Any fiber needed should come from food—so eat beans.**

Colon cleansing;

Is described, as the mechanical irrigation (flushing or washing) of the entire six feet of the colon. This is sometimes necessary when the buildup in the colon causes toxic effects as seen in inflammatory response (Crohn's disease, irritable bowel disease, celiac disease, and even gastric reflux or GERD), resulting in decreased colon function. Colon cleansing; **should only be performed, by a qualified clinic or an alternative physician, who is certified and skilled in the practice of colonics.** This procedure, **should never be performed, during an inflammatory episode** since the inflammation in the colon will cause gaps in the intestinal wall (leaky gut) and absorption of those toxins back into the circulating system rather than the passage out of the body via the colon.

There are several types of detoxification that that are not recommend.

Since they actually counter the functions your body is working to improve. These forms of detoxification can be dangerous when used improperly.

The use of diuretic over-the-counter oral bowel cleansers.

This includes those herbals containing, liquorish root or whole senna, are designed to increase fluid loss along with aggressive stimulation of the entire intestinal tract (**laxatives**). These forms can decrease body weight through dehydration and will upset the delicate balance of minerals and bacteria in the intestinal tract. This can lead to malabsorption syndrome (loss of vital nutrients), acute dehydration, and severe mineral imbalances (loss of vital electrolytes, like potassium). It can affect the balance of body hormones and bone structure and the function of the nervous system. In severe cases, it can cause death from acute loss of potassium and heart failure. **The use of this form of detoxification, is often seen, in people who suffer from eating disorders (anorexia and bulimia) and is definitely not recommended.**

Fasting;

Placing the body in starvation mode **for extended periods of time** to force toxins from the body, is also not recommended. Removing fuels from the body between seven at night and nine in the morning and adding exercise will force the fat cells to relinquish their contents (ketosis). The toxins released on a daily basis, can be removed, with less aggressive measures (as mentioned earlier in this chapter).

Fasting or starvation for longer than twenty-four hours at a time requires delicate balancing to keep the fuel or blood sugar (glucose) level above sixty.

When true fasting occurs, the blood sugar will drop, and must be monitored to prevent it from dropping below fifty. A blood sugar below thirty can result in coma or death. This practice is only used when the desired result is rapid full ketosis and conversion of the body from a poly-glucose burner to a fat burner.

Natural ketosis can slowly be increased to full ketosis without this effect. Aggressive fasting requires routine and frequent blood and urine monitoring, and it should only be attempted, with the assistance of a medical professional who is well versed in this field. **In other words, intermittent fasting for up to twenty hours at a time is acceptable and can be quite efficient for weight loss purposes, but extended periods of starvation require strict monitoring.**

Intermittent juice fasting;

Is fasting for extended periods of time with the use of fruit juices to maintain blood glucose levels. Fasting will prompt the fat cells to release their toxins, but maintaining a fast with fruit juices only introduces fructose back into the liver where the undesirable by-products, are then reproduced. **So, someone who fasts on fruit juice will replace their lost belly fat with new belly fat. Obviously, this is not a recommended strategy.**

In conclusion;

Detoxification in one or two simple forms is usually all that is needed for most people when losing weight or working to improve overall body function. The use of a spa or sauna with body massage and mild exercise three or more times a year will not only detoxify, but will relax, and improve overall function as well as emotion.

We can also look at detoxification as a preventative measure, keeping toxins out to improve overall health, can be done by anyone. We can follow the old saying; **"an ounce of prevention is worth a pound of cure".**

CHAPTER 17

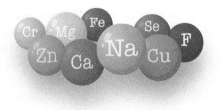

Minerals

The basic elements necessary for every living structure on earth

Without minerals, the human body would be a cold, soggy, nonfunctional mass.

Without balanced minerals, we could not move fluids and nutrients in and out of every cell membrane, we cannot form digestive enzymes or stomach acid, which delivers nutrition. Without balanced minerals, we cannot form cell membranes or cell walls, which gives us **form.** Without balanced minerals, we cannot form bone, which gives us **structure.** Without balanced minerals, we cannot contract or relax muscle tissue, which gives us **movement.** Without balanced minerals, we cannot move electrical charges across nerve tissue, giving us **physical as well as mental function. In short, without structure, form, movement, along with physical and mental function, the body would be a nonfunctioning mass.**

Remember your biochemistry lesson?

We learned there are two of the basic elements required for cell function: potassium and sodium. These, are classified, as ionic minerals (water-soluble minerals that can carry an electric charge; salts). They are only two of the **seventy-eight minerals** that are a vital part of the essential chemical reactions within your body. These reactions create structure, metabolism (utilization of fuels), and function. Keep in mind, **Vitamins, cannot be absorbed or utilized by the body, without the presence of these balanced minerals.**

Minerals are found in fresh water, in ground deposits where oceans once existed, and in the ocean itself, where all ionic minerals are found in salt form.

The ocean contains a supersaturated solution of all the minerals found in mammals, including humans, in perfect balance and concentration, with the exception of sodium, which is more concentrated in ocean water than in humans. We need to drink fresh water to maintain functional life, and **fresh water contains fifty-five of those necessary minerals**. Our bodies are 72 percent water, and the remainder is composed of minerals as solid structure. **Seventy-eight minerals in perfect balance and specific concentrations make up the remaining 28 percent of the body's composition.** When we alter these specific concentrations of minerals within the body, we shift a delicate balance that can have a devastating effect on our health.

Minerals are divided into two groups, macro or major elements and trace or minor elements.

These groups are separated by the quantities needed in the body. Major minerals, those required in substantial amounts (milligrams) as opposed to trace minerals that are necessary in a very small amounts (micrograms). The most important are the most abundant or the major or macro minerals.

To the human body, minerals are precious gems.

The body will not waste even the smallest amount unless it is forced to. Like a squirrel with too many nuts, the body will store minerals and recycle them until they can no longer be used. When the mineral balance in the body becomes altered, some minerals will be lost via the kidneys in an attempt by the body to rebalance. As a result, some tissues may be damaged due to hording.

Element	Symbol	Percentage in Body
Oxygen	O	65.0
Carbon	C	18.5
Hydrogen	H	9.5
Nitrogen	N	3.2
Calcium	Ca	1.5
Phosphorus	P	1.0
Potassium	K	0.4
Sulfur	S	0.3
Sodium	Na	0.2
Chlorine	Cl	0.2
Magnesium	Mg	0.1
Trace elements include boron (B), chromium (Cr), cobalt (Co), copper (Cu), fluorine (F), iodine (I), iron (Fe), manganese (Mn), molybdenum (Mo), selenium (Se), silicon (Si), tin (Sn), vanadium (V), and zinc (Zn).		less than 1.0

Calcium

Calcium is most abundant mineral in the human body at 1.5 percent of total body elements.

The first thing people think about when they hear the word calcium is bones. The thought has been programmed into us by nutritional advocates and conventional medicine for years: "Got milk?"

Unfortunately, our bones are not purely made of calcium, and **the improper consumption of calcium will actually cause more damage to bones rather than helping.**

When the body is young and developing, the use of calcium found in unprocessed sea salt, unprocessed milk, and organic vegetables will maintain structure. And when stress is added in the form of exercise, then bones can restructure.

As the body matures, the changing levels found in association with a decrease of male and female hormones—and the decrease in thyroid hormones—will influence the ability of the bones to restructure, losing the ability to remain flexible and strong. Unfortunately, we have been bombarded by the health industry into believing that high doses of calcium will prevent bone loss. **This is not true.** Today, **the excessive use of large amounts of calcium** in all processed foods, including double-fortified milk, which is even being promoted for children, **could result in bone damage as well as multiple bone fractures.**

Bones are actually composed of twelve minerals: potassium, magnesium, calcium, manganese, silica, iron, zinc, selenium, boron, phosphorus, sulfur, and chromium. **Without the proper combination (in proper balance) of these minerals, bones will not form.** A diagnosis of osteoporosis or osteopenia simply means that you are **mineral deficient**. The severity of the deficiency can be measured by hair tissue analysis (see chapter 4). Calcium is only one of those minerals, and although it is important, it is still required in a balanced form. If an overabundance of calcium occurs in the body, then that delicate balance is altered. As an example; a research study, performed by Walter Willett, PhD, chairman of the Department of Nutrition at Harvard School of Public Health and T. Colin Campbell, professor emeritus of nutritional biochemistry at Cornell University, showed that: "Boosting calcium intake to the currently recommended levels will not prevent fractures and even suggested that it may, in fact, weaken bones resulting in fracture".

Contrary to popular opinion, we do not store calcium in our bones;

Ninty Eight percent of the calcium we consume becomes a part of bone structure. While two percent is utilized for function at the cellular level. Calcium works much like potassium as its ion moves in and out of the cell wall, causing increased electrical activity in neurons and muscles, this is called **excitosis.** Vitamin D is an essential element in the maintenance of calcium in bone structure. Calcium binds with other elements to facilitate the formation of clots in the blood. Calcium is also essential in a systematic series of steps that cause muscle contractions. When the outer layer of bone dies, **which is a part of normal function**, the calcium in that layer breaks down and this calcium, is reabsorbed into bone, or shuttled to the kidneys for disposal, and this appears to be the only natural way we lose calcium.

The parathyroid gland (in the neck on either side of the thyroid gland) could 'lovingly be called' our 'squirrel'. This gland regulates calcium levels by increasing absorption of calcium from the intestinal tract, decreasing calcium loss through the kidneys. As a result, there is more calcium in the circulating system. For a clear diagram of this process, refer to chapter 18 and the discussion on vitamin D. There, you will find a diagram of the pathway for calcium and the direct effect of vitamin D.

Calcium levels in the blood may be deceiving since not all calcium remains in blood.

The blood's calcium level may remain normal while the other tissues of the body may have too much. Protein has a special bond with calcium as a carrier, and it has been shown that high-protein diets will draw calcium from the circulation, creating this 'squirrel-like' behavior. This is seen when over-supplementation is done and hording results (too much protein or calcium). Like that squirrel with too many nuts, excess calcium becomes stored in all kinds of soft tissues ('just in case'). This includes joints between bones, glands, and lymphatic nodules, including the thyroid gland, ends of bones, and even on dry surfaces (plaque) lining the arterial walls. On bones, these become calcified nodules (bone spurs), which is another good reason to minimize your protein intake.

Studies have found a protein that mimics parathyroid hormone, which has been found in fairly large amounts in various tissues of newborns, their mothers, and nursing mothers' milk. It's even seen in smaller amounts in adult tissues. This may be a form of calcium balancing in the infant while the immature parathyroid gland is still developing, providing calcium in sufficient quantities to form the bone matrix since bone is also still developing. **This protein, is not found in infant formula, which is another good reason to nurse your baby.**

In a continual attempt to balance one mineral, the body will inadvertently cause the loss of other minerals.

The increase or excess of protein in the circulating blood will also cause a loss of minerals via the kidneys. Excess calcium will attempt to create balance with magnesium (pulling magnesium from muscles and soft tissues), creating a magnesium deficiency. That deficiency will cause, among other problems, suppression of adrenal function (adrenal glands located on the side of kidneys that regulate kidney function), and since the adrenal glands cause re-absorption of sodium and potassium in the kidneys, it follows that the needed sodium and potassium are then lost in the urine (another deficiency). This affects the sodium pump (loss of sodium and potassium), and the cells begin to die. This causes a decrease in the production of thyroid hormones (including the parathyroid), which can result in decreased calcium and a decrease in mineral re-absorption in bones and loss of formation of stomach acid. **As you can see, this cascade can become a form of tumbleweed, growing larger and affecting multiple organs. It all comes from excess use of just one mineral or element and a loss of balance.**

Healthy food sources of calcium are;

Unrefined milk and milk products, including cheeses, salmon, sardines, vegetables, broccoli, mustard greens, turnip greens, kale, bok choy, spinach, beans, and legumes. Children need twelve to sixteen ounces of whole raw milk daily, along with three to four servings of healthy organic vegetables daily. Adults need eight to ten servings of healthy organic vegetables daily. Please refer to the tables, charts, and graphs for a list of foods.

Supplementation of human calcium levels is not necessary if the daily intake of milk and/or vegetables is sufficient and unrefined sea salt is used.

If supplementation with calcium is necessary, **never consume more than one gram (one thousand milligrams) daily,** including calcium consumed in your food. Calcium is added to a large variety commercially produced food, and all milk products are fortified with calcium. Please read your ingredient labels carefully and avoid as much additional calcium as possible.

Recommended Dietary Allowance (RDA) for Calcium			
Life Stage	Age	Males (mg/day)	Females (mg/day)
Infants	0-6 months	200 (AI)	200 (AI)
Infants	6-12 months	260 (AI)	260 (AI)
Children	1-3 years	700	700
Children	4-8 years	1,000	1,000
Children	9-13 years	1,300	1,300
Adolescents	14-18 years	1,300	1,300
Adults	19-50 years	1,000	1,000
Adults	51-70 years	1,000	1,200
Adults	71 years and older	1,200	1,200
Pregnancy	14-18 years	-	1,300
Pregnancy	19-50 years	-	1,000
Breast-feeding	14-18 years	-	1,300
Breast-feeding	19-50 years	-	1,000

USDA Food Database/RDA

How do I know if I'm getting too much calcium?

Excess calcium storage is seen as crystallized calcium (bone spurs) in the fingers, hands, feet, and toes. There is a loss of joint function or stiffness in the joints and palpable (by feel) firm, non-painful, nodules in the neck and thyroid glands. Calcium deposits and spurs can also be seen on x-rays and scans (usually seen on the spine or in deeper tissues such as the arteries). **Oxidized cholesterol (oxysterols) will increase the deposits of calcium in the arterial walls (see chapter 13).**

One added note, on the use of osteoporosis pharmaceuticals.

If you are using them or if you are considering them, a suggested word of caution. These drugs have no viable long-term studies connected to their use. But over a two-year period of use, they have been found to cause increased fractures, seen as shattered bone, and these fractures do not heal. They can also cause a slow and progressive loss of circulation to the bone, resulting in aseptic necrosis (bone death without infection). This is frequently seen in the jaw, which begins to literally crumble—and the teeth fall out. Look to your total body mineral content and hair mineral analysis, proper balance of vitamin D levels, and the use of weight-bearing exercise before using that prescription.

Phosphorus

The second most abundant mineral element, weighing in at 1 percent total body content is phosphorus.

Healthy food sources of phosphorus are organic meat, fish, poultry, eggs, bone, and bone meal or bone soup. Please refer to tables, charts, and graphs for a list of foods.

This element is necessary for cellular function (inside the cell) and the maintenance of body fluid pH (acid base balance), and it is found in the formation of human bone. Calcium and phosphorus will bind together to form a matrix or base on which the other ten minerals will crystallize, creating strong, flexible, healthy bone. It is also a main ingredient and end-product of the formation of adenosine triphosphate (energy) produced within every cell.

Again, caution needs to be taken when understanding this element.

This element is found in foods that contain protein, but it is not bonded to protein. In very minute amounts, it is also found in protein-containing plants like brown rice or peas, but it is not bound to the protein. Since phosphorus is not bonded, the body can absorb this as a free element. Rather than breaking a bond in the liver, it will bond to lipids in the liver. The lipids (cholesterol) act as a carrier, and phosphorous will be released from its bond during lipid metabolism. It is also found in moderate amounts in bone and bone meal (bone soup).

So now you ask; How much?

If the daily diet, contains sufficient healthy protein (see chapter 10), than the intake of phosphorus will also be sufficient. **Supplementation with phosphorous—as seen in such products in calcium/phosphorus combinations—is not recommended.** This combination is already bonded and can go straight to the tissues, which can lead to hardening of soft tissues, like tendonitis, and can sometimes mistaken for calcification. It will also cause severe diarrhea and block the body's ability to absorb and use iron, calcium, magnesium, and zinc, which will lead to malabsorption syndrome, with tissue and bone damage. **As long as sufficient healthy protein, is consumed, this mineral never needs to be supplemented.**

Potassium

The third most abundant mineral in the human body, weighing in at 0.4 percent of the total body minerals, is potassium.

Healthy food sources include meat, unprocessed milk, fresh fruit, and vegetables. Please refer to tables, charts, and graphs for a list of foods.

This mineral plays an important role in muscle contractions and nerve transmissions (the other side of the sodium pump). In that same positive to negative flow of ions (see chapter 1), the potassium will also cause balance and result in muscle relaxation. It's that balance between the sodium ions and the potassium ion that maintains the cell wall integrity and allows an electrical current as seen in nerve tissue. All wrapped around the cell's capacity to produce APT (energy) and push out the sodium ions in exchange for the potassium. The adult recommended daily allowance of potassium is two grams daily (two thousand milligrams daily).

Any potassium supplementation should be done under a physician's guidance.

Too much can cause heart attacks. As an example, the surgeon in the operating room wants to work on the heart, but in order to do that, he must stop its movement. The patient is placed on a heart-lung bypass machine to keep the circulation going, and the heart is injected with potassium. This is the same potassium that is used to stop the heart in lethal injections.

Too much potassium (hyperkalemia) can be seen in renal failure, excess or uncontrolled use of supplements, tissue trauma, and burns. Symptoms include tingling of the hands and feet, muscular weakness, temporary muscle paralysis, which can progress to irregular heartbeat (arrhythmias), and cardiac arrest.

Pharmaceuticals that tend to prevent natural potassium loss with a resulting increase in potassium levels are;

Potassium-sparing diuretics, blood pressure drugs (ACE inhibitors or beta blockers), non-steroidal anti-inflammatory drugs (Advil, Motrin, Indomethacin), NSAIDs, and the anticoagulant heparin.

Too little potassium (hypokalemia);

Can result from prolonged vomiting or diarrhea, use of diuretics (drugs that increase the urinary output), and some forms of kidney disease. Symptoms include fatigue, muscle weakness and cramps, intestinal paralysis (ileus), bloating, abdominal pain, and constipation. This can also result in abnormal heart rhythms (arrhythmias), which can be fatal.

Generally, pharmaceuticals that can cause a dramatic decrease in potassium levels in the body are;

Those that cause an increase in potassium loss in the kidneys, seen as diuretics, decongestants, bronchodilators (to open the airway), high-dose antibiotics, licorice, and caffeine. The end result is not enough potassium.

A majority of the population never needs to supplement with potassium. The use of sea salt and the adequate intake of a balanced diet with sufficient organic meat (or milk) and vegetables, with an occasional banana, will keep the body within the necessary limits for healthy function.

Sulfur

Sulfur is the fifth most abundant mineral in the human body, comprising 0.3 percent of total body mineral elements.

Since we have already discussed sulfur at length, we will not go into great detail here. Healthy food sources are organic eggs, meats, seafood, poultry, wild-caught fish, unprocessed milk, and a variety of legumes. Refer to chapter 15 for further information, tables, charts, and graphs for sulfur-containing food.

Supplementation with sulfur may be necessary—given its wide implications in health and cellular function and the encroachment of illness provided by the American diet.

Sodium

The sixth most abundant mineral element in the human body, comprising 0.2 percent of total body minerals is sodium.

This mineral is used by all the cells in the body. We need sodium as a major component in making stomach acid to break down proteins. We need sodium to facilitate the movement of fluids and nutrients in and out of the cell (the sodium pump). This same pump principle is more aggressively used in our nervous system. Which is seen as an ion exchange, at high speed, on the outside of the cell, creating a form of electric current down neurons at high speed. This creates electrical function of the nerve without cellular damage, while maintaining the cell structure at the same time.

This particular element is **found naturally in unprocessed sea salt crystals**. Table salt is only sodium and chloride and not in chemical balance to our body chemistry. And not a recommend form of salt in any diet. This is also the form of salt found in almost all processed foods and fast foods in large quantities, and it can be devastating to healthy mineral balance, creating disease progression with increasing obesity, hypertension, and multiple mineral imbalances. **Table salt is not recommended.**

Some small amounts of natural sodium can be found in unprocessed milk, meats, vegetables, and seafood. Sea salt crystals are a combination of major and trace minerals in basic equal balance to the human body, and liberal use of this source is highly recommended. **Be sure to get sea salt that has color—gray, black, red, or pink—since this indicates the presence of unprocessed minerals. If salt is white, it has been processed.**

Magnesium

Magnesium, the seventh most abundant mineral element in the human body, weighs in at 0.1 percent of total elements.

Food sources are nuts, seeds, legumes, green, leafy vegetables, seafood, chocolate, artichokes, foods containing high levels of chlorophyll, and unfiltered hard water. Please refer to tables, charts, and graphs for a list of foods. It appears that our ever decreasing mineral balance in our soil has now created magnesium deficiency throughout our population. As a result **this is one element that should be considered as a supplement in all diets.**

Much like potassium, this mineral creates balance to that sodium pump and relaxes muscle tissue. It also plays a role in the production of ATP (energy within the cell). Magnesium is attracted to calcium, and they deplete each other when either is in excess. When blood calcium levels are in excess, it will draw the magnesium from the muscle tissue, creating a magnesium deficiency. This magnesium is usually lost through the kidneys. It is difficult to develop a magnesium excess since this mineral is readily balanced and filtered out by the kidneys. High doses are rare but can occur, and when they do, it will draw calcium from the tissues, causing a calcium loss.

Magnesium also plays a role in the formation of multiple enzymes in the body, including those involved in the formation and replication of DNA and RNA (our biological code).

Recent research shows, that magnesium also aids in brain health by decreasing neuro-excito stimulation caused by glutamine in the brain (by blocking glutamine at the cellular level). It has been demonstrated, in studies that magnesium can lower blood pressure in a dose-dependent manner. It is used in the treatment of mild hypertension (high blood pressure), preeclampsia, and eclampsia in pregnancy (uncontrolled hypertension during pregnancy and childbirth). It is also used, in therapy to decrease calcium levels throughout the body as seen in atherosclerosis (calcification in arteries). Magnesium levels are not traditionally measured (blood tests) by modern science, but people who suffer from kidney disease or alcoholism tend to have difficulty maintaining a mineral balance and often suffer from a magnesium deficiency. These people need their magnesium levels maintained by their doctors.

How do you know if you are low in magnesium?

The basic place to look is in your body's responses. Low magnesium levels are seen in such symptoms as migraines, muscle numbness, muscle twitching, nerve tingling, muscle spasms, and muscle cramps.

Excess calcium and the presence of calcium deposits throughout the body are not necessarily an indication of magnesium deficiency.

They are calcified formations and do not affect the blood calcium levels. An elevated blood calcium level appears to be the factor that draws magnesium from muscle tissues. Studies have found that those calcium deposits can also be reduced by increasing magnesium intake.

It is difficult, if not impossible,, to overdose on magnesium from food, since healthy kidney function will maintain a normal balance. Too much magnesium can result in an upset stomach or diarrhea.

High-dose supplementation, found in oral doses of milk of magnesia (oral laxative) or Epsom salts (used as an oral laxative), are not recommended. They can cause sudden high doses, resulting in toxicity. Toxicity can be seen; as nausea, vomiting, low blood pressure, confusion, cardiac arrhythmias, and even death.

Below, you will find various forms of supplementation in magnesium.

All forms come in a variety of doses since they contain varying amounts of magnesium. Follow the label instructions on whatever type you choose to use. Most require one to two doses daily. Absorption will vary, and your symptoms (headaches, muscle numbness, or twitching) should be your guide. If your kidneys are healthy, vary your dosage according to symptoms—and only increase as response improves as seen in decreased symptoms. Back off if upset stomach or diarrhea occur. **Oxide is the most common form, and, taurate and theonate are the newest and show promise.**

- **Magnesium Threonate:** Newest of supplements, studies show improved absorption.
- **Magnesium Glycinate:** A chelated form of magnesium, good absorption and bioavailability, may aid in sleep.
- **Magnesium Oxide:** A non-chelated form with 60 percent elemental magnesium content, tends to soften stool.
- **Magnesium Malate:** A new form of supplement, bonded to maltic acid, appears to be more absorbable, has pain relief, muscle relaxation, and laxative properties.
- **Magnesium Taurate:** It is made by combining magnesium and taurine (an amino acid), a protein bond that has calming effects on muscles and the brain.
- **Magnesium Chloride/Magnesium Lactate:** It absorbs as well as the oxide form, but it contains only 12 percent elemental magnesium.
- **Magnesium Carbonate:** It contains 20–45 percent elemental magnesium (found in chalk) and has antacid properties.
- **Magnesium Citrate:** It is bonded to citric acid, contains up to 16 percent elemental magnesium, and has laxative properties.

- **Magnesium Sulfate/Magnesium Hydroxide**: It is found in laxatives and contains 42 percent elemental magnesium. **Use caution since it can cause a magnesium overdose.**
- **Magnesium Aspartate**: It is bonded to L-Aspartate. This neuro-excitory element causes neuro-excitation (as seen in glutamine response). **Use with <u>extreme caution</u> since it may cause central nervous system damage and demyelination of nerves.**

Trace Minerals;

All minerals in descending order of concentration found in sea salt:

Magnesium, chloride, potassium, sulfur, sodium, boron, bromide, calcium, carbonate, silicon, nitrogen, selenium, phosphorus, iodine, chromium, iron, manganese, titanium, rubidium, cobalt, copper, antimony, molybdenum, strontium, zinc, nickel, tungsten, germanium, scandium, tin, lanthanum, yttrium, silver, gallium, zirconium, vanadium, beryllium, tellurium, bismuth, hafnium, terbium, europium, gadolinium, samarium, cerium, cesium, gold, dysprosium, holmium, lutetium, erbium, ytterbium, neodymium, praseodymium, niobium, tantalum, thorium, thallium, rhenium, and other minerals found in seawater

The concentrations of sea salt minerals do not quite match the descending order of concentrations found in the human body.

Why?

If we compare the lists,

We find that the highest concentration of minerals in sea salt is magnesium, whereas calcium is actually eighth in descending order of concentrations. Our bodies stockpile and store calcium—like a 'squirrel' with too many nuts. Under normal conditions, we do not dispose of calcium. As a result, we require less intake of calcium to maintain balance.

On the other side of that coin, our kidneys continually filter and attempt to balance the magnesium in the blood. As a result, we actually need higher levels of magnesium in our diets to maintain the low concentration found in the blood and maintain balance as well as electrical function of nerves and muscle tissue.

Iron is classified; as a trace mineral and is found in unprocessed sea salt as number sixteen in descending order. It is only necessary in very small quantities, but it is vital for the transport of oxygen in our bodies. **Most people who supplement with iron are actually deficient in the three minerals that make up stomach acid: sodium, potassium, and chloride.** Stomach acid is necessary for the breakdown of proteins that contain iron. If you are not using sea salt, you cannot form healthy stomach acid or break down proteins. If you cannot break down proteins, you will become iron deficient (as seen in iron-deficiency anemia).

Recent studies show the use of **iodine** as an effective treatment of hypothyroid disease (a low-functioning thyroid). In the United States, the recommended daily allowance of iodine is 150 micrograms, but Japan suggests two thousand to three thousand micrograms. Iodine has shown improvement in thyroid function. It, has also been suggested that iodine can be useful in the prevention of breast cancer. Care must be taken with iodine supplements (read your labels) since it is formulated from seaweed, and many of the supplements come from Japan where radiation contamination is present. **Look to other areas of the world—like the Norwegian coast— for your seaweed iodine supplements.**

Sulfur is number four in the descending order of sea salt concentrations. It is actually equal to the body's need to create balance. We utilize sulfur in large quantities throughout the body. If our vitamin D levels are too low, we will lose sulfur through the kidneys. Medical science places little or no importance on the role of sulfur in our bodies. As a result, it is not recommended as a supplement by medical science.

If we alter the balance found in natural sea salt.

It will cause an imbalance of mineral concentrations in our bodies, which leads to organ malfunction, illness, and disease. **So, do you really need that** calcium supplement? If so, are you getting enough magnesium? And if you supplement with vitamin D, are you getting enough magnesium?

Trace minerals are an important factor in the total balance of the body's minerals, and these minerals can found in foods grown in healthy soil and natural sea salt. Remember, there is a distinctive difference between sea salt and table salt (see chapter 4). Table salt contains only sodium and chloride (you can't make stomach acid out of it), which will cause an imbalance in minerals and result in loss of protein (low stomach acid), loss of iron, body fluid retention, and hypertension (high blood pressure). This is the main reason why doctors restrict salt (table salt) intake, which is found in most processed foods, which causes even more imbalances of the minerals in the body. **The answer here is the liberal use of sea salt (all the needed minerals in a balanced form) in all diets and a serious reduction or restriction of processed foods in all diets.**

A major portion of our total mineral intake, in balanced form;

Comes from unrefined natural sea salt in the crystal form (grind it as you use it), used liberally in the diet. The remainder of our mineral intake comes from produce grown in soil (fruits and vegetables). In 1992, the Earth Summit reported "a noted decline in the mineral content of the soils in North America by 85 percent." In 1999, a study by Rutgers University, concluded that "the mineral content of commercial produce was less than 16 percent compared to vine-ripened organic produce."

Today, eighteen years later, we can see that we have literally bankrupted our soil, and since the mineral content of our foods determines the vitamin content, we can safely say that commercial produce has almost no nutritional value. **A large percentage of the American population is probably mineral deficient. Today, the loss of mineral density results in multiple mineral imbalances in men, women, and poorly nourished children.**

We all need unrefined sea salt in our diets. Your mom was right,—eat your veggies (preferably organic ones).

CHAPTER 18

Vitamins and Supplementation

There has been increasing public debate, in regard to the use of supplements as a part of a healthy diet.

The FDA, the pharmaceutical industry, and the federal government clearly state that supplements are of little value—and the American diet supplies enough vitamins and minerals in food alone.

If we look at the nutritional value of the vegetables in the 'American diet', we can see an enormous gap in quality and quantity.

Most Americans eat little or no vegetables on a daily basis. When you compare the vitamin and mineral content of today's produce, it is sorely lacking. As a result, It is recommended that if you want to receive all of your required nutrients from food alone, you will need to eat eight to ten servings of vegetables, juice vegetables or ferment vegetables daily. We have already mentioned that organic vegetables are much higher in nutrient content, but you still need eight to ten servings a day to meet the standards set by the American Nutrition Board and the American government. Juicing your vegetables means just vegetables. Fruit is Mother Nature's desert (containing fructose), and should be used in tiny amounts (for flavoring only).

There's always room for improvement.

Whether you are already in good functional health or fighting disease, the use of whole plant-source vitamins and minerals is definitely worth considering. And there is agreement with the general consensus, that Chemically produced vitamins provide little or no value to the 'American diet'.

Conventional and alternative medical physicians generally agree;

That poor nutrition, poor eating habits, and the ingestion of multiple prescription medications, over a prolonged period of time, can cause increased immune system damage, loss of proper organ and hormone function, which lays the foundation for multiple diseases, and a shortened life span.

Before we embark on the subject of nutritional supplementation.

Keep in mind that you can consume large amounts of vitamins that will slip through your system without being recognized or utilized if you do not have the proper balance of minerals in your system first. **Minerals can supply some function in the body alone, without any other nutrient, but vitamins and essential fatty acids (as found in vitamin E) cannot be absorbed or utilized without the presence of balanced minerals.**

If you are already on a supplementation regime or considering the use of supplements, look to your mineral balance first. The liberal use of natural, unrefined sea salt in its crystalline form (grind it as you use it) is the recommendation here. When looking for the correct form of salt, look for a crystal that still has color. It can be gray, black, pink, or red, but the color tells you that the crystal is still in the natural mineral form and has not been refined. For those of you who have problems with bone mineral density or are suffering from illness related to excess calcium, please refer to chapter 17 and the section on calcium. You may need to consider hair mineral analyses (covered by most insurance companies) or a more aggressive mineral replacement in the form of concentrated minerals until your total mineral content improves. Whatever you do, keep in mind that vitamins do not work without the presence of balanced minerals.

A majority of health problems start with poor digestion or a poorly functioning digestive tract.

There are, so many substances that can interfere with proper function, and absorption of nutrients. People who are attempting to improve their health need to correct, any, and all problems involving digestion. This includes avoiding foods that cause inflammation of the colon wall, the increase and maintenance of proper fluids and balanced minerals, and an increase and maintenance of a wide variety of high-count probiotics or friendly bacteria in the digestive tract. Once the colon is functioning efficiently and effectively, what you eat will move through your system in twenty-four hours or less. It will be soft, brown, and easy to pass. Now your supplements and vitamins will work!

There are several ways to acquire nutrients:

Natural vitamins found in food, concentrated natural vitamins found in fermented foods, and synthetic or chemically derived vitamins. Look towards the natural forms for two major reasons. The body does not recognize synthetic forms, and as a result, they are poorly utilized,—if at all. The natural forms, whole food source vitamins or whole vitamins are derived, directly from organic foods, usually from fermented forms, which gives you the entire vitamin complement. For example, when the body uses vitamin C from food, the natural cofactors, coenzymes, and phytonutrients in the food work with that vitamin and will be recognized, absorbed, and fully utilized by the body. A **synthetic** vitamin is simply - **formulated to mimic the true element,** without the other cofactors that make it a functional vitamin in the body.

When we look at vitamins, we must include water-soluble and fat-soluble forms.

Most fat-soluble vitamins work in the body by reacting with oxygen or oxygen-containing compounds, producing a functional action either outside or inside the cell. Vitamins must have those cofactors and other compounds, including phytonutrients, which contain oxygen as well as minerals to produce their desired effect(Remember; it takes a community). This effect, can be found in whole food source vitamins.

With chemically processed vitamins, the lipids contained in them (like vitamin E) are put through a process called esterification.

Yes, the lipid is extracted and whole, but in order to place it on the market and prevent it from becoming oxidized and rancid, the process of esterification is used. This is the combining of alcohol and an acid to yield an ester and water (the removal of the oxygen), thus preventing the vitamin (ester) from reacting to oxygen and oxidizing. This process results in the preservation of the shelf life of the vitamin (it will last forever). Now this ester found in commercially produced vitamin E and other lipid based vitamin mixes cannot react with the natural oxygen found in healthy cofactors in the body. Without that needed reaction, with oxygen compounds, the vitamin - itself, is basically, useless—**another good reason to use only whole food-based vitamins with their natural cofactors and phytonutrient compounds.**

The best form of mixed whole food-source vitamins, is found in liquid.

This consists of **fermented organic vitamins in their original forms**— with no chemical or heat processing. In this form, you get the vitamin and all of its cofactors in a directly absorbable state—and you can be confident you are getting your money's worth.

For this reason it is strongly recommended that you consider the use of supplementation with whole food vitamins along with a change in healthier dietary habits to regain a healthy, active immune system. If you are fighting an illness or recovering from one, the increased use of vitamins will help rebuild and repair most of the damage that exists.

On both sides of the conventional and integrative coin, we find agreement as to the use of vitamins and supplements, but controversy still exists as to the dosages and their therapeutic values.

Vitamin C

Vitamin C is also marketed, as Buffered C, Ester-C, and liposomal vitamin C.

This is a water-soluble vitamin that is not made by the human body. Please refer to tables, charts, and graphs for food charts. Found in fruits and vegetables, it is required for the body to synthesize (make) collagen (our connective tissue). This vitamin is an important structural component of blood vessels, tendons, ligaments, and bones. Vitamin C is also necessary for the body's manufacture of neurotransmitters (hormones and enzymes that act as electrical conductors in the nerves) that are critical to brain function.

Vitamin C plays a direct role in the transport of poly-glucose between fat and tissue cells for conversion to energy (ketosis).

This is a highly effective antioxidant (prevents cellular oxidation or destruction), protecting indispensable molecules and proteins of the body including RNA and DNA (our genetic chain). Vitamin C is known to regenerate vitamin E from its oxidized form, thus the action and function of Coenzyme Q-10 are increased with the presence of sufficient vitamin C. This vitamin is regulated by the kidneys, which can reabsorb vitamin C when the circulating blood levels are low. Also bone and muscle tissue can uptake and utilize moderate amounts of vitamin C. This vitamin has been the subject of countless studies, and is still, not fully understood. Vitamin C has been shown to have protective capabilities with heart disease, cataracts, lead toxicity, hypertension, and even the common cold. **With all its functions, one might think vitamin C is the miracle cure, but you must remember that 'it takes a community'.**

How does the body respond to vitamin C?

When considering vitamin C and its effects, it appears to have a very wide net in regards to structures and functions that it plays a role in. But the one that appears the most responsive is the **immune system**. We need to take a closer look at this system because vitamin C is just one piece that completes the puzzle for proper function of this system.

Inflammatory Response and Immune Response

The immune system is a key area where vitamin C does its best work.

So, let's look at this system, why it is so important, and what happens when a foreign bacteria or virus enters the body.

You have noticed many times throughout this book the use of the term inflammatory response. Not all inflammatory response within the body is countered by the immune system in the same way that a bacterial or viral infection is countered.

For example;

Let's say you take a nose-dive off your bicycle, twist your ankle, and end up with several nasty bruises, the response you get from your immune system is different from what you would get if you ended up with open wounds or a broken bone.

With that sprained ankle and bruises, we get tissue trauma and swelling.

That is the body's attempt to isolate the injured area. This sets off a chain reaction in the body. An increase in histamine in the area of the wound signals and attracts the release of white blood cells and platelets, entering the wound area. The platelets stop bleeding (formation of clots), and the white blood cells (WBCs) stabilize the wound. Over a period of time (hours), this inflammatory response signals the release of cholesterol sulfate, which enters the area to heal damaged tissue (cellular repair—scar tissue is composed of cholesterol), while macrophages (our trash compactors—found among WBCs) eat the dead cellular tissue so it may be disposed of via the lymphatic system (through the circulation or the gallbladder). As the swelling slowly recedes, we heal.

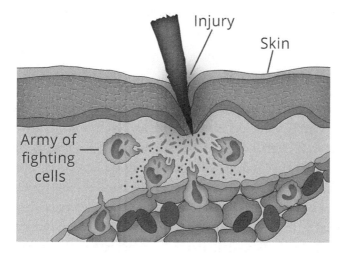

But if a wound or broken bone is open to the air.

The presence of cuts, scratches, or open wounds will allow bacteria in the air and on the skin can invade the wound. In this case, the response is different and more aggressive. When foreign invaders enter the body, it triggers not only the release of histamine, but also cytokines, and interferon. These signaling enzymes that stimulate the release of more specialized white blood cells—B cells and T Cells—along with macrophages, ROS (reactive oxygen species) and glutathione.

Think of any invading microbe, be it bacteria or virus, as an antigen, the army of invaders.

The function of ROS or reactive oxygen species is seen in enzymes, and is activated by vitamin C. These enzymes break down foreign material by oxidation, exposing the antigen for destruction by' macrophages' (our trash compactors), along with 'B cells', and 'T cells'. **The end- result of this oxidation comes from those enzymes and vitamin C, and the end-products are oxygen and hydrogen peroxide.** Gultathione neutralizes the reaction and the macrophages simply eat the antigen, making it possible (safe) for it to be shuttled back through the lymphatic system for disposal. Leftover pieces of antigen are attacked by 'B cells' that actually produce antibodies (formed by copying the DNA of that antigen), targeting and killing specific antigens. 'T cells' attach directly to antigens (like little bombs with suction cups) so they can be destroyed.

By the way;

That white material that drains from an open wound is simply dead bacteria mixed with WBCs and lots of macrophages. Not to worry, you need to get rid of that stuff, "better out than in". If you put small amounts of hydrogen peroxide in that wound, it will increase ROS, increasing the bacteria-killing factor or oxidation and cleaning the wound even faster. Once clean, cholesterol sulfate can come in to heal the wound. Please remember, that commercial hydrogen peroxide at just three percent, is damaging to eyes and should never be swallowed. Better yet, an increase in the consumption of vitamin C during illness or injury is a good option. This way your immune system can get a boost in doing it's job.

So what happens when the bacteria, virus, or invading factor is in overwhelming numbers or resistant?

Then the body (immune system) brings out the big guns. The inflammatory response will progress from minutes to hours, and the soldiers of our immune system will respond. The big guns are the' killer cells'. Some of the white blood cells made by the body—specifically 'B cells' and 'killer cells'—actually contain a memory (the DNA of previous infectious agents or antigens). This memory, can be called '**antibodies**'. They know which armies they have fought before and remember how to defeat that army if it returns. We call this '**acquired immunity**'. If you have had a contagious disease before, your chances of its full return are slim as long as your immune system remains healthy.

Killer cells are specialized cells that can literally engulf, kill, and dissolve foreign substances (DNA that does not belong).

They can distinguish between our own DNA and the cells that do not contain our DNA, like tumors and cancer cells. All WBCs develop in the marrow or center core of our long bones. Specialized cells like 'T cells', 'B cells', and 'killer cells' can also develop in the area of connective tissue just below the reticular bed of our skin and are stored in the spleen.

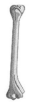

Bone Marrow
The yellow tissue in the center of your bones that is responsible for making white blood cells that become lymphocytes

Spleen
The largest lymphatic organ in the body. It contains white blood cells that fight infection or disease

Vitamin C, has been shown to stimulate and activate the function of white blood cells.

We see increasing, progressive steps to counter injury—from minor to major. And as each battle ensues, the size of the army and its arsenal grows to match, meet, and take down its opponent. **This system is very effective when kept in proper function.**

Conventional medicine promotes the conservative use of vitamins, although there are instances when high-dose therapy of specific vitamins, is recommended. The debate over the use of vitamin C in the treatment of cancer is still ongoing, but it has been agreed that the use of high-dose oral vitamin C in combination with intravenous (in the vein) administration of pharmaceutical-dose vitamin C can be used as an adjunct to conventional cancer therapy and has been shown to have positive results. The use of vitamin C in these instances is at very high doses: ten grams (ten thousand milligrams) a day intravenous for ten days followed by ten grams a day orally indefinitely. One gram equals one thousand milligrams, and one milligram equals one thousand micrograms.

High-dose vitamin C, is recommended by integrative medicine, whereas conventional medicine continues to use the Food and Nutrition Board of the Institute of Medicine recommended daily allowances (RDA). The RDA recommends doses of vitamin C that range from fifty milligrams daily for children to 120 milligrams daily for adults.

Recommended Dietary Allowance (RDA) for Vitamin C			
Life Stage	Age	Males (mg/day)	Females (mg/day)
Infants	0-6 months	40 (AI)	40 (AI)
Infants	7-12 months	50 (AI)	50 (AI)
Children	1-3 years	15	15
Children	4-8 years	25	25
Children	9-13 years	45	45
Adolescents	14-18 years	75	65
Adults	19 years and older	90	75
Smokers	19 years and older	125	110
Pregnancy	18 years and younger	-	80
Pregnancy	19 years and older	-	85
Breast-feeding	18 years and younger	-	115
Breast-feeding	19 years and older	-	120

Table 1 USDA Food Database/RDA

Studies have found that disease prevention with the use of vitamin C begins at four hundred milligrams daily and ranges upward to five and ten grams daily.

Most integrative medicine physicians recommend four to five grams (five thousand milligrams) of vitamin C in divided doses of 2,000 to 2,500 milligrams twice daily for patients during illness or recovery from illness. The RDA established tolerable upper intakes of vitamin C at two thousand milligrams per dose to prevent the only side effect of gastrointestinal irritation and diarrhea, which resolves with temporary discontinuation or reduction in dosage.

To date, there is no reliable scientific evidence that large amounts of vitamin C (up to ten grams a day) are toxic or detrimental to health.

The recommended dose of whole-source vitamin C is four hundred milligrams daily for the average adult and 120 milligrams for the average child. If you take vitamin C supplements, 'buffered ascorbic acid' contains sodium and calcium (114 milligrams calcium per thousand milligrams of ascorbic acid and 131 milligrams of sodium per thousand milligrams of ascorbic acid). People find the buffered form to be less irritating to the gastrointestinal tract. Also, there are no published studies to date that show Ester-C is different from other commercial vitamin C supplements in usability or function within the body. While studies are now in process, showing liposomal vitamin C as more absorbable and less irritating to the intestinal wall.

The B Vitamins

The B vitamins include;

Thiamine (vitamin B1), riboflavin (vitamin B2), niacin (vitamin B3), pantothenic acid (vitamin B5), vitamin B6, biotin, folic acid, and vitamin B12, which are all water-soluble. No studies to date have shown any of the B complex vitamins to be toxic. However, there is a safety concern regarding the long-term use of very high (above five hundred milligrams per day) doses of vitamin B6 and high-dose use of niacin. **The largest supplementation (fortification), of synthetic B vitamins, is found in breads and cereals. These are processed foods, that contain gluten, add to this the fact that fortification comes from genetically altered and synthetic additives and you can see why these are not recommended foods.**

When you think of B vitamins, think about the brain.

It appears that all the B vitamins work in concert with each other for multiple functions throughout the body, but the one organ that receives the most community effect from vitamin B is the brain. Our neurological system and its multiple hormone functions, are stimulated and enhanced by the presence of B vitamins.

Proactive Health Education

Each of the B complex vitamins appears to interact or depend on the others for absorption and function within the body.

Particularly folic acid, biotin, B3, B5, B6, and B12. This complement of vitamins has been found beneficial in the treatment of a large variety of problems, including cancer, heart disease, and Alzheimer's disease. If we look at fetal development, we see that these vitamins play a direct role in the formation of fetal tubes (the basic components for the original formation of our nervous system). Without these B vitamins, these tube formations become defective, giving rise to neurologic birth defects.

This combination of B vitamins appears, to be directly connected to the formation of steroid hormones and neurotransmitters. These vitamins are, also directly connected to the formation and strength of DNA and RNA (our basic gene code).

Throughout the rest of the body, these vitamins continue to work together for the protection and prevention of liver damage from toxins, the formation and strength of red and white blood cells, and increased strength and function of the immune and hormonal systems with the added benefit of decreased cholesterol and triglycerides within the blood, keeping a balance.

Let's take each of these valuable vitamins and look at their functions and the body's basic needs.

Thiamine, Vitamin B1

Thiamin is necessary for the function of coenzymes.

Along with niacin, it aids in the breakdown and synthesis of fatty acids that are necessary for brain hormone function. Deficiency can be seen in severe neurological disorders (Alzheimer's), gastrointestinal disorders, fluid retention, and congestive heart failure.

The richest forms of thiamine, are found in legumes (beans and lentils), nuts, lean pork, and yeast. Please refer to tables, charts, and graphs for a list of foods.

Thiamin, is derived from bacterial breakdown in the colon.

You need healthy, active bacteria for the formation and absorption of this vitamin. Anticonvulsants or seizure medications, diuretics (drugs to increase renal flow), and alcohol consumption all decrease thiamin levels in the body.

Recommended Dietary Allowance (RDA) for Thiamin			
Life Stage	Age	Males (mg/day)	Females (mg/day)
Infants	0-6 months	0.2 (AI)	0.2 (AI)
Infants	7-12 months	0.3 (AI)	0.3 (AI)
Children	1-3 years	0.5	0.5
Children	4-8 years	0.6	0.6
Children	9-13 years	0.9	0.9
Adolescents	14-18 years	1.2	1.0
Adults	19 years and older	1.2	1.1
Pregnancy	all ages	-	1.4
Breastfeeding	all ages	-	1.4

Table 5 USDA Food Database/RDA

It is generally believed that three to five daily servings of a variety of legumes, green peas, nuts, spinach, raw milk, lean pork, and yeast will meet the thiamin need.

Riboflavin, Vitamin B2

Riboflavin, vitamin B2;

Is found in most organic plant and animal foods, meat, eggs, milk, poultry, and vegetables. Please refer to tables, charts, and graphs for a list of foods. Riboflavin is necessary for the metabolism and absorption of vitamin B6, folate, niacin, and iron. Remember, 'it takes a community'!

This vitamin has a direct relation to the reduction of cataract formation in the eyes. It is a key factor in the function of folate (also known as folic acid) in the body, and has been shown to have a direct relation to migraine headaches. Vitamin

B2, is also linked to preeclampsia and eclampsia (uncontrolled hypertension) in pregnant women. **Classified as an antioxidant, it is critical in the formation of glutathione, our reactive oxygen controller (the master controller).**

Deficiency is often seen in skin rashes, oral redness, and swelling. This may progress to malabsorption disorder with the loss of essential nutrients for tissue and bone function. During pregnancy, this vitamin is essential.

People taking anticonvulsants, anti-malarial drugs, antidepressants, chemotherapy, or chronic alcohol consumption will have a decreased availability of riboflavin in the body.

Recommended Dietary Allowance (RDA) for Riboflavin			
Life Stage	Age	Males (mg/day)	Females (mg/day)
Infants	0-6 months	0.3 (AI)	0.3 (AI)
Infants	7-12 months	0.4 (AI)	0.4 (AI)
Children	1-3 years	0.5	0.5
Children	4-8 years	0.6	0.6
Children	9-13 years	0.9	0.9
Adolescents	14-18 years	1.3	1.0
Adults	19 years and older	1.3	1.1
Pregnancy	all ages	-	1.4
Breast-feeding	all ages	-	1.6

Table 7 USDA Food Database/RDA

A varied diet should supply 1.5–2.0 milligrams of riboflavin daily for the average adult, and as such, **it does not need to be supplemented.**

Niacin, Vitamin B3

Food sources include;

Yeast, meat, red fish (tuna or salmon), poultry, legumes, seeds, organic milk, and green, leafy vegetables. Please refer to tables, charts, and graphs for a list of foods. Niacin is **essential for the formation of brain hormones.** It is required for the proper metabolism of tryptophan (found in meat), which forms the hormone melatonin (our sleep-regulating hormone). Sixty milligrams of tryptophan will yield one milligram of niacin. **The coenzyme formed by niacin is essential in the transfer of electrons during oxidation (oxidation reaction or redox cycles) and requires vitamin B6, B2, and iron to become active.** Again, 'it takes a community'! This vitamin is essential for the breakdown of fats, proteins, and alcohol and the structural formation of fatty acids and cholesterol in the liver.

Nicotinamide is the derivative of niacin used in the body to form the needed coenzymes. None of these forms of niacin are related to nicotine found in tobacco.

The presence of normal levels of tryptophan prevents rejection of the fetus during pregnancy, making this is an essential element during pregnancy.

The most common symptoms of niacin deficiency are seen in dermatitis (skin rash and flushing), diarrhea, and dementia (functional mental instability). Early schizophrenia presents with these signs and has been treated as a niacin deficiency with some success.

Niacin can be toxic to the liver in large doses. Upper limits have been set for safe supplementation.

Tolerable Upper Intake Level (UL) for Niacin	
Age Group	UL (mg/day)
Infants 0-12 months	Not possible to establish*
Children 1-3 years	10
Children 4-8 years	15
Children 9-13 years	20
Adolescents 14-18 years	30
Adults 19 years and older	35

*Source of intake should be from food and formula only.

Table 9 USDA Food Database/RDA

Most people who eat a varied diet that includes the minimum daily amount of needed protein **do not need to supplement with niacin.**

People using L-tryptophan for sleep need to stay below twenty milligrams to avoid liver damage. While high-dose supplementation with niacin may be necessary, these instances need to be, strictly regulated by a medical professional.

Recommended Dietary Allowance (RDA) for Niacin			
Life Stage	Age	Males (mg NE*/day)	Females (mg NE/day)
Infants	0-6 months	2 (AI)	2 (AI)
Infants	7-12 months	4 (AI)	4 (AI)
Children	1-3 years	6	6
Children	4-8 years	8	8
Children	9-13 years	12	12
Adolescents	14-18 years	16	14
Adults	19 years and older	16	14
Pregnancy	all ages	-	18
Breast-feeding	all ages	-	17

*NE, niacin equivalent: 1 mg NE = 60 mg of tryptophan = 1 mg niacin

Table 2 USDA Food Database/RDA

The average niacin intake is thirty milligrams daily for adult men and twenty milligrams daily for adult women.

Pantothenic Acid, Vitamin B5

Food sources rich in pantothenic acid include;

Liver, kidney, yeast, egg yolk, broccoli, avocado, split peas, sweet potato, fish, shellfish, chicken, raw milk, raw yogurt, legumes, and mushrooms. Please refer to tables, charts, and graphs for a list of foods.

This is an essential component of coenzyme A, which is vital for multiple reactions throughout the body. Coenzyme A, is needed for generating energy from fats into sugars within the cell (ketosis). It is a contributor to the formation of cholesterol, steroid hormones, the neurotransmitter 'acetylcholine', and the brain hormone 'melatonin'. It is also required for the synthesis of hemoglobin (the element that carries oxygen in red blood cells) from iron. Coenzyme A is also essential in the formation of lipids in the liver, thst become cholesterol sulfate, which forms cell walls, including those in the brain (myelin sheaths).

Pantothenic acid deficiency, has only been seen in severe cases of starvation.

Symptoms are headache, fatigue, insomnia, painful numbness, and burning of the feet and hands.

Some small studies have found that panthine (a derivative of pantothenic acid) has been successful in decreasing the serum (in the blood) cholesterol with little or no side effects.

Not enough studies exist to formulate a recommended daily allowance for vitamin B5, instead, an adequate intake was established.

Adequate intake (AI) for Pantothenic Acid			
Life Stage	Age	Males (mg/day)	Females (mg/day)
Infants	0-6 months	1.7	1.7
Infants	7-12 months	1.8	1.8
Children	1-3 years	2	2
Children	4-8 years	3	3
Children	9-13 years	4	4
Adolescents	14-18 years	5	5
Adults	19 years and older	5	5
Pregnancy	all ages	-	6
Breast-feeding	all ages	-	7

Table 3 USDA Food Database/RDA

Pantothenic acid, is not known to be toxic in humans, but diarrhea can occur at doses above ten to twenty grams a day. Remember that one thousand milligrams is equal to one gram.

Intestinal bacteria in the colon produce their own pantothenic acid.

It has been suggested that humans can absorb pantothenic acid and biotin produced by intestinal bacteria. And again, we see that 'it takes a community'!

Since no true guidelines have been set, it has been suggested that people who eat a well-balanced diet of meats and vegetables would meet the basic intake standards. At the time that this suggestion was made, our vegetable sources were still at moderate levels of vitamin and mineral content. Minimum protein and two to three vegetables constituted 'balance'. **Unfortunately, now that vegetable intake needs to be six to eight servings to constitute 'balance'. Consider juicing?**

As a final note;

The use of birth control pills containing estrogen and progesterone will decrease the absorption of pantothenic acid in the intestinal tract.

Vitamin B6, Pyridoxine

Food sources of vitamin B6 are;

Found in plants and animals containing healthy dietary proteins. Please refer to tables, charts, and graphs for a list of foods.

This particular vitamin, must be obtained from food since the human body cannot synthesize it.

The basic coenzyme that is used by the human body is PLP (pyridoxal 5—phosphate), and it plays a vital role in one hundred different chemical reactions inside and outside the cell. Its functions include aiding in the release of glucose inside the cell for needed energy.

This coenzyme plays a direct role in the production of neurotransmitters such as serotonin, dopamine, norepinephrine, and gamma-aminobutyric acid (GABA). It also aids in the formation of heme from iron for hemoglobin.

Dosage should be limited if supplementing.

Long-term high-dosage usage of B6 is associated with sensory neuropathy (pain and numbness of the extremities). For this reason, the food and nutrition board of the institute of medicine placed an upper limit of one hundred milligrams per day. This vitamin can also block the steroid hormone (estrogen, progesterone, and testosterone) reception within the cell and may result in functional steroid hormone loss.

Deficiency in vitamin B6 can be seen in neurological symptoms of irritability, depression, and confusion, and seizure activity has been seen in infants and children. Other signs of deficiency, mimics that of riboflavin deficiency with oral swelling, redness, and ulcerations of the mouth and corners of the skin of the mouth.

Since increased dietary protein is directly related to B6 consumption, B6 consumption can be calculated by protein intake.

Since women have recommended healthy protein intake of forty-five to fifty-five grams a day, the calculation would read grams of protein times .02 milligrams of B6. This yields 0.9 milligrams to 1.1 milligrams of B6 daily. For men, it would yield 1.1 milligrams to 1.3 milligrams of B6 daily.

Recommended Dietary Allowance (RDA) for Vitamin B$_6$			
Life Stage	Age	Males (mg/day)	Females (mg/day)
Infants	0-6 months	0.1 (AI)	0.1 (AI)
Infants	7-12 months	0.3 (AI)	0.3 (AI)
Children	1-3 years	0.5	0.5
Children	4-8 years	0.6	0.6
Children	9-13 years	1.0	1.0
Adolescents	14-18 years	1.3	1.2
Adults	19-50 years	1.3	1.3
Adults	51 years and older	1.7	1.5
Pregnancy	all ages	-	1.9
Breast-feeding	all ages	-	2.0

Table 4 USDA Food Database/RDA

Despite multiple studies to provide a need for B6 supplementation, little evidence has surfaced to give credence to its need beyond that of basic neurological function. **Since this element is directly tied to the proteins used for these functions, we can safely say that supplementation with B6 is not necessary as long as the minimum healthy protein is used.**

Anti-tuberculosis medications, penicillamine (a metal chelator), and antiparkinsonian drugs all bind to B6 and create a functional deficiency. High-dose vitamin B6 has been found to decrease the efficiency of anticonvulsants.

Biotin, Vitamin H, Vitamin B7, or Coenzyme R

This water-soluble vitamin is bonded to protein with a sulfur bond.

High food sources are egg yolk, liver, and yeast as the richest forms, but it is also found in fish, poultry, dairy, and some vegetables. Please refer to tables, charts, and graphs for a list of foods.

This element is necessary;

For the synthesis of fatty acids (ketosis) and the production of glucose inside the cell, from sources other than sugars (ketone bodies). This element is necessary for the body to convert fat back to sugar inside the cell (fat metabolism or ketosis). It provides an essential step in the breakdown of leucine (an essential fatty acid), dietary cholesterol (sterols), and other odd chain fatty acids (containing an odd number of carbon molecules).

Deficiency can be seen;

In signs of hair loss and scaly, red rash around the eyes, nose, mouth, and genital area. Neurologic symptoms can be seen as numbness and tingling in the extremities, depression, lethargy, and hallucinations.

Prolonged consumption of raw egg white will decrease biotin levels since egg white contains avidin (a biotin-binding enzyme) that blocks absorption of biotin. Individuals with a long-standing biotin deficiency may develop immune system impairment and increased susceptibility to bacterial and fungal infections.

The body requirement for biotin is increased during pregnancy, causing an unrecognized deficiency to form in the mother. Deficiency is also seen in liver disease, particularly in cirrhosis of the liver from heavy metal exposure or alcohol consumption.

In 2004, an assay was performed, by J. Food Compost Analysis; using the ability of avidin to bind to biotin (the sulfur-bonded protein).

In this study, even minute amounts of biotin were discovered in a wide variety of foods, including meats, fish, poultry, vegetables, and nuts. This study appears to be more accurate and more encompassing than those foods previously published as high in biotin.

Biotin exists in foods as protein-bound form called 'biocytin'. Release of this protein (which still contains its sulfur bond) by intestinal bacteria allows for the absorption of biotin. **We must then conclude that intestinal function** and sufficient bacteria in the intestinal tract have a direct impact on the absorption of this vitamin. Are you beginning to see how important healthy intestinal bacteria are?

Reduced levels of biotin, are seen in people using anti-seizure medications over long periods of time—in adults as well as children. In long-term use of sulfa drugs—not to be confused with the organic mineral, sulfur, which is found naturally in the body. Sulfa drugs bind to sulfur and prevent absorption, which results in deficiency.

Adequate Intake (AI) for Biotin			
Life Stage	Age	Males (mcg/day)	Females (mcg/day)
Infants	0-6 months	5	5
Infants	7-12 months	6	6
Children	1-3 years	8	8
Children	4-8 years	12	12
Children	9-13 years	20	20
Adolescents	14-18 years	25	25
Adults	19 years and older	30	30
Pregnancy	all ages	-	30
Breast-feeding	all ages	-	35

Table 5 USDA Food Database/RDA

The Food and Nutrition Board found "insufficient scientific evidence" to recommend an RDA on biotin.

Instead, an adequate intake level was established. This AI assumes that an average intake of thirty-five to sixty-five micrograms would meet the daily requirement.

The need for studies on biotin and its effect on the body remain to be met since little or no research exists. Present recommendations conclude that a varied diet should meet the adequate intake level. If supplementation is necessary, **liquid supplement that contains biotin from natural whole**

foods is recommended. Biotin is a sulfur-bonded protein, and since we, as a population, are sulfur deficient, it would make sense to look to protein foods that contain sulfur. Please refer to the charts and grafts, in the back of the book for more information on sulfur-containing foods and sulfur supplementation.

Folic Acid, Folate

Most synthetic supplements, are referred to as folic acid, but 'folate' and 'folates' are the true chemical term for this vitamin.

Food sources of this vitamin are found in green, leafy vegetables. The term **foliage** gave us the name folate. A wide variety of raw, green, leafy foods includes lettuce, spinach, chives, parsley, asparagus, lentils, and beans. Please refer to tables, charts, and graphs for a list of foods.

This vitamin is necessary for proper DNA replication, and it is required for the breakdown and bonding of methionine (protein) to sulfur to form SAM (S-Adenosylmethionine, a sulfur-bonded protein). This particular vitamin requires vitamin B6 and B12 to produce SAM (see chapter 16).

In order to understand the chemical relationship between methionine and B vitamins, we need to take a closer look at one end- product of methionine biosynthesis: homocysteine.

Homocysteine

This non-protein amino acid is derived from biosynthesis (made by the body) of the sulfated amino acid methionine.

Methionine breaks down during ATP (energy) production inside the cell to yield SAM, which formulates the neurotransmitters norepinephrine and epinephrine. During this process, homocysteine (a by-product) breaks away. This same homocysteine can be recycled back into methionine with the aid of B vitamins (folate and B12).

This element, has been shown to have a direct and indirect relationship with a wide variety of functions and related diseases.

The blood levels of homocysteine in the body are used to measure immune function or 'inflammatory response' and the risk of heart and neurological diseases. Men appear to have a slightly higher limit for homocysteine levels in the body, but since this element lowers your immune system's capabilities, achieving lower target numbers should be your goal with an average blood range of 45nmol/l to 130nm/l. With age, the body experiences higher stress levels and vitamin B deficiencies. These two factors (increased stress and vitamin B deficiency) will make homocysteine levels higher.

If we look closely at its formation, we see that it has a direct relationship to B vitamins, particularly B6, B12, and folate. **A deficiency in any or all these vitamins will result in elevated homocysteine levels and a decrease in immune function.** Uncontrolled levels of homocysteine in the body act much like free radicals, creating cellular damage by oxidation (oxidative stress).

If you want to make a comparison of function, **B vitamins are a form of master controller of homocysteine.** The presence of B vitamins controls the levels of homocysteine in the body and reduces the damage from oxidative stress, which can affect multiple systems, including the brain and the heart.

Now back to folate;

Folate, is directly connected to the production of healthy (normal size) red blood cells in the bone marrow.

A deficiency in folate can cause the formation of enlarged, abnormal red blood cells (megaloblastic anemia). This can result in the loss of oxygen-carrying capacity of red blood cells. The symptoms are fatigue, weakness, and shortness of breath. This is the same anemia that can be caused by B12 malabsorption (loss of protein breakdown in the stomach due to poor hydrochloric acid production—got sea salt?). **As we can see, B12 and folate have a very close, interlinked relationship; one cannot function without the other.**

Folate in the body has a direct effect on women during pregnancy.

This vitamin is essential for fetal cell growth, especially in neuro tube formations (the basic formation of our nervous system). These defective formations are also seen in other cellular defects involving heart and limb formations. One study found that low folate levels during pregnancy were associated with an increased risk of premature birth, miscarriage, and preeclampsia (uncontrolled blood pressure during pregnancy). It has never been indicated in any study, but it is generally believed that vitamin B12 may also play a significant role in these problems. **For this reason, all women of childbearing age should maintain a sufficient level of folate (above four hundred micrograms daily) and as already mentioned, folate cannot function without B12.**

Recommended Dietary Allowance for Folate in Dietary Folate Equivalents (DFE)			
Life Stage	Age	Males (mcg/day)	Females (mcg/day)
Infants	0-6 months	65 (AI)	65 (AI)
Infants	7-12 months	80 (AI)	80 (AI)
Children	1-3 years	150	150
Children	4-8 years	200	200
Children	9-13 years	300	300
Adolescents	14-18 years	400	400
Adults	19 years and older	400	400
Pregnancy	all ages	-	600
Breast-feeding	all ages	-	500

Table 6 USDA Food Database/RDA

Therapeutic doses of nonsteroidal anti-inflammatory drugs (NSAIDS) will decrease folate absorption. Methotrexate (arthritis medication) is a folate antagonist and will create deficiency. Anticonvulsant drugs also display anti-folate activity and block absorption of folate, resulting in deficiency. Other drugs in this class (blocking absorption of folate) include trimethoprim (an antibiotic), pyrithiamine (an antimalarial), triamterene (a blood pressure medication), sulfasalazine (a treatment for ulcerative colitis), and high-dose contraceptive birth control pills.

Vitamin, B12

This is the largest structure chemically of all the vitamins and the one B vitamin that contains a metal ion (cobalt).

Vitamin B12 is part of an essential cofactor in the synthesis of methionine (protein— one of the major building blocks dependent on folate for function). **Without B12 and folate, we cannot produce methionine from homocysteine.**

Only bacteria, can synthesize or make vitamin B12 (got bacteria?).

It is also present in animal products such as meat, poultry, fish, and shellfish. For vegan diets, it can be found in fermented forms of beans and vegetables and algae like chlorella and mushrooms.

Remember this is a heat-sensitive vitamin, which means no pasteurization and minimal heat with cooking. Also, these foods should be organic with no pesticides or herbicides that kill bacteria. Please refer to tables, charts, and graphs for a list of foods.

B12 is necessary for;

The biochemical reaction that produces energy from fats and protein, the metabolism for the formation of our myelin sheaths (the protective coating on our nerve cells), and the formation of neurotransmitters. **Please keep in mind the steps required to burn (metabolize) protein.** First, the body needs to utilize all the glucose and glucose stores (ketone bodies), and then the body utilizes all fats and fat stores (again more ketone bodies). When all the glucose and fats are gone, then and only then, does the body begin to utilize (burn or metabolize) protein for energy. **If our proteins (minimum required only), are not being used as fuel, than they become the foundation healthy cholesterol that produce myelin sheaths and neurotransmitters.**

Strict vegetarian and vegan diets have one major problem: a lack of vitamin B12. These people need to supplement, but the problem with supplementation with synthetic vitamin B12 is that it is derived from GMO sources (genetically altered bacteria is definitely not recommended). This is where fermented foods come in handy. Fermented beans and vegetables can provide B12, and algae products like chlorella and mushrooms provide healthy sources of B12.

B12 also provides the enzymes that are required for the formation of hemoglobin.

The body actively works to break down and absorb B12 from the digestive tract. The acid in the stomach releases or frees up the protein containing this enzyme, then pancreatic enzymes from the gallbladder release or break away the B12 from the protein for synthesis by our biologics and absorption in the small intestine, 'got bacteria'? People who suffer from malabsorption of B12 have a decrease in stomach acid production, which prevents that primary breakdown. No matter how much pancreatic enzyme you produce, that B12, is still trapped inside that protein. **This problem can usually be countered with mineral balance and improvement in the intestinal function overall. This means,'got sea salt', 'got bacteria'?**

Also, the use of acid reduction medications (Zantac, Prevecid, Tagamet, and proton-pump inhibitors), will cause a loss of B12 absorption. The use of anticonvulsants, sulfa drugs (not to be confused with sulfur), antibiotics, and birth control pills containing progestin and/or estrogen will cause decreased absorption and use of B vitamins. B12 deficiency, can be seen in iron-deficiency anemia or elevated homocysteine levels. **Megaloblastic anemia (large, immature red blood cells), is the result of either decreased vitamin B12, a folate deficiency, or both. This also means, 'got sea salt and bacteria'?**

The clinical symptoms of B12 deficiency include;

Numbness and tingling in the arms and more frequently the legs, difficulty walking, memory loss, dementia (loss of cognition), and mood changes. These are slow and gradual symptoms and are not necessarily completely reversible with B12 treatment, especially if these symptoms have occurred for years.

Folate and B6 are necessary for the prevention of neuro tube defects during pregnancy;

B12 is a part of that requirement. These vitamins must work together to keep our neurological system in proper functional order. **During pregnancy and childbearing years, these vitamins, are a must, but use fermented forms only, any form of syntheticis is not recommended.**

Without B12, our nerve protection or myelin sheath cannot form. The diseases involved in this area of damage include Alzheimer's disease, ALS, depression, cognitive disorders, and birth defects.

The recommended daily allowance will meet the guidelines set down by the Food and Nutrition Board.

Recommended Dietary Allowance (RDA) for Vitamin B$_{12}$			
Life Stage	Age	Males (mcg/day)	Females (mcg/day)
Infants	0-6 months	0.4 (AI)	0.4 (AI)
Infants	7-12 months	0.5 (AI)	0.5 (AI)
Children	1-3 years	0.9	0.9
Children	4-8 years	1.2	1.2
Children	9-13 years	1.8	1.8
Adolescents	14-18 years	2.4	2.4
Adults	19-50 years	2.4	2.4
Adults	51 years and older	2.4*	2.4*
Pregnancy	all ages	-	2.6
Breast-feeding	all ages	-	2.8

Table 15 USDA Food Database/RDA

Studies vary, but almost all the relevant studies show active response above forty micrograms per day.

That is where you should start. Healthy children should get up to two micrograms per day, and healthy adult men and women should get four to five micrograms per day. Those who are looking to improve health should start at fifty micrograms. Pregnant women should start at one hundred micrograms, and those who are over fifty should start at one hundred to four hundred micrograms. There is no toxicity with this vitamin, and response appears to improve at the dose increases, and this does not work without folate.

Organic, whole, and synthetic vitamins should not contain corn or corn by-products, soy or soy by-products, or GMOs. Those elements only contribute to more health problems. **Most vitamin B12 supplements are derived from GMO sources, which are not recommended.** With vegetables, eat them raw, juice them, or ferment them, and use whole, organic-source vitamins.

All B vitamins work together.

Vitamin B12 supplementation activates the function of folate (folic acid), and sufficient supplementation of folate acts as part of the chain in the breakdown and absorption of vitamin B12; one cannot function without the other. This also appears to be true for the other B vitamin complements. They appear to work together to enhance or activate each other. For example, vitamin B5 is necessary for the formation of neurotransmitters and acts as a carrier protein along with biotin and niacin for the synthesis and utilization of fatty acids in the body as well as the brain. Please refer to tables, charts, and graphs for full B vitamin needs with RDA and integrative medicine.

For patients with vitamin B12 malabsorption problems, the injectable form of B12 can be used at one milligram monthly. Oral or sublingual absorption (under-the-tongue tablets or liquid) is also available in five hundred micrograms and one thousand micrograms. These products should have no corn or soy in their ingredients, and Malabsorption, can be corrected (see chapter 4).

Vitamin A

This vitamin has been 'lovingly called' the eye vitamin.

This, is a fat-soluble vitamin that requires sufficient dietary fat (healthy fat) to function. But its implications for health reach further and need more attention. Only whole food vitamins are recommended, and when it comes to vitamin A, this is very important. **Please note that the body has its own**

control mechanisms when it comes to the function and usability of this vitamin.

Plants contain carotenoids, some of which are precursors for vitamin A (alpha-carotene, beta-carotene, and beta-kryptoxanthin). Yellow and orange vegetables contain significant quantities of carotenoids. Green vegetables also contain carotenoids with the pigment masked by the green of chlorophyll.

Eggs and dairy also contain animal-converted carotenoids in the form of retinol. Beta carotene and other carotenoids can be converted in the body to retinol and its related compounds (retinoids). Please refer to tables, charts, and graphs for food chart.

The word **retinol** refers to the retina (the lining or wall in the back of the eye). Retinol is the main compound necessary for vision. In order to understand this vitamin and its functions, we need to look closely at how our eyes function.

Eye Anatomy and Chemistry

Retinol, is transported to the retina, the nerve layer that lines the surface of the inside and back of the eye. It contains rods and cones, the receptors for color and light. Retinol is delivered to the eye via the circulating blood, the retinol collects and is **stored in surface layers of the retina (the inside wall of the eye)**. This retinol is esterified by the body (the oxygen component is removed), leaving retinol esters that can remain in storage indefinitely. This form of esterification is done by the body and is not a part of food processing. When needed, the absorption of light into the eye will trigger these esters to be broken down and bond to compounds, including zinc, to form (11-cis-retinal). That will again allow oxidation, which binds with a protein called opsin to form the visual pigment in the rods (visual receptors) of the eye. This pigment is known as visual purple.

This rapidly repeating process with the presence of light will generate or create a cascade of events that form an electrical signal to the optic nerve. This impulse is transferred to the brain where it is interpreted as vision.

The Retinol Cycle

Once this cycle is completed the zinc, is utilized, **this retinal is converted back to retinol and reabsorbed into the retina** (inside wall of the eye) for esterification and storage to be used again. **Thus, we store and recycle our retinol from vitamin A to maintain eye function and health.**

Beta-carotene and other carotenoids, can be converted in the body to retinol and their related compounds called retinoids. This form of vitamin A, is known to affect gene transcription (DNA and RNA formation) and the production of growth hormones. These are often referred to as provitamin A carotenoids.

Retinoids and their related compounds (retinol, retinal, and retinoic acid), produced from carotenoids **by the body**, are essential elements required for the formation of limbs, heart, eyes, and ears during fetal development. It is also essential for the formation of red blood cells from stem cells in the fetus, during pregnancy, and is essential for the formation of hemoglobin (the oxygen carrying unit in red blood cells) with iron, in adults as well as fetuses.

Several independent studies have shown that vitamin A works in conjunction with zinc and iron at the cellular level. This is particularly important during infection since the combination appears to reduce the severity and length of illness, especially in cases of respiratory infections or disease. When levels of vitamin A decrease, the frequency and duration of infection will rise. This appears to be the same with immune function.

The surface cells of the skin and mucus membranes (the cells that line the urinary tract, digestive tract, and airways, including eye, ear, nose, and throat) are our first line of defense from infection. Vitamin A is a necessary part of maintaining the structure and function of these cells, but more research is necessary to pinpoint vitamin A function in this area. The correlation is there, but the mechanism is still unknown. A decrease in function of these structures is associated with vitamin A deficiency. **If frequent, prolonged infections, such as the flu or colds are a problem, you might need more beta-carotene (more eggs, milk, and butter!) in your diet.**

The most prominent deficiency of vitamin A is seen in the eyes.

Inadequate retinol available to the retina results in impaired dark adaptation (night blindness). A mild vitamin A deficiency will result in changes in the tissues in the corners of the eye (conjunctiva), which are called 'Bitot's spots'. This can progress to severe vitamin A deficiency over an extended period of time and can result in dry eye (xerophthalmia). This can progress to changes in the cornea (the clear covering over the eye) with ulcers, scarring, and eventual blindness.

The body has its own control mechanisms when it comes to the function and usability of vitamin A.

There are two forms of vitamin A available, and you should be careful with which one is in your vitamin mix. **Provitamin A** is highly recommended, as opposed to **preformed vitamin A.**

All retinol compounds (preformed vitamin A—synthetics) have been found to cause birth defects.

And the side effects (birth defects) have been reported months after discontinuing any retinol therapy. **Any woman in her childbearing years should avoid preformed vitamin A.**

It has also been noted that high doses of vitamin A, containing an excess of 1,500 micrograms of preformed vitamin A daily, are directly associated with osteoporotic fractures (bone density or acute bone mineral loss). It appears that preformed vitamin A blocks the function and absorption of vitamin D, which is so vital to mineral re-absorption in bones.

The use of vitamin A supplements for skin treatments, which contain vitamin A analogs (preformed vitamin A) such as Retin-A (used by young women for skin rejuvenation) and Accutane (used by young adults for acne), should not be used with vitamin A supplementation since it will cause toxicity and birth defects. **Preformed vitamin A is usually labeled as vitamin A acetate, retinol acetate, vitamin A palmitate, or retinol palmitate and can be**

found in many multivitamin supplements. Read your labels—these are not recommended.

Pharmacologic treatment with preformed vitamin A of such diseases as retinitis pigmentosa, acute pronyelocytic leukemia, and various skin diseases should be attempted with strict medical supervision only.

The breakdown and absorption of vitamin D can only exist in the presence of vitamin A.

Retinol (preformed vitamin A) used as a form of supplementation actually blocks the breakdown and absorption of vitamin D. Read your labels! Vitamin A supplementation should only be in the form of beta-carotene, at a minimum of three thousand micrograms (five thousand international units). This includes the intake of vitamin A in the form of added fruits and vegetables with rich red, yellow, and orange pigments.

To date, no toxic results, or damage, has been noted with the use of vitamin A as beta-carotene. With provitamin A or beta-carotene, it has been shown that you can eat carrots until you turn orange—and you will still have no signs or symptoms of adverse effects. So, use provitamin A (beta-carotene), and not preformed vitamin A, **again we can see the difference between a synthetic and the 'real deal'.**

Due to multiple problems associated with the use of preformed vitamin A, many vitamin companies have reduced their preformed vitamin A in their supplements to 750 micrograms (2,500 international units) to prevent 'detectable' side effects. **The research suggests that this form of vitamin A is too destructive to the human body, and any form of preformed vitamin A, should be strictly avoided.**

To sum it up;

The body recognizes beta-carotene and its carotenoids and will easily convert them to the needed vitamin A (retinol) throughout the body. Preformed vitamin A (vitamin A palmate and vitamin A acetate) is not!

The use of preformed vitamin A only causes damage—**so be aware and eat your colorful vegies!**

Vitamin D and A

Fifty percent of the American population is vitamin D deficient.

For this reason the blood test for 25- hydroxyl vitamin D should be performed on adults as well as children. Science has been found, in related tests that the absorption benefits of vitamin D start in the intestinal tract. **The breakdown and absorption of this vitamin can only exist in the presence of vitamin A.** It has also been found that retinol (preformed vitamin A), used as a form of supplementation, actually blocks the breakdown and absorption of vitamin D. For this reason, **vitamin A supplementation should only be in the form of beta-carotene.**

Vitamin D – The Sunshine Vitamin

There are very few vitamins that need supplementation, vitamin D is one of them.

In the past six to eight years, the research on vitamin D has literally skyrocketed. We now know more about the use and effects of vitamin D in the human body than we know about the use and effects of our own body cholesterol. What we have found gives vitamin D more than just credit for bone formation and strength. **It appears that our cellular structure, muscle function, and even our immune system are affected by the presence of vitamin D.**

Found in white blood cells, that are known to activate 'T cells' and 'B cells' (our army of fighting soldiers).

Research has now tagged this vitamin as a preventative, at acceptable blood levels, for multiple forms of cancer. It, has also been shown to boost the overall function of the immune response, aid in maintenance of mineral balance, improve muscle function and neurologic function.

Dietary vitamin D (from food sources) is a fat-soluble vitamin (there must be healthy fat in the diet to break it down for use) that actually enhances the absorption of minerals (calcium, iron, phosphorous, and zinc) from the intestinal tract. **The presence of aluminum in the diet (found in unfermented soy) will block the absorption of both vitamin D and these minerals.**

Rickets is the term used for severe vitamin D deficiency.

This, is normally seen in children and is described as 'demineralization' or 'soft bone'. In adults, it is called; **osteomalacia.**

Bone forms in the body using twelve minerals.

The base of the matrix that these minerals bind to, comes from a combination of calcium and phosphorous in a two-to-one combination. **Rickets is a lack of phosphorous** (one of the minerals found in sea salt and healthy protein foods) to create balance with calcium and form that matrix. **Vitamin D influences the calcium to phosphorous balance and increases the absorption of this matrix into bone as well as re-absorption back into bone.**

Recent research has uncovered a very interesting problem that we evidently overlooked when considering the effects of this vitamin.

Two statements that have been proven as false: **newborn and pediatric rickets is rare in this country, and adult rickets (osteomalacia), is also rare.** In order to understand this problem, we need to take a closer look at the pathway that vitamin D takes through the body.

The Pathway of Vitamin D

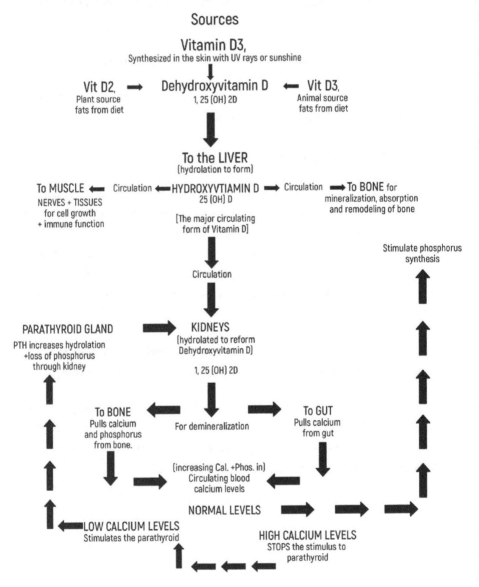

Sources

Vitamin D3,
Synthesized in the skin with UV rays or sunshine

Vit D2,
Plant source
fats from diet
→
Dehydroxyvitamin D
1, 25 (OH) 2D
←
Vit D3,
Animal source
fats from diet

To the LIVER
(hydrolation to form)

To MUSCLE ← Circulation ← **HYDROXYVTIAMIN D** → Circulation → **To BONE** for
NERVES + TISSUES   25 (OH) D   mineralization, absorption
for cell growth   and remodeling of bone
+ immune function
[The major circulating
form of Vitamin D]

Circulation

PARATHYROID GLAND → **KIDNEYS**
PTH increases hydrolation   (hydrolated to reform
+loss of phosphorus   Dehydroxyvitamin D)
through kidney
                            1, 25 (OH) 2D

Stimulate phosphorus
synthesis

To BONE ← For demineralization → **To GUT**
Pulls calcium   Pulls calcium
and phosphorus   from gut
from bone.

(increasing Cal. +Phos. in)
Circulating blood
calcium levels

NORMAL LEVELS

LOW CALCIUM LEVELS   **HIGH CALCIUM LEVELS**
Stimulates the parathyroid   STOPS the stimulus to
                                  parathyroid

Vitamin D2, is found in plant fats (sterols). Vitamin D3 is found in animal fats and can also be synthesized in the skin with exposure to sunlight. Both of these forms become dihydroxy-vitamin D or 1, 25 (OH) 2D. This element bonds to proteins and is processed in the liver (hydroxylated or broken down) to become hydroxyvitamin D or 25 (OH) D. **This is the major circulating form, of vitamin D, that creates all the positive effects on bone, muscle, brain, and immune health.** This circulating form can pass into the kidneys where it can be reversed or hydrolated back to dihydroxy-vitamin D or 1, 25 (OH) 2 D. This loop (reversal), is tightly - regulated by the parathyroid gland in an attempt to maintain that two-to-one calcium-to-phosphorous balance. This gland is stimulated by low levels of calcium in the blood.

Two factors you must remember here;

Dihydroxy-vitamin D or 1, 25 (OH) 2 D will actually pull calcium and phosphorous from bone, causing demineralization. Where as Hydroxyl-vitamin D or 25 (OH) D will actually force calcium and phosphorous back into bone causing re-mineralization or bone modeling. We need, **both** for proper bone growth and strength.

And without healthy function of the liver, kidneys, and parathyroid gland, this balance of bone structure and maintenance will not occur properly.

When hydroxyl-vitamin D is high (fifty to seventy nanograms per milliliter) from healthy liver production (hydrolation), this offsets the destructive effects of dihydroxy-vitamin D, thereby preventing excessive bone loss, loss of immune and neurologic function, and depletion of skin function. **In other words, the higher the vitamin D (hydroxyl-vitamin D), the better.** This is particularly true for people who are fighting any form of illness, and that is why, this is one of the few vitamin supplements recommend for everyone.

Excess dihydroxy-vitamin D or 1, 25, (OH) 2 D, will pull calcium from bone, causing demineralization of bone or soft bone and eventual rickets. This, is seen in adults as osteomalacia. The use of calcium carbonate preparations, usually seen during pregnancy, will pull phosphorous from available bone matrix formation, causing demineralization of bone. Excess dihydroxy-vitamin D, is also seen in liver failure. In liver failure, the loss of formation of hydroxyvitamin D results in loss of matrix formation and restructuring of bone.

Excessive consumption of products containing aluminum (unfermented soy and vaccination adjuncts) will block the absorption and use of vitamin D and calcium in the body. **This is a good reason to read your labels, never ingest unfermented soy, and have a thorough understanding of the use and value of any immunizations.**

Again we see why our liver health is so important.

It is the one place where the body converts dihydroxy-vitamin D to hydroxyl-vitamin D, and that is the form of vitamin D that the body needs in large quantities to keep us healthy.

Infantile rickets starts before the infant is born.

Children are born with 60–70 percent of the mother's vitamin D level. To date, general research, has estimated, that the average vitamin D level of childbearing women in the United States is eighteen to twenty nanograms per milliliter, which is well below the required levels for normal health (fifty to seventy nanograms per milliliter). This indicates a severe vitamin D deficiency or adult rickets (osteomalacia), and it **is not rare** in this country. Infants born to these mothers have vitamin D levels at approximately ten to fourteen nanograms per milliliter (the safe level for newborns is thirty to fifty nanograms per milliliter), this is also rickets and **not rare** in this country.

Unfortunately, rickets has no outward symptoms.

Dr. David Ayoub, radiologist and instructor at Southern Illinois University School of Medicine and fellow researcher, has discovered some very old medical literature, which describes head sweating as the only known sign of rickets. If a child has heavy perspiration at night, especially around the head and neck, enough to soak the sheets, then a severe deficiency of vitamin D is probably the culprit, and blood tests, are warranted to resolve the problem.

Although there are no symptoms in adult vitamin D deficiency, there appears to be a strong association between common gastric reflux symptoms (dyspepsia, constipation, and bloating) and the deficiency. It appears, that muscle weakness of those muscles lining the digestive tract (esophagus, stomach, and intestines) are more prominent in those people with vitamin D deficiency, which aids in the production the reflux symptoms.

All people (young and old) should have their vitamin D (25 dihydroxy-vitamin D) level tested, and know their vitamin D levels.

First at birth, then every three months until the proper level is achieved with supplementation (including sunshine), and every two to three years after appropriate levels have been established in the body.

Vitamin D during pregnancy is very important.

All, pregnant women should be tested. Their vitamin D levels, should be adjusted to meet or exceed fifty nanograms per milliliter, so that the infant can be born with a level of at least thirty nanograms per milliliter. This is not optimum, but it is the minimum for healthy birth and development. This is the sunshine vitamin—so sun exposure first and supplementation second.

During pregnancy, women should avoid antacids, especially calcium carbonate preparations like Tums or Rolaids, since calcium carbonate binds with the phosphorous in the body, preventing bone matrix formation, **resulting in soft bone and infantile rickets in both mother and infant**. For years, doctors have recommended calcium carbonate as a calcium builder (also found in some calcium supplements—please read your labels), not realizing that these preparations do just the opposite of what they were intended. As a result, these women suffered from demineralization of bone, which progresses to fractures, osteomalacia, and osteoporosis.

Another reason why infant formulas are not recommended.

Most infant formulas contain soy and palm olein, a synthetic supplement designed to mimic palmic acid that is found in breast milk.

This olein, like soy, blocks the absorption of calcium through the gut. **All studies** on palm olein to date show definitive lower bone mass in **all test subjects**. Mothers, please breastfeed your babies for at least six months and move straight to raw cow or goats milk from there.

Recent studies show strong scientific evidence that vitamin D can be helpful for psoriasis (a chronic inflammatory skin disease), and vitamin D3 appears to control skin cell growth.

The skin can produce vitamin D with exposure to UV rays from the sun. Sun exposure (sun bathing) three times weekly, can be sufficient. Remember, no sun block or other chemical preparations on the skin since they can alter skin cell growth and result in skin cancer. Limit sun exposure to ten to forty minutes at a time and then cover up or get out of the sun. Some doctors are now using safe tanning beds for the treatment of multiple skin conditions with positive effects of new cell growth and elevated levels of vitamin D.

The current recommendation for supplementation is;

Thirty-five international units of vitamin D3 (natural vitamin D) per pound of body weight. This is the daily dose required for the healthy individual to maintain good health. To find your minimum required level, multiply your weight in pounds times thirty-five. If you weigh 180 pounds, you need 6,300 international units daily ($35 \times 180 = 6,300$) as the 'minimum daily dosage' for a healthy individual. **This is the new standard for children and adults.** Scientists now believe that proper supplementation of vitamin D, should be guided by lab tests (blood tests). The daily, recommended values by the American Nutrition Board appear to fall far short of that requirement for healthy individuals. **Everyone must know and keep a record of their vitamin D level.**

Please note;

A blood level below fifty nanograms per milliliter is classified; as a vitamin D deficiency. If you are already taking vitamin D at the time of testing, and you are found to be deficient, **you need to adjust your intake from that level**. If you are taking five thousand international units of vitamin D, and your blood tests show your level at twenty nanograms per milliliter, you will need to increase your dose to fifteen thousand international units to bring the level up to fifty nanograms per milliliter to maintain a normal healthy level. You will need to adjust higher if you are ill or recovering from an illness. Dosage needs to be adjusted, by blood test results, two to four times the first year and once a year thereafter. This level needs to remain high to maintain good health, prevent illness, and maintain bone strength and structure. **So, know your vitamin D level and get out in the sun.**

25-Hydroxy Vitamin D: New Values for All Ages

25- HYDROXY VITAMIN D New Values For All Ages	
Deficient Levels	< 50 ng/ml
* Optimal Levels	50 to 70 ng/ml
** Required During Illness	70 to 100 ng/ml
Excess	> 100 ng/ml

Research reflects the belief that vitamin D, beta-carotene, vitamin C, and vitamin K work together in a symbiotic relationship, much like the B vitamins.

They each function with the aid of the other. Again, '**It takes a community**'!

Vitamin K

Vitamin K, is produced by the bacteria in the gut.

It is found in fermented foods and fermented vegetables, cheeses, and Japanese fermented food called 'natto'. **Vitamin K1 is needed to prevent the formation of clots in the circulating blood.** Keep in mind that people who are deficient in vitamin D or who have rickets tend to have elevated levels of blood clot formation. This explains traumatic injury at birth as well as arterial ruptures with bleeding in the brain (sometimes seen mistakenly as shaken baby syndrome). **Vitamin K2 is needed for the calcium-phosphorus matrix formation, and keeping calcium in bone.**

Since this is also a fat-soluble vitamin, it requires healthy fats, in the diet for absorption along with vitamin D. Supplementation, with vitamin K2, is only recommended for those suffering from bone disease, rickets, osteomalacia, and osteoporosis. There is no known toxicity of vitamin K2, and this vitamin, is well tolerated at high doses. **This is a good reason to juice and ferment your own vegetables (high amounts of vitamin k2, are found in fermented foods).**

Please refer back to chapter 11 and the use of fats in the diet. Plant sterols are extremely important in the proper function of all cellular tissues. For this reason, all diets should be based on a minimum of 50 to 60 percent raw vegetables. This gives you the precious fats missing in the American diet and all the necessary whole-chain vitamins, calcium, and cofactors. **So, learn to ferment and juice your vegetables.**

CHAPTER 19

GMO's: The Nightmare Come True

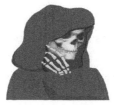

The following material is presented to you as a story, it's not necessarily a happy story, but it's the vision that can be seen of our future, **if we continue on our present path**. By simply looking at what science has told us so far, and following the path that research has set down. With any problem, whether it is an ailment or disease, the resolution lies in finding and correcting the cause. In this story, the cause would be genetically altered foods.

If we were eating the wholesome foods that were available fifty years ago, the elimination of toxins would be simple. But unfortunately, we live in the age of 'modern science', which basically means; genetically modified organisms or GMO's.

By definition;

The combining genes from different organisms is known as 'recombinant DNA technology', and the resulting organism is said to be **"genetically modified", "genetically engineered", or "transgenic"**. GM products include medicines and vaccines, foods and food ingredients, feeds, and fibers. According to the FDA and the United States Department of Agriculture (USDA), more than forty plant varieties have completed all

the federal requirements for commercialization.

Several very large biotech corporations have literally changed the foods we eat by changing the **genetic structure** of corn, soy, sugar beets, sweet corn, rice, honey, canola and vegetable oil, tomatoes, potatoes, squash, papaya, and cotton. GMO's can be found in almost all commercially produced foods on the market today. This includes milk products via animal feed and even vitamins.

The theory behind GMO's was to improve food production by eliminating the need for herbicides and pesticides during plant growth, thereby producing a higher yield of crops to supposedly, "feed the masses."

Genetic modification; introduces a foreign gene from a pesticide and/ or herbicide into the plant's gene.

As a result, the plants become toxic to insects and weeds, creating a 'living pesticide or herbicide'. **Once created, this process was not reversible**. In 1997, this was successful for the first generation of insects. The insects evolved and became resistant to the toxins, and the weeds developed their own resistance and became even more difficult to eradicate. This resulted in an increased use of even stronger pesticides and herbicides. The industry that produces the crop seeds also produces the additional pesticides and herbicides—a win-win situation for the biotech industry. And we can plainly see the driving force behind all of this is not the improvement of health or feeding the masses; instead, it is the filling of the pocketbook.

Tinkering with DNA requires selective, refined, long-term studies and scientific verification for safety.

Unfortunately, the USDA in all its wisdom did not require testing to prove that these "Franken-crops" are not harmful to animals or humans. They graciously allowed the industry to sell these crops to not only the animal feed industry but the American food market as well.

Today, there is still, no independent testing required by the USDA or the FDA to prove the safety of these crops.

You would think that if the crop failed in its intended use, that this experiment in Franken-foods would end. Instead, it prompted the use of multiple foreign genes (stacked traits) consisting of, not only other plant genes, **but bacteria, viruses, and even human genes,** implanted into the seeds with no knowledge of what the crops could do to our animal or human population when consumed. **Today, the United States does not require any toxicological studies on any genetically altered crop to determine adverse effects and safety. Europe requires ninety-day studies on single-trait crops but not stacked traits.** In actuality, it takes months of detailed studies to determine safety and identify any possible illnesses. Once these Franken-crops are planted, the mold has been cast—**and the process cannot be undone.**

In order to tell this story, we need to understand the evolution of animal and man.

Each species has its own rate of evolution. The honeybee produces several generations of its own species in one year, but microorganisms like bacteria will produce thousands of generations in one year. The cow; has a life span of twenty years and will produce three to four generations in that time. Pigs, normally live five to ten years and produce three to four generations in their lifetime. But, it takes forty to sixty years for the human population to create three or four generations.

Microorganisms will adapt and change their structure and even their DNA to survive. Small insects will also be able to adapt because these living entities multiply and can change in a very- short period of time (from hours to months). Larger animals and humans take years—even centuries—to adapt and change for the purpose of survival.

If we use this as a form of comparison, we might be able to look down the road and see the future for humans in this 'Franken-food' experiment.

There are some who will say that as humans, we can change anything with science.

This statement, may be true to some extent, but at what cost? What price will we ultimately pay before we see the mistakes that were made? Can we correct the error? It appears the price may be too high.

If we look at what science has given us so far, we might be able to put some of the pieces of this puzzle together.

Keep in mind, we do not have independent studies to verify any safety in the use of these Franken-foods. It's interesting to note that every independent test found, that has been conducted anywhere, throughout the world, has been either destroyed, discontinued, or discredited by members of the biotech industry or government officials. **You would think that if these foods are as safe as the GM industry states they are, they would welcome independent opinion and research as a form of validation of their work. Unfortunately, this is not the case.**

First, let's look, at what science tells us so far.

So far our safety requirements in this country have been limited to what is called a 'comparative study'.

This means, that the manufacturer of the GM foods can declare safety by comparing the GM crop structure with that of a non-GM crop. **In other words, if it looks like a duck, then it will quack the same—and therefore**

it is safe. Regulations, have been written into these 'safety guidelines', that require **no further testing past this point,** and even these comparisons have been bypassed, according to the same GM producers. The proteins of some GM plants are **too difficult to extract from the plant** for the purpose of comparison, and a **'substitute protein'**, has been used for this comparison instead. Now they are using a **'wooden duck' instead of the real duck, and it still looks like a duck so it should quack the same; therefore, no further testing is necessary.**

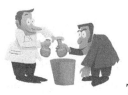

This is not science by any stretch of the imagination.

The following studies, span over the past seventeen years, since genetically modified crops were introduced into this country.

T. Netherwood and J. Heritage (2004)

A human study using GM soybean meal found that GM DNA survived processing and was discovered in human digestive tracts. The same DNA in the soybean, was found in human gut bacteria. This gene transfer from plant to bacteria was called **horizontal gene transfer.** The **bacteria was alive and functional,** which raises the question of possible development of complex nutritional-host interaction (**a living pesticide factory in human**

intestines) and **new strains of antibiotic-resistant mega-bacteria with resulting human infection and disease.** The GM industry dismissed this study as "not genetically relevant," and no further studies were conducted.

Poulsen (2007)

A feeding trial on rats fed GM rice found significant differences as compared to non-GMO rice. There were *distinctive* **differences in blood chemistries, a positive immune response (possible indication of allergens), and altered gut bacteria, with the female rat organs were significantly heavier.** This was classified by the GM industry as "not considered as adverse." The researchers requested further studies to draw long-term conclusions, but none were funded, and no further studies were done.

Schroder (2007)

A study on GM rice-fed rats found significant differences compared with those fed non-GMO rice. Conclusions found **23 percent higher levels of coliform bacteria (disruptive bacteria) in the digestive tracts**. The reproductive organs were also heavier. Overall, **they concluded "possible**

toxicological findings" in the GM rice. The GM rice had changed its composition with respect to mineral, amino acid, total fat, and protein content. One amino acid was markedly higher (histidine). **So, it's not a duck (it did not pass comparative study),** but the GM producer dismissed the findings as "not genetically relevant." No further research was done.

Kroghslo (2008)

This study found that rats fed GM Bt rice (Bt = pesticide gene) discovered a Bt-specific immune response in the test and the control groups. The

conclusion was that all test subjects had inhaled particles of powdered Bt-toxin from the feed, which was not the route of use for this study. The unexpected **allergic reaction to the Bt-toxin (negative**

response) caused, the study to be dropped and new feeding parameters to be recommended.

Austria (2008)

The Austrian government published a study on GM corn-fed mice with **smaller size and fewer babies per litter, the death rate in the mice was twice that of the control group,** which, was fed non-GMO corn. An additional note, was made that unexpected deaths in adult mice were determined to come from **cancer.** Not long after the study began, the supplier of the rat food abruptly changed its formula to include GM soy in all its foods, thus ending any further research due to contamination of the test feed. But it was noted that within two months of that time, **the infant rat mortality skyrocketed to 55.3 percent.**

Russia 2010

A study, was performed at the Institute of Ecology and Evolution of the Russian Academy of Sciences with the National Association for Gene Security. Russian biologists Alexey V. Surov and Irina Ermakova tested hamsters and rats with diets based on GM Soy Roundup Ready (a higher potency Bt toxin designed to tolerate the use of large amounts of bacterial toxin spray known as bacillus thuringiensis). Dramatic changes in reproductive health were found, **including increased infant mortality rates, increased birth defects, and third-generation sterility.** Preliminary reports were published and made public, but before the final results could be published, they were vilified, their labs were 'mysteriously' destroyed, samples were stolen, and written research was burned. No one yet has attempted to verify their research. Dr. Surov said, "Without the details of these tests we cannot pinpoint the true cause of these reproductive disasters."

Quebec, 2011

This **human study** detected significant levels of the insecticidal protein,

Cry1Ab, which is only present in GM Bt Crops, circulating in the blood of sixty-nine women (pregnant, non-pregnant, and their fetuses) The percentage of Cry1Ab protein was as follows: **93 percent in maternal blood, 80 percent in fetal blood, and 69 percent in non-pregnant blood.**

How the protein got into the blood, was not clarified. Was it the result of horizontal gene transfer? Did the women have a living pesticide factory in their intestinal tracts? **These are unanswered questions, and there was no testing done in these areas.** But the true question that needs to be asked is; **Should this toxin be there at all? And what impact could it have on future generations?**

We are biologic creatures, and we have a responsibility to protect animal life. In doing so, we also protect ourselves. Warm-blooded or cold-blooded, it makes no difference, we are all affected by the environment in the same ways.

If we eat the same foods, we may have the same problems.

Italy (2009)

A team of independent scientists conducted a follow-up study using the raw data (released after a lawsuit) from three of Monsanto's own ninety-day rat feeding studies using GM corn varieties. The results **found signs of toxicity in the liver and kidneys as well as toxic effects on the heart, adrenal glands, spleen, and blood of all the test subjects.**

Europe (2007)

Twenty-three farmers reported their pigs had reproductive problems when fed GM Bt corn. **Pigs became sterile, had false pregnancies, or gave birth to bags of water.** Similar complaints were made about **cows and bulls becoming sterile.** GM Bt corn was also the feed of choice during a large-scale death of cows, horses, water buffaloes, and chickens.

India (2006 and 2007)

An incident of sheep grazing on Bt cotton plants found 25 percent of the herd dead within five days. Postmortem showed **death due to high toxin intake with liver and kidney failure.** A small feeding study using Bt cotton was done following the incident. This study **resulted in 100 percent death within thirty days.**

The GM industry tells us that if there is no change in structure, then there is no need for safety testing. It may indeed look like a duck, but it may not quack the same. This in itself, is enough to warrant testing, and without testing, what do we look for? We are already surrounded by diseases, that we have not found the cause, let alone, the cure for. GMOs have been in our food for the past seventeen years. **Are they already a part of today's problems with increasing diseases?** The connections can be seen, and we can say **yes!**

The prime example would be in high-fructose corn syrup, a product of GMO corn that is found, in almost every processed food in this country. This is the leading cause of metabolic syndrome or syndrome X (obesity, heart disease, and diabetes). Is this a monkey wrench we don't need? - Yes! - GMO corn belongs in the gas tanks of our cars—and not in our mouths. One added footnote; a recent increase in the use of corn in gasoline was found to produce irreparable damage to car engines. **We need science to give us the answers, and that means testing.**

What do we see?

If we continue on the present path and keep GM ingredients in our foods—without knowledge or safety testing—**the muddy waters of illness, disease, and death will become deeper and colder.**

Let's recap;

And look at what the actual science has shown us over the past seventeen years. We see evidence of **'horizontal gene transfer'** of active (live) DNA in gut bacteria and an increase in **harmful bacteria.** Evidence of increased **allergic-type responses** resulting in **malabsorption syndrome, osteoporosis, marked liver and kidney disease, and various forms of cancer involving all these organs.** Evidence of the actual Bt gene (bacillus thuringiensis), **a living pesticide and known toxin,** found in the blood of pregnant women and their fetuses.

What does this tell us, and what do we see?

If our diets remain unchanged, we can see a marked increase in diseases associated with malabsorption syndrome (failure to absorb proper nutrients for growth and development) and the accompanying dietary deficiencies, including osteoporosis and neurological diseases, especially in the pediatric and geriatric populations. **Then ten years from now, the statistics for childhood and geriatric disease and deaths will dramatically rise.** These are our venerable populations; the young have undeveloped immune systems and bodies, and the elderly have immune systems, that are already compromised.

Genetic changes are unpredictable.

But we do know that the human species is very slow and poor when it comes to naturally adapting to environmental changes. These adaptations could take as much as eighty to one hundred years, which would encompass three to four generations.

If GMOs continue at their present pace.

Hidden in all of our processed foods, without knowledge or safety testing, then, **in forty years, we can see a dramatic decrease in our population due to damaged reproductive organs and decreased number of births.** For those who appear to survive, we see compromised immune systems with persistent **chronic illnesses, including allergic responses, autoimmune diseases, and liver and kidney disease—and overall dramatically shorter life spans.**

In eighty years, We can see a new generation that will have to rely on test-tube babies for the next generation.

This new generation will have malformed reproductive organs and will be sterile. As a result, the population will drop dramatically, and only those who can afford test-tube genetic development of the next generation will survive. And at that time, if the foods we eat remain genetically altered, then **one hundred**

years from now, humankind as we know it, may no longer exist.

Granted, this extreme picture, was posed to make you stop and

think.

Is this possible? Yes!

It is possible, and it may be our new reality if the GM industry goes unchecked. Without any outside safety controls to protect our health, we are left, venerable to any and all the insults that are so freely provided by this GM industry through our food.

Now you ask, what can I do?

First, each and every adult in this country needs to take one step back, return to a healthy diet and lifestyle, and use bondable versus non-bondable, to get there. You are in control—and you must make the changes.

Vote for GM labeling **on all foods in this country.**

And stop eating foods that contain GM ingredients. Until we have a law that enforces GM labeling, it is recommended that you buy only those foods that bear the "USDA 100 Percent Organic label." Look for verified "Non-GMO Project" seals—and avoid products containing soybeans, canola, cottonseed, corn, and sugar from sugar beets. Buy the products that, are listed in the non-GMO shopping guide, found on the internet.

Remember, over thirty thousand products in this country have GM ingredients.

Read all labels and do not buy products with GMO ingredients.

This sends a clear message   to the product manufacturers that we do not want GMOs in our food. Join the Institute for Responsible Technology and utilize the Non-GMO Shopping Guide (www.NongmoShoppingGuide.com), (www.HealthierEating.org), and join the tipping point. Keep yourself and your family healthy. Do not consume these toxic foods, especially if you have any unexplained illness or allergy.

Outside, independent safety testing will only come -

After we unite and force our legislators to make the appropriate changes in our laws and changes in the structure of our federal agencies, including the elimination of lobbies to ensure proper enforcement of new regulations and laws. Each and every person is urged to join the Alliance for Natural Health, a nonprofit organization that fights for natural health for the general public at the government level, protecting our needs and our basic rights to good health through legislation, as a governmental watchdog. Their work can only succeed with the voice of all the people.

This nightmare can change.

But it takes every individual to make a concerted effort, and this effort **must start now.** It's time to stop looking over our shoulders at past mistakes and start changing what we see now. **GMOs do not belong in our food.** Do not buy any products that contain them!

The following is a list of those foods that are presently produced by the GM industry, this list has been provided by the United States Department of Agriculture (USDA):

Rapeseed;

This vegetable oil was developed for resistance to certain pesticides, these rapeseed cultivars were devised to be free of erucic acid and glucosinolates. Gluconsinolates, which were found in rapeseed meal leftover from pressing, are toxic and prevented the use of the meal in animal feed. In Canada, double-zero rapeseed was developed. The crop was **renamed "canola" (Canadian oil) to differentiate it from nonedible rapeseed.**

Honey;

Honey can be produced from GM crops. Some Canadian honey comes from bees collecting nectar from GM canola plants. **This has shut down exports of Canadian honey to Europe.**

Cotton;

Resistant to certain pesticides, it is considered a food because the oil can be consumed. The introduction of genetically engineered cotton plants has had an unexpectedly effect on Chinese agriculture. The so-called Bt cotton **plants that produce a chemical that kills the cotton bollworm have reduced the incidence of the pest in cotton fields and in neighboring fields of corn, soybeans, and other crops.**

Rice;

Genetically modified to contain high amounts of vitamin A, rice **containing human genes** is to be grown in the United States. The broken theory behind GM rice is that, rather than ending up on dinner plates, the rice will make human proteins useful for treating infant diarrhea in the developing world.

Soybean;

Genetically **modified to be resistant to herbicides,** soy foods include soy beverages, tofu, soy oil, soy flour, and lecithin. Other products include breads, pastries, snack foods, baked products, fried products, edible oil products, and special purpose foods.

Sugarcane;

Made resistant to certain pesticides, a large amount of sweeteners in processed food actually come from corn—not sugarcane or beets. **Genetically modified sugarcane, is regarded so badly by consumers at the present time that it could not be marketed successfully.**

Tomatoes;

They, are designed for a **longer shelf life** and to prevent a substance that causes tomatoes to rot and degrade.

Corn;

Resistant to certain pesticides, corn oil, flour, sugar, or syrup may also be included in snack foods, baked goods, fried foods, edible oil products, confectionery, special purpose foods, and soft drinks.

Sweet Corn;

Is, genetically **modified to produce, its own insecticide.** Officials from the FDA have said that thousands of tons of **genetically engineered sweet corn have made their way into the human food supply chain—even though the produce, has been approved only for use in animal feed.** Recently, Monsanto, a biotechnology food producer, said that about half of the USA's sweet corn acreage, has been planted with genetically modified seed.

Canola;

Canola oil may include edible oil products, fried foods, baked products, and snack foods.

Potatoes;

Atlantic, Russet Burbank, Russet Norkatah, and Shepody potatoes may be in snack foods, processed potato products, and other processed foods.

Flax;

More and more food products contain flax oil and seed because of its excellent nutritional properties. **No genetically modified flax is currently grown.** An herbicide-resistant GM flax was *introduced in* 2001, but it was soon taken off the market because European importers refused to buy it.

Papaya

The first virus-resistant papayas, were commercially grown in Hawaii in 1999. Transgenic papayas now cover about one thousand hectares—three quarters of the total Hawaiian papaya crop. Monsanto donated technology to Tamil Nadu Agricultural University, Coimbatore, for developing a papaya resistant to the ringspot virus found in India.

Squash (Yellow Crookneck);

Some zucchini and yellow crookneck squash are also GM, but they are not popular with farmers.

Red-Hearted Chicory (Radicchio);

Chicory (Cichorium intybus var. foliosum) is popular in some regions as a salad green, especially in France and Belgium. Scientists developed a genetically modified line of chicory containing a gene that makes it male sterile, simply facilitating the production of hybrid cultivars. **Today, there is no genetically modified chicory on the market.**

Cottonseed oil;

Cottonseed oil and linters may be included in blended vegetable oils, fried foods, baked foods, snack foods, edible oil products, and small goods casings.

Tobacco;

Vector has a GMO tobacco being sold under the brand of **Quest cigarettes** in the United States. It is engineered to produce little or no nicotine.

Meat;

Meat and dairy products usually come **from animals that have eaten GM feed.**

Salmon;

Genetically altered salmon has been cleared for sale in the US.

Peas;

Genetically modified peas created immune responses in mice, suggesting that they may also create serious allergic reactions in people. The peas had been **inserted with a gene from kidney beans, which creates a protein that acts as a pesticide.**

Vegetable Oil;

Most generic vegetable oils and margarines used in restaurants and in processed foods in North America are made from soy, corn, canola, or cottonseed. **Unless these oils specifically say "non-GMO" or "organic," it is probably genetically modified.**

Sugar beets;

They may be in any processed foods containing sugar.

Dairy;

About 22 percent of cows in the United States are injected with **recombinant (genetically modified) bovine growth hormone (rbGH).**

Vitamins;

Vitamin C (ascorbic acid) is often made from corn, and vitamin E is usually made from soy. Vitamins A, B2, B6, and B12 may also be derived from GMOs. Vitamin D and vitamin K may have carriers derived from GM corn sources, such as starch, glucose, and maltodextrin. **This is a good reason to use whole, plant-based, organic vitamins.**

CHAPTER 20

A Question of Personal Choice

The true effect of Statin drugs on your body

In the past thirty years, we have evolved into a fast-paced, highly technical, modern society. We move at an ever-increasing pace, eat on-the-go meals, fuel ourselves with caffeine and sugar, and communicate with cell phones and computers. We drive at lightning speeds to high-stress jobs, we eat poorly—if at all—sit for hours at a time, and use tobacco products. When it comes to addressing our poor health or even health maintenance, we 'take a pill'. In today's society, an increased emphasis, is placed on health maintenance or disease prevention. Our present medical system, is only designed to address illness once it occurs. Your doctor will give you a yearly health physical and write a prescription or two to treat those lab values that are not quite at an acceptable range. This is the closest you will get to health maintenance—the rest, is left up to you.

How do we learn our personal health care?

Most of us start with what our parents teach us as we grow up. We diligently follow their lead, which is what they learned from her parents, until we learn that crossing our eyes and making those funny faces will not cause permanent damage. In school, we learn what STD's are and how to practice personal hygiene. The rest of our education consists of bits and pieces of information along the way. We depend on our physicians to 'maintain our health', but the era of the true 'family physician', who would encourage and coach us in lifestyle changes for maintenance of good health, is long past. We are left with a pat on the back and a prescription in hand, as we walk out of his door. For a majority of the population, this means that we fill the prescription and continue our lives as usual, until illness strikes and the good doctor steps back into our lives to 'treat the illness', and unfortunately, this happens more often than it should.

There is a wide variety of teaching materials available to us that can offer guidance in our daily health, but what about that prescription in your hand? There is that 'ticker tape style' form of information that comes with the drug that's supposed to warn you about all the problems that might occur and the symptoms you should look for, but a majority of the population never reads it. Of the thousands of drugs on the market in this country, there are a few, that should have more than just a warning label.

Forewarned is forearmed.

The goal here is to arm you with more knowledge about some of the most popular and dangerous prescription medications in use in this country today. Your doctor only writes the prescription. He or she doesn't swallow the pills. You are the one who must decide, whether or not, to take the medication in question, and that little 'ticker tape' of information is nowhere near clear enough.

This brings us to the drug in question, which actually is a family of drugs called statins (cholesterol-lowering drugs). The five top competitors in this group are Lipitor (atorvastatin)—the leader in this competition—Zocor (simvastatin), Mevacor (lovastatin), Prevachol (pravastatin), and Crestor (rosuvastatin). Recently, it was estimated, that sixteen million Americans take a daily dose of Lipitor, making it one of the most popular drugs in the country. It is widely advertised as safe and effective by its producer and marketer. Pfizer is the world's largest pharmaceutical company and derives a major portion of its income from this drug.

Statin drugs, are prescribed at a staggeringly high rate. They, are doled out like candy to children by cardiologists as well as every other medical specialty, including gynecology. The production and sales of statin drugs in this country have become a competitive, uncontrolled frenzy with pharmaceutical promotions and unsupported claims. Such rivalry has put the fast-food industry's sales of on-the-go meals to shame.

The American Heart Association lists the six risk factors for heart attack: high blood pressure, use of tobacco (smoking), diabetes, gender (male), family history of heart disease, and high blood cholesterol. One-third of this nation's population has an elevated serum cholesterol level, according to IMS health (a pharmaceutical market research group). Thirty years ago, a male who possessed at least two of these risk factors and had a cholesterol level of 250 or greater, would have been placed on a diet and exercise program. A statin drug would only be added if that diet program was ineffective after six months. Twenty years ago, that number dropped to 240 with only one risk factor. With the publication of the 2001 federal cholesterol guidelines, the number was again, reduced to 200. Somewhere along the line, the trusted diet and exercise recommendation, was dropped—and females were added to the list.

In the past year, the pharmaceutical industry has suggested that this treatment number be reduced again to 180 and that everyone—even those who are otherwise healthy—should be treated with statins. The federal government and the insurance industry have given the pharmaceutical industry their blessings. To date, there are no true measurements to determine where to draw the line when it comes to cholesterol. **The present data, being used to measure the 'normal' cholesterol, was determined by the FDA in 2001, following a review of clinical trial results and recommendations, which were funded by and supplied to them by the pharmaceutical companies, who were seeking the approval of their form of statin drug for commercial sales.**

Since heart disease is the number one cause of death in this country, it would only make sense that we aim our health efforts at preventing its occurrence. Today's physicians do not have the time to study and research all the new drugs flooding the market. As a result, they have learned to depend on the drug companies to do that research and provide guidance when it comes to use, dosage, and effects of their drugs.

There are some physicians in this country, who prescribe statin drugs only rarely and in extreme circumstances, unfortunately, these doctors are themselves, rare. Most doctors tend to jump in with both feet, ordering a statin drug, rather than recommending diet and exercise, which is safer and has a wide variety of long-term benefits beyond simply lowering cholesterol, including lower blood pressure and prevention or elimination of diabetes.

When it comes to **negative effects**, which are usually referred to as **side effects, all statin drugs create the same effects** to varying degrees (according to brand and dosage).

Before we can understand statin drugs and their side effects, a more thorough understanding of their direct effect on the human body is necessary.

A majority of the tissues that form our vascular and nervous systems, including the brain, are made of cholesterol. In fact, more than 30 percent of the dry weight of our brain is cholesterol. Cholesterol is the main constituent of cell membranes throughout the body, making our cells water-resistant. It, is a key player in the production of hormones; that facilitate growth, development, stress response, and memory. The circulating cholesterol in the bloodstream plays several other key roles. It is an integral part of the function of the body's immune system. Blood cholesterol also transports nutrients, stimulates enzyme production, and repairs tissues. All scar tissue in the body contains high levels of cholesterol. Structure found, within each cell's membrane (outer coating) are called **lipid rafts.** They are also made of cholesterol, acting as both protection of the cells' protoplasm and transporter for multiple nutrients, enabling cell function (see chapter 13).

We need to ask; what is truly a normal cholesterol level and when do we cross into dangerously high or low serum concentrations?

The number we use as a guide is only a measurement of the free cholesterol circulating in the bloodstream. **Dangerously low cholesterol levels are rare, but they, are now seen - frequently in those under statin therapy.** Before the advent of statin therapy, high cholesterol, was treated with diet changes and exercise. This is still the proven and effective therapy, but the changes in lifestyle must be permanent.

We derive cholesterol from plants and animals. It, is synthesized (in the liver) from acetyl Co-A through the HMG-Co-A -reductase enzyme. It, is absorbed and utilized by molecular chain reaction to form three unique molecular substances: **cholesterol, dolichol, and ubiquinone.**

Dolichol is a part of the necessary chain in the formation of DNA proteins, resulting in genetic body programming. Without dolichol, the DNA sequence chain becomes broken. This may be the reason why all the pharmaceutical companies that produce statin drugs clearly state that these drugs, should not be taken by pregnant women or those who can become pregnant. They do not include males who produce the sperm. Genetic body programming is inherent and predetermined in **all single cells, including the egg and the sperm**, and does not occur after pregnancy.

Ubiquinone, which is also known as coenzyme Q-10, is the key ingredient necessary for all cell respiration, cell membrane integrity, nerve conduction, and muscle integrity. Of all the muscles in the body, the heart produces the highest energy demand by virtue of its oxygen consumption via cell respiration, utilizing the largest portion of available coenzyme Q-10 in the body.

All statins work the same way within the human body.

They block the production of HMG-Co-A-reductase enzyme in the liver. This is the enzyme needed for that molecular chain reaction, which produces **cholesterol, dolichol, and ubiquinone.** With the introduction of statin drugs, this chain reaction is broken, creating a loss of structural components of the cell's membrane.

Once the circulating blood cholesterol is below that level, which is needed by each individual human body to maintain its own cell membrane integrity and function (the body's normal level), a new chain reaction begins with the slow degradation of the cell membrane, culminating in eventual necrosis and cell death. Loss of cholesterol robs the structure of its protective membranes, progressive cell wall oxidation, with resulting cell wall rupture and cell death (see chapter 13). This is seen on the cellular level—**in all tissues**. Once the cells die, they liquefy into the tissue bed. Unnoticed, this reaction continues, with slowly expanding microscopic loss of tissue, eventually producing symptoms. **In some areas of the body, these tissue losses are permanent—even if the blood cholesterol returns to the body's normal level. This new chain reaction, ending in cell death, can occur anywhere in the body, including the heart.** Keep in mind that the molecular reactions explained here are a part of complex biochemistry. The microscopic substances and their reactions remain unchanged, but a broader view, has been given here to facilitate better understanding.

As a result, of aggressive advertising, we have learned that the presence of an elevated cholesterol level is a risk factor for heart disease, which can lead to a heart attack. But 'heart disease', encompasses a multitude of physiological problems, and the presence of cholesterol plays a very minor role. **To date, there is no research to prove that the presence of an elevated serum cholesterol (somewhere above 180) is a direct cause of a heart attack.** Recently, a new campaign for statin use has surfaced, stressing the reduction of plaque formation to prevent heart attack (plaque and blood platelets are a necessary constituent of normal blood clot formation). **The only studies in this area, show no direct correlation between the formation of plaque and elevated serum cholesterol.**

In our efforts to become 'heart healthy', the use of statin drugs have contributed to the development of 'heart failure', **diagnosed as statin-induced diastolic dysfunction**, which is the loss of significant function of the muscle composing the heart wall. It often leads to congestive heart failure, which is a life-threatening condition, usually controlled with the use of diuretics and digoxin. Digoxin is a drug that causes slow and forceful contraction of the heart, but this drug may be **poorly effective due to the statin-induced preexisting damage to the muscle wall.**

Today, it is a common practice for physicians to start patients on statin drugs after a heart attack, regardless of the patient's cholesterol level. It, is assumed that elevated serum cholesterol is present; therefore, actual testing for base levels before medicating is not usually done. We can see the true cause of heart damage in lethal oxysterols (see chapter 13).

But what about those who take this drug?

For those who take statin drugs, the loss of microscopic areas of tissue throughout the body may go completely unnoticed. The recommended lab studies that are used to measure or detect any possible side effects of statin drugs do not become elevated until long after significant symptoms begin. If you understand the statin-induced chain reaction that leads to cellular necrosis and cell death, the symptoms that develop as side effects will be more than clear.

In their efforts to make the sales of statin drugs more appealing, the pharmaceutical industry has made broad statements that stress the word **safe**—and side effects are noted as minor problems. **Along with headaches, nausea, unexplained fevers, and insomnia, which may all be a result of the microscopic tissue necrosis (cell death), we can add myopathy, renal failure, liver damage, polyneuropathy, retinal hemorrhages, brain hemorrhages, and infertility.**

The most common complaint, seen in all studies is that of, 'muscle pain or weakness' (myopathy), which is easily dismissed, by physicians and treated with anti-inflammatory drugs. One study on statin side effects, currently being conducted, by Dr. Beatrice Golomb, a neurobiologist at the University of California at San Diego, notes that 98 percent of those using Lipitor experienced some form of muscle problem. She also noted that those who had more active lifestyles, experienced more muscle pain than those who live more sedentary lifestyles. **As muscle activity increases, the demand for coenzyme Q-10 (cell respiration) also increases. The statin-induced microscopic loss of tissue and loss of coenzyme Q-10 ultimately result in increased muscle pain.**

After loss of muscle function, the serum creatinine phosphokinase (recommended blood test used to detect liver damage) becomes elevated; which indicates a condition known as '**rhabdomyolysis**'. This **skeletal muscle injury** is defined: as muscle cell necrosis (death) and release of intracellular contents, resulting in myoglobinuria (blood in urine), eventual renal failure, as well as multiple electrolyte imbalances in the body. This diagnosis requires hospitalization with aggressive treatment, and can be life-threatening. **The tissue damage is permanent and can occur in any muscle, including the heart.**

'**Renal failure**', myoglobinuria, can be a result of rhabdomyolysis or simply the result of direct microscopic tissue loss within the kidneys with rupture of the vessels in the renal tubules (kidney filters). **Again, this necrosis is permanent, leading to permanent loss of kidney function.**

'**Liver damage**' is only noted with laboratory studies or after the appearance of 'jaundice' (yellow discoloration of eyes and skin). The loss of microscopic areas of tissue in the liver can destroy its intricate functions. The liver is actually the largest gland in the body, and it is second only to the brain for its multiple functions. To date, there are no studies to verify the fact that this microscopic necrosis in the liver causes permanent damage. The extent of individual damage, as seen beyond that of elevated liver enzymes, in all known studies is also unverified. However, we do know that failure of only one or two of the liver's multiple functions can lead a wide variety of diagnosed problems, such as diabetes, aggressive infections, and renal insufficiency. **The body cannot afford liver damage (see chapter 6).**

'**Polyneuropathy**', which is also known as '**peripheral neuropathy**', is marked by symptoms described as tingling, numbness, and weakness in the hands and feet and occasional difficulty walking. The fibrous coating on nerve cells is primarily composed of cholesterol. This coating is necessary for the passage of electrical activity across the cell's surface. **It has been documented that small nerves can regenerate and repair after damage, but only if the required cholesterol and coenzyme Q-10 are in sufficient quantities in the circulating bloodstream.**

'**Retinal hemorrhages**' are defined as the rupture of blood vessels of the retina, resulting in loss of vision (blindness). The pharmaceutical industry has no written warnings in reference to this condition or side effect, stating that the percentage of occurrence is too low, to be considered as a risk factor when taking statin drugs.

'**Brain hemorrhages**' present with a variety of symptoms, including amnesia, progressive memory loss, insomnia, depression, and emotional instability. Such symptoms may ultimately result in an Alzheimer's disease or a stroke diagnosis. All of these symptoms result in decreased cognitive activity (mental function or memory) to varying degrees.

Dr. Golomb has noted that a decrease in cognitive activity occurred in 15 percent of all the patients taking statin drugs in her study. The pharmaceutical industry denies any connection to the use of statin drugs and memory loss or cognitive impairment. Although, many questions have been raised, several published clinical trials, which did not examine cognitive response directly, provided data showing a total figure that combined all cognitive changes as 0.5 percent of recorded side effects. These clinical trials, were small and may not represent the present total population of statin drug users, but it was enough information for the pharmaceutical industry to again state that this percentage is too low to be considered a risk factor for taking statin drugs.

'**Infertility**' is seen as decreased sperm motility (independent, spontaneous movement) and can only be found on direct examination, which is not one of the recommended tests for managing statin use. Doctors will only run this examination when a couple is seeking assistance with infertility.

Who should take statin drugs?

Children and young adults don't need cholesterol management. Their bodies are able to balance themselves with the assistance of a proper diet and good physical activity. Adults between the ages of twenty and fifty are of childbearing age and should not use statin drugs, including men and women. Low tissue levels of coenzyme Q-10 are associated with decline in energy levels and metabolism with resulting cell structure and DNA damage. **Every study has found no decrease in risk factors for heart attack in women when using statin drugs—no matter their age. This means women will not benefit from these drugs.**

Those over fifty should not take statin drugs since this group already has an increased risk of 'hypocholesterolemia' (severe low cholesterol). This is due to age-related decreased energy metabolism and the subsequent decreased production of cholesterol as well as coenzyme Q-10. Their normal cholesterol levels are progressively decreasing from the levels they may have had in their younger years. And they may still be above the pharmaceutical industry and the FDA's recommended 'normal'. **The risk to this group is much higher; unfortunately, many of the symptoms and diseases of the elderly are never associated with the use of statin drugs.**

When assessing the risks, we must consider the statements made by researchers in the Honolulu Heart Program's clinical trial of 2001. Their data accords with previous findings that show an increased mortality in people over the age of fifty with low serum cholesterol. **Long-term persistence of low serum cholesterol concentrations actually increases the risk of death**. These clinical trial results support the findings that those with low cholesterol have a poor outlook when compared with those over fifty who have higher concentrations of serum cholesterol. **The data suggests that individuals with a low serum cholesterol—below two hundred maintained over a twenty-year period—will have the worst outlook for all causes of mortality.**

So, who is left?

Statin drugs, were originally designed to be used only as augmentation to non-pharmacologic interventions that fail—and only on a short-term basis of eight to twelve weeks. When statins are used without the necessary lifestyle changes and the drug is discontinued, the body's cholesterol will return to its original level. That has prompted physicians to continue the drug and even increase the dosages. Today, we see long-term use of statin drugs as the standard, which is encouraged by the pharmaceutical industry.

When considering the use of statin drugs and other causes of mortality, we must also include cancer. Clinical trials have not addressed this disease. Cancer cells grow slowly and are difficult to detect, requiring more than six years of study with a cost that would be prohibitive for clinical trials. A

CARE study (clinical trials) in 2000 **noted an increase in breast cancer of 1500 percent in women taking statin drugs.** Without the defenses provided by the immune system, we can develop cancer and other aggressive, infectious diseases. The pharmaceutical industry does recognize and makes note of the fact that **statin drug use lowers the immune system.** Using this logic, they have recommended that statin drugs be used for the treatment of inflammatory arthritis and transplant patients, a population with an already depleted immune system.

The subject here is the use of statin drugs and their effect on this country. Over the past thirty years, heart disease has been the leading cause of death in the United States. Although the percentage of those deaths has dropped, the overall percentage of all causes of death has equally dropped. During that same period, new diseases and increasing death rates have occurred, such as diabetes and Alzheimer's disease. Ten years ago, Alzheimer's disease, was not listed as one of the top ten causes of death in this country. In 2006, Alzheimer's disease took the position of number six on that list, and it has been steadily rising ever since. There has also been an impressive rise in diseases affecting our pediatric population including cancer, birth defects, and neurological disorders such as autism.

There is no way to tell if the use of statin drugs over the past thirty years by such an overwhelming number of our population has created more problems than it has solved. Have, future generations been damaged? Have we inadvertently increased disease and death in our older (over fifty) population? **By clinical studies; it has been shown, that the use of statin drugs has not significantly enhanced the prevention of heart disease.**

We are now left with a prescription in hand and the ultimate question;

Does the benefit of using statin drugs outweigh the risks?

Or, do the risks now outweigh the benefits?

Since this article was written, and published in 2009, research science has discovered a direct link between the development of congestive heart failure, degenerative neurological damage, and the use of statin drugs.

Recent research has resulted in lawsuits claiming a direct link of statin use and diabetes.

New guidelines promoted by the American Heart Association recommend statin use for life—without further testing, without dietary changes, and to any age population. Should these recommendations ever be followed? - Or does the idea of cholesterol control need to be eliminated? **See chapter 13 for a more thorough understanding of cholesterol and its function in the body.**

In Conclusion

It's unfortunate, but we cannot narrow the answers to our health problems to just 'one thing'. But it can be said that the combination of everything you have just read is actually the answer. '**It takes a community**'; this means that the components of each and every chapter have a definitive effect on your health. This also means that it takes a thorough understanding of the use of each element, sea salt, probiotics, fuels (bondable versus non-bondable), healthy protein, healthy fats, whole vitamins and minerals, and a healthy functioning liver to handle it all and maintain good, long-lasting health— without any of the destructive diseases associated with metabolic syndrome.

In today's society, we base good health on proper nutrition, but most nutritionists and some nutrition experts in this country only understand the basics of what can be called '**synthetic nutrition**', which is largely promoted by the food industry. This industry involves large corporations that sell processed foods.

This book emphasizes the 'interpretation of good health' with proper nutrition, which encompasses the use of **basic, natural, real foods** and not synthetically derived substitutes that are called 'food'. Nor does it involve the use of chemicals to grow food.

We need to understand that our bodies know exactly what to do in order to keep us healthy, and each organ will work hard to provide everything the body needs to accomplish that. The human body is an amazing functioning unit, bent on survival, whether you want it or not. **And this entire scenario of how your health evolves is completely dependent on <u>what you eat!</u>**

You can say that genetics has dealt you a bad hand, but genetics only loads the gun. **It's what you eat that pulls the trigger.**

Approximately 90 percent of the food in this country is processed, from fast food to frozen meals right down to that glass of milk. The processing (manipulating foods with chemicals and heat) literally destroys the true nutrition found in natural foods. And when nutrients are destroyed, we replace them with a synthetic version and try to convince ourselves that it works just as well. It may mimic the actions of the true element—protein, fat, vitamin, or mineral—but the body knows better and will not utilize it the same way or even utilize it at all. And in some cases, that synthetic food will actually cause direct disease.

Think about it;

When this country consumes a diet of 60–70 percent or more 'synthetic foods', can we expect to remain healthy for very long? Children today are showing signs and symptoms of metabolic syndrome as early as six years of age, and children who start that young do not live very long. Today, young adults are giving birth to malnourished infants with rickets. These children have a poor start in life, but the parents also succumb to illness, disease, and death long before they should.

The point here; is '**we are not synthetic**', and this uncompensated mass experiment in synthetic food, junk science, and death by malnutrition needs to stop. This country has more 'food' than any country in the world, but this endless supply of 'cheap food' has no nutrition. It will never give the body what it needs, and as a result, we are all starving and developing disease, "Water, water everywhere — and not a drop to drink."

In the final analysis, all the decisions about your health, are really **left up to you.** There are plenty of people out there, who will try to convince you that their "enriched," "enhanced," "fortified foods" are "good for you." After all, it, is approved by one organization or another and "proven by science", so that synthetic, chemical, and genetically altered ingredient "won't hurt you," and it "just tastes so good." **The plain truth is, that your body can't use any of it to function—it needs the real deal.**

In this age, we can push mechanics and electronics into the future at light speed, but our bodies are still stuck in the earliest stages of evolution. Unless we can find a way, to convert the entire body into a synthetic version of itself, at that same light-speed pace, we will not survive.

Why would we want to change such a marvelous functioning unit?

It's true, we as scientists and researchers are still learning how the human body really works, yet medical science is ready and willing to jump in with both feet to change things. We still don't know all the intricate details of this marvelous body, and the research tends to show, that light-speed change will continue to make things worse rather than better.

There is no magic cure, no fountain of youth, no magic beans to change us back to good health, but we do have healthy organic foods, and with this book, you now have the basics.

The word carbohydrate does not appear anywhere in this book. They are not considered to be a part of any diet. This word is simply an overused term that describes sugars, starches, non-bondables, and nonessential nutrients that are simply not healthy and do not contribute to healthy body function. The body does not recognize what, up to now, has been classified: as carbohydrates. Bondable versus non-bondable encompasses this entire spectrum that utilizes the flow of insulin in the body. To change the way you look at these terms, think of carbohydrates as non-bondable, and vegetables that contain natural sugars (glucose) as bondable. Fructose is a natural sugar found in fruit, but unless it is the whole food, it is classified: as a non-bondable.

The use of bondable versus non-bondable foods will lead to improved liver function and decreased incidence of illness and disease. The use of sea salt and probiotics (fermented foods) will improve digestive function. The incorporation of healthy balanced plant and animal sources of fats along with a minimum healthy protein intake (forty-five to sixty-five grams)—from both plant and animal sources and a minimum of 50 percent raw food that incorporates vitamin and mineral sources—will get you started. **Now add exercise, water, plenty of sleep, and stir.**

This will return the overall function of the body back to being the 'lean, mean', 'bent on survival machine' it was designed to be. Now that you understand how the organs of the body function with the foods you use, **you can change how you look at food, improve your health, and live a longer, happier life.**

Tables, Charts, and Graphs

The following tables are derived from information provided by the Department of Human Nutrition, Deakin University Australia, the USDA Food Composition Database, the Natural Health Research Institute, and the American College of Nutrition.

These foods encompass only those foods that are a part of a natural organic diet and follow bondable versus non-bondable teaching with only healthy fats and proteins listed. Nutrient content such as vitamins and CoQ-10 are also available in some instances in these lists and in the chapters involving vitamins and minerals (chapters 17 and 18).

The use of processed foods is not advocated, but if you need to use some of these types of foods in your diet, please read your labels and make sure that you exclude those added ingredients and chemicals that can cause direct damage to your body. These include soy, corn, grains and gluten, whey, artificial ingredients and sweeteners, vegetable oils, and GMOs.

Remember; we are not 'synthetic', and artificial or synthetic foods just don't work in the body. We need the real deal!

Use these graphs and charts as a guide for healthier eating. Incorporate the basic caloric-need calculations as a guide to keep you in or below your estimated needs for dietary changes, such as fat increase or weight loss, using bondable fuels only.

If you wish to measure the general caloric need of your body at your present or future weight, use this calculation:

Women: weight (or desired weight) x 3.95 + 825 = caloric limit for that weight

Men: weight (or desired weight) x 5.3 + 879 = caloric limit for that weight

No calculations are needed for children. Their diets should always be the same: no sweet drinks of any kind, water (filtered- reverse osmosis) and raw milk only, minimum healthy proteins (forty grams), and plenty of healthy fats and organic vegetables.

The Building Blocks of a Healthy Life

 The Healthy Organic Diet

<u>Sugars</u>
<u>Fruit /Chocolate</u>
<u>Milk / Cheese /Yogurt</u>
<u>Eggs /   Raw or Cooked</u>
<u>Beans /Legumes / Nuts / Seeds</u>
<u>Olive Oil   /   Butter   / Coconut Oil</u>
<u>Fish /   Seafood /   Red Meat / or   Poultry</u>
<u>Juiced or Raw   Vegetables   Lightly cooked</u>

- vegetables = eight to ten servings daily
- fish, seafood, red meat or poultry = minimum of four to six ounces daily
- oils/butter = one-to-one ratio, 1 teaspoon animal to 1 tablespoon plant
- beans, nuts, and seeds = ½ cup daily (unprocessed and raw)
- eggs (raw or lightly cooked) = one to two daily
- raw milk, cheese, and yogurt = adults one and children three servings daily

- fruit, chocolate (Mother Nature's desert) = one to two ounces
- sugars = trace amounts only

No grains, processed foods, vegetable oils, and fried foods. For sauces and gravies, use your meat drippings or bone soup. Try garbanzo bean, coconut, cassava or almond flour—and only use 100 percent stevia with liquids or baking or very small amounts of sugar.

Drink half your weight in ounces of water daily, and use coffee, beer, and wine sparingly. If you must have breads, try sprouted grains that have small amounts of gluten.

Healthy Foods, Fats, and Proteins

Organic Meats Grass fed	Saturates fat Content	Omega 3 Content	Sulfur Content	COQ-10 Content	Protein Content
Beef	H		M	H	H
Chicken	H		M	H	H
Eggs	H		H (yoke)	L	H
Turkey	H		M	M	H
Bison	H		M	M	H
Organ Meats	H		H	L	H
Pork	H		M	L	H
Organic Milk products					
Goats Milk (Raw)	H		H	M	M
Cow's Milk (raw)	H		H	M	M
Hard Cheese (raw)	M		M	L	M
Yogurt (raw)	M		M	L	M
SEAFOOD Wild Caught Only					
Salmon	H		H	L	H
Oysters	M		H	0	M
Lobster	H		H	0	H
Crab	H		H	0	H
Deep salt water fish	M		L	0	M
NUTS AND SEEDS Organic and Raw					
Chocolate (dark)	H		M	0	M
Almonds	L		M	0	M
Walnuts	H		M	0	M
Macadamia	H		0	0	M
Cashews	L		M	0	M
Sesame seeds	M		M	0	M
Flax seeds	H		0	0	0

Healthy Plant-Sourced Proteins

Food Source	Protein Level	Mineral Level		Vitamins
Pumpkin	Moderate	Moderate		B, K and E
Asparagus	Moderate	Low		K and A
Cauliflower	Low	Low		High B Vit's
Peanuts (raw)	Moderate	High		B and E
Green Beans	Moderate	Moderate		A, B, C, D, E, and K
(Mung Bean Sprouts)				
Almonds	High	Moderate		Vit E
Spinach	High	Moderate		A, K and B
Broccoli	High	Moderate + Ca		B vit's and C
Green Peas	High	Moderate		B, C, E, and K
Brown Rice	High	Moderate		B Vit's

Healthy Foods Fat Content

Scale

L = (↓ 2 Gm) M = (3 to 5 Gm) H = (5 to 10 Gm) H+ = (↑ 10 Gm) H++ =(↑50 Gm)
per 100 Gm food

Milk and Milk Products

MILK RAW	
Human	M
Goat	H
Cow	H

Organic Cheeses

Camembert	H+
Cheddar	H+
Cottage	L
Cream	H+
Blue	H+
Edam	H
Parmesan	H+
Stilton	H+
Swiss	H+
Plain Yogurt	L

Nuts and Seeds

Almonds	H++
Brazil	H++
Cashews	H+
Chestnuts	L
Coconut	H++
Hazel nuts	H+
Macadamia	H++
Peanuts	H+
Pistachio	H+
Walnuts	H+
Sunflower	
Sesame	

OTHER FOODS

Olives	M
Avocado	H

Vegetables contain little or no fat content, but they do contain sterols, a type of fat that acts as a foundation for cell wall formation, which is highly sensitive to extreme heat and cold. Think of sterols as natural cofactors for fats—just like those natural cofactors and coenzymes found in foods that work with vitamins. These natural forms of cofactors work with their partner elements to aid in their full function inside the body.

Fish are relatively low in fat content with the exception of salmon, sardines, and tuna, which have low-to-moderate fat content.

Butter, beef drippings and lard all contain 80–100 percent fat.

The most valuable food you can eat is the organic pastured egg.

The **egg is high in fat, high in protein, contains high levels of sulfur as well as high levels of vitamins, minerals, and antioxidants for daily health.** In essence, it is truly the 'perfect food'. Egg white contains protein and fat, but the yolk contains higher levels as well as all the vitamins, minerals (including sulfur), and antioxidants, so don't throw that yolk away. Eat the whole egg, at least one to two eggs every day. And this advise goes for every member of the family. Never eat powdered eggs; they become lethal oxysterols, causing direct damage to your cholesterol in your circulating system and eventually your heart.

Sulfur-Containing Foods

Sulfur Containing Foods
Scale
L = 10 Gm, M= ↑ 20 Gm, H= ↑ 40 Gm, H+ ↑ 100 Gm, / 100 Gm of food

Meats		Milk and Milk Products	
Eggs (yokes)	H+	**Cheese Organic;** whole, unprocessed	
Beef Fat	L	Cheddar	H
Beef	H+	Cottage	0
Chicken	H+	Cream Cheese	0
Pork	M	Parmesan	H
Lamb	0	Stilton	H
Turkey	0	Swiss	0
Organ Meats	H	**Milk; Organic unprocessed**	
Rabbit	M	Cow	M
Bison	M	Human	0
Veal	H	Goat	0
Fish; unprocessed, wild caught		**Nuts and Seeds; (raw) unroasted, unsalted**	
Crab	H+	Almonds	M
Lobster	H+	Brazil	H
Shrimp	H+	Chestnuts	L
Scallops	H+	Coconut	M
Oysters	M –H	Hazel Nuts	M
All Salt Water Fish	M –H+	Peanuts	H
All Fresh Water Fish	L –M	Walnuts	M
Nuts and Seeds, (raw) unroasted, unsalted		**Vegetables**	
Cashews	0	Cucumber	L
Macadamia	0	Egg Plant	0
Pistachio	0	Endive	H
Chocolate	H	Garlic	H
Coffee	M	Leeks	H
Vegetables Raw, little or no cooking		Lentils	H
Artichoke	L	Lettuce	0
Asparagus	L	Mushrooms	H
Bamboo Shoots	0	Onions	H
Green Beans	L	Parsley	0

Broad Beans	M		Parsnips	M
Kidney Beans	M		Peppers	0
Mung Beans	H		Red Potato	M
Beets	L		Pumpkin	L
Broccoli	0		Radishes	H
Brussel sprouts	H		Spinach	H
Cabbage	H		Corn	0
Carrots	L		Sweet Potato	M
Cauliflower	0		Tomato	L
Celery	L		Turnip	L
Chickpeas	H		Yam	0

Sulfur Containing foods continued

Fruits, Whole, Raw and unprocessed

Apple	L		Pear	L
Apricots	H+		Pineapple	L
Avocado	L		Prunes	M
Banana	L		Raisins	M
Black Cherries	L		Rhubarb	L
Cantaloupe	L		Strawberries	L
Cherries	L		Watermelon	0
Dates (dried)	M		Figs (dried)	M
Grapes	L		Grapefruit	L
Lemon	L		Olives	M
Nectarine	L		Mandarin	0
Mango	0		Orange	L
Black Currents	M		Guava	0
Peach	M			

Food Value Tables for Vitamins and Minerals

Calcium

Healthy food sources of calcium are unrefined milk and milk products including cheeses, salmon and sardines, vegetables, broccoli, mustard greens, turnip greens, kale, bok choy, spinach, beans, and legumes. For children, twelve to sixteen ounces of whole raw milk daily, along with three to four servings of healthy organic vegetables daily, and for adults, eight to ten servings of healthy organic vegetables daily.

Food	Serving	Calcium (mg)	Servings needed to equal the absorbable calcium in 8 oz of milk
Milk	8 ounces	300	1.0
Yogurt	8 ounces	300	1.0
Cheddar cheese	1.5 ounces	303	1.0
Pinto beans	1/2 cup, cooked	45	8.1
Red beans	1/2 cup, cooked	41	9.7
White beans	1/2 cup, cooked	113	3.9
Tofu, calcium set	1/2 cup	258	1.2
Bok choy	1/2 cup, cooked	79	2.3
Kale	1/2 cup, cooked	61	3.2
Broccoli	1/2 cup, cooked	35	4.5
Spinach	1/2 cup, cooked	115	16.3
Rhubarb	1/2 cup, cooked	174	9.5

USDA Food Database

Those foods marked in gray are not recommended unless they are derived from whole organic sources and are not pasteurized, homogenized, contain no gluten, or are not processed with sugars.

Supplementation of human calcium levels is not necessary if the daily intake of milk and/or vegetables is sufficient and unrefined sea salt is used. If supplementation with calcium is necessary, never consume more than one gram (one thousand milligrams) daily, for total intake, including calcium in your food. When we think of the use of calcium in the diet, we must keep in mind that calcium is added to a large variety commercially produced food, and all milk products are fortified with calcium. **Please read your ingredient labels carefully and avoid as much additional calcium as possible.**

Potassium

The third most abundant mineral in the human body, weighing in at 0.4 percent of the total body minerals, healthy food sources include; meat, unprocessed milk, fresh fruit, and vegetables.

Food	Serving	Potassium (mg)
Banana	1 medium	422
Potato, baked with skin	1 medium	926
Prune juice	6 fluid ounces	528
Plums, dried (prunes)	1/2 cup	637
Orange juice	6 fluid ounces	372
Orange	1 medium	237
Tomato juice	6 fluid ounces	417
Tomato	1 medium	292
Raisins	1/2 cup	598
Raisin bran cereal	1 cup	362
Artichoke, cooked	1 medium	343
Lima beans, cooked	1/2 cup	485
Acorn squash, cooked	1/2 cup (cubes)	448
Spinach, cooked	1/2 cup	420
Sunflower seeds	1 ounce	241
Almonds	1 ounce	200
Molasses	1 tablespoon	293

USDA Food Database

Those foods marked in gray are not recommended unless they, are derived from whole, organic sources and are not pasteurized, homogenized, contain no gluten, or are not processed with sugars.

Magnesium

The seventh most abundant mineral element in the human body, weighing in at 0.1 percent of total elements, food sources are nuts and seeds, legumes, green, leafy vegetables, seafood, chocolate, artichokes, foods containing high levels of chlorophyll, and unfiltered hard water.

Food (100 grams)	Magnesium Content (mg)
Seaweed, agar, dried	770 mg
Coriander leaf (spice), dried	694 mg
Pumpkin seeds, dried	535 mg
Cocoa, dry powder, unsweetened	499 mg
Basil, dried	422 mg
Flaxseed	392 mg
Cumin seed (spice)	366 mg
Brazil nuts, dried	376 mg
Parsley, freeze dried	372 mg
Almond butter	303 mg
Cashew nuts, roasted	273 mg

- **Magnesium Threonate**: Newest of supplements, studies show improved absorption.
- **Magnesium Glycinate**: A chelated form of magnesium, good absorption and bioavailability, may aid in sleep.
- **Magnesium Oxide**: A non-chelated form with 60 percent elemental magnesium content, tends to soften stool.
- **Magnesium Malate**: A new form of supplement, bonded to maltic acid, appears to be more absorbable, has pain relief, muscle relaxation, and laxative properties.
- **Magnesium Taurate**: It is made by combining magnesium and taurine (an amino acid), a protein bond that has calming effects on muscles and the brain.
- **Magnesium Chloride/Magnesium Lactate**: It absorbs as well as the oxide form, but it contains only 12 percent elemental magnesium.
- **Magnesium Carbonate**: It contains 20–45 percent elemental magnesium (found in chalk) and has antacid properties.
- **Magnesium Citrate**: It is bonded to citric acid, contains up to 16 percent elemental magnesium, and has laxative properties.
- **Magnesium Sulfate/Magnesium Hydroxide**: It is found in laxatives and contains 42 percent elemental magnesium. Use caution since it can cause a magnesium overdose.
- **Magnesium Aspartate**: It is bonded to L-Aspartate. This neuro-excitory element causes neuro-excitation (as seen in glutamine response). Use with extreme caution since it may cause central nervous system damage and demyelination of nerves.

Vitamin C

Vitamin C, also marketed as Buffered C, Ester-C, and liposomal vitamin C, is a **water-soluble vitamin that is not made by the human body.**

Food	Serving	Vitamin C (mg)
Orange juice	¾ cup (6 ounces)	62-93
Grapefruit juice	¾ cup (6 ounces)	62-70
Kiwifruit, gold	1 fruit (86 g)	91
Orange	1 medium	70
Grapefruit	½ medium	38
Strawberries	1 cup, whole	85
Tomato	1 medium	16
Sweet red pepper	½ cup, raw chopped	95
Broccoli	½ cup, cooked	51
Potato	1 medium, baked	17
Spinach	1 cup, raw	8

Table 7 USDA Food Database

Items in gray are not recommended unless whole, organic, and unprocessed.
Found in fruits and vegetables, it is required for the body to synthesize
(make) collagen (our connective tissue). This vitamin is an important
structural component of blood vessels, tendons, ligaments, and bone.
Vitamin C is also necessary for the body's manufacture of neurotransmitters
(hormones and enzymes that act as electrical conductors in the nerves) that
are critical to brain function. Vitamin C plays a direct role in the transport of
poly-glucose between fat and tissue cells for conversion to energy (ketosis).

B Vitamins, Think Brain;

Vitamin B1 or Thiamine

The richest forms of thiamine, are found in legumes (beans and lentils),
nuts, lean pork, and yeast.

Food	Serving	Thiamin (mg)
Lentils (cooked, boiled)	1/2 cup	0.17
Green peas (cooked, boiled	1/2 cup	0.21
Long-grain, brown rice (cooked)	1 cup	0.19
Long-grain, white rice, enriched (cooked)	1 cup	0.26
Long-grain, white rice, unenriched (cooked)	1 cup	0.04
Whole-wheat bread	1 slice	0.10
White bread, enriched	1 slice	0.23
Fortified breakfast cereal (wheat, puffed)	1 cup	0.31
Wheat germ breakfast cereal (toasted, plain)	1 cup	1.88
Pork, lean (loin, tenderloin, cooked, roasted)	3 ounces*	0.81
Pecans	1 ounce	0.19
Spinach (cooked, boiled)	1/2 cup	0.09
Orange	1 fruit	0.11
Cantaloupe	1/2 fruit	0.11
Milk	1 cup	0.10
Egg (cooked, hard-boiled)	1 large	0.03

*3 ounces of meat is a serving about the size of a deck of cards

Table USDA Food Database

Those foods marked in gray are not recommended unless they, are derived from whole, organic sources and are not pasteurized, homogenized, contain no gluten, or are not processed with sugars. Enriched and fortified means chemical vitamins have been added.

It is generally - believed that three to five servings of a variety of these foods (legumes, green peas, nuts, spinach, raw milk, lean pork, and yeast) daily will meet the thiamin need.

Riboflavin and vitamin B2

Found in most organic plant and animal foods, meat, eggs, milk, poultry, and vegetables.

Food	Serving	Riboflavin (mg)
Fortified, wheat, puffed cereal	1 cup	0.22
Milk	1 cup (8 ounces)	0.45
Cheddar cheese	1 ounce	0.11
Egg (cooked, hard-boiled)	1 large	0.26
Almonds	1 ounce	0.29
Salmon (cooked)	3 ounces*	0.13
Halibut (Greenland, cooked, dry-heat)	3 ounces	0.09
Chicken, light meat (roasted)	3 ounces	0.08
Chicken, dark meat (roasted)	3 ounces	0.16
Beef (ground, cooked)	3 ounces	0.15
Broccoli (boiled)	1/2 cup chopped	0.10
Asparagus (boiled)	6 spears	0.13
Spinach (boiled)	1/2 cup	0.21
Bread, whole-wheat	1 slice	0.06
Bread, white (enriched)	1 slice	0.09

*A 3-ounce serving of meat is about the size of a deck of cards.

Table USDA Food Database

Those foods marked in gray are not recommended unless they are derived from whole organic sources and are not pasteurized, homogenized, contain no gluten, or are not processed with sugars. **Fortification with B2 comes from genetically altered foods**.

A varied diet should supply 1.5 to 2.0 milligrams of needed riboflavin daily for the average adult, and as such, it does not need to be supplemented.

Niacin, Vitamin B3

Food sources include yeast, meat, red fish (tuna or salmon), poultry, legumes, seeds, organic milk, and green, leafy vegetables.

Food	Serving	Niacin (mg)
Chicken (light meat)	3 ounces* (cooked without skin)	7.3-11.7
Tuna (light, canned, packed in water)	3 ounces	8.6-11.3
Turkey (light meat)	3 ounces (cooked without skin)	10.0
Salmon (chinook)	3 ounces (cooked)	8.5
Beef (90% lean)	3 ounces (cooked)	4.4-5.8
Cereal (unfortified)	1 cup	5-7
Cereal (fortified)	1 cup	20-27
Peanuts	1 ounce (dry-roasted)	3.8
Pasta (enriched)	1 cup (cooked)	1.9-2.4
Lentils	1 cup (cooked)	2.1
Lima beans	1 cup (cooked)	0.8-1.8
Bread (whole-wheat)	1 slice	1.3
Coffee (brewed)	1 cup	0.5

*A 3-ounce serving of meat is about the size of a deck of cards.

Table USDA Food Database

Those foods marked in gray are not recommended unless they are derived from whole organic sources and are not pasteurized, homogenized, contain no gluten, or are not processed with sugars.

Most people who eat a varied diet that includes the minimum daily amount of needed protein do not need to supplement with niacin. **People using L-tryptophan for sleep need to stay below the twenty milligrams dosage to avoid liver damage.** While high-dose supplementation with niacin may be necessary, these instances, need to be strictly regulated by a medical professional.

Pantothenic Acid (Vitamin B5)

Food sources rich in pantothenic acid include liver, kidney, yeast, egg yolk, broccoli, avocado, split peas, sweet potato, fish, shellfish, chicken, raw milk, raw yogurt, legumes, and mushrooms.

Food	Serving	Pantothenic Acid (mg)
Fish, cod (cooked)	3 ounces	0.15
Tuna (light, canned in water)	3 ounces	0.18
Chicken, cooked	3 ounces	0.98
Egg (cooked)	1 large	0.61
Milk	1 cup (8 ounces)	0.83
Yogurt	8 ounces	1.35
Broccoli (cooked)	1/2 cup (chopped)	0.48
Lentils (cooked)	1/2 cup	0.63
Split peas (cooked)	1/2 cup	0.58
Avocado, California	1 whole	1.99
Sweet potato (cooked)	1 medium (1/2 cup)	0.88
Mushrooms (raw)	1/2 cup (chopped)	0.52
Lobster (cooked)	3 ounces	0.24
Bread, whole wheat	1 slice	0.19

Table USDA Food Database

Those foods marked in gray are not recommended unless they are derived from whole organic sources and are not pasteurized, homogenized, contain no gluten, or are not processed with sugars.

Since no true guidelines have been set, it has been suggested that people who eat a well-balanced diet of meats and vegetables would meet the basic intake standards.

Vitamin B6 (Pyridoxine)

Food sources of vitamin B6, are found in both plants and animals containing healthy dietary proteins.

Food	Serving	Vitamin B_6 (mg)
Fortified cereal	1 cup	0.5-2.5
Banana	1 medium	0.43
Salmon, wild, cooked	3 ounces*	0.48
Turkey, without skin, cooked	3 ounces	0.39
Chicken, light meat without skin, cooked	3 ounces	0.51
Potato, Russet, baked, with skin	1 medium	0.70
Spinach, cooked	1 cup	0.44
Hazelnuts, dry roasted	1 ounce	0.18
Vegetable juice cocktail	6 ounces	0.26

Table USDA Food Database

Those foods marked in gray are not recommended unless they are derived from whole organic sources and are not pasteurized, homogenized, contain no gluten, or are not processed with sugars. **Fortified vitamin B6 comes from genetically altered foods**. Since this element is directly tied to proteins, we can safely say that supplementation with B6 is not necessary.

Biotin (Vitamin H, Vitamin B7, or Coenzyme R)

This is a water-soluble vitamin, bonded to protein, using a sulfur bond. High food sources are egg yolk, liver, and yeast as the richest forms, but it is also found in fish, poultry, dairy, and some vegetables.

Food	Serving	Biotin (mcg)
Yeast	1 packet (7 grams)	1.4-14
Bread, whole-wheat	1 slice	0.02-6
Egg, cooked	1 large	13-25
Cheese, cheddar	1 ounce	0.4-2
Liver, cooked	3 ounces*	27-35
Pork, cooked	3 ounces*	2-4
Salmon, cooked	3 ounces*	4-5
Avocado	1 whole	2-6
Raspberries	1 cup	0.2-2
Cauliflower, raw	1 cup	0.2-4

*A 3-ounce serving of meat is about the size of a deck of cards.

Table USDA Food Database

Those foods marked in gray are not recommended unless they are derived from whole organic sources and are not pasteurized, homogenized, contain no gluten, or are not processed with sugars.

Today, the need for studies on biotin and its effect on the body, remain to be met since little or no research exists. A varied diet should meet the adequate intake level. If supplementation is necessary, a liquid supplement that contains biotin from natural whole foods is the recommendation here. **During pregnancy, biotin supplementation is recommended.**

Folic Acid (Folate)

Most synthetic supplements, are referred to as folic acid, while folate and folates are the true chemical term for this vitamin.

Food sources of this vitamin are found in green, leafy vegetables. The term **foliage** gave us the name folate, a wide variety of raw green, leafy foods including lettuce, spinach, chives, and parsley.

Food	Serving	Folate (mcg)
Fortified breakfast cereal	1 cup	200-400
Orange juice (from concentrate)	6 ounces	83
Spinach (cooked)	1/2 cup	132
Asparagus (cooked)	1/2 cup (~ 6 spears)	134
Lentils (cooked)	1/2 cup	179
Garbanzo beans (cooked)	1/2 cup	141
Lima beans (cooked)	1/2 cup	78
Bread	1 slice	20 (Folic acid)*
Pasta (cooked)	1 cup	60 (Folic acid)*
Rice (cooked)	1 cup	60 (Folic acid)*

Table USDA Food Database

Those foods marked in gray are not recommended unless they are derived from whole organic sources and are not pasteurized, homogenized, contain no gluten, or are not processed with sugars.

All women of childbearing age should maintain a sufficient level of folate (above four hundred micrograms daily), and folate cannot function without B12.

Vitamin B12

This is a heat-sensitive vitamin, which means no pasteurization and minimal heat with cooking. Also, these foods should be organic with no pesticides or herbicides that kill bacteria.

Food	Serving	Vitamin B_{12} (mcg)
Clams (steamed)	3 ounces	84.0
Mussels (steamed)	3 ounces	20.4
Crab (steamed)	3 ounces	8.8
Salmon (baked)	3 ounces*	2.4
Rockfish (baked)	3 ounces	1.0
Beef (cooked)	3 ounces	2.1
Chicken (roasted)	3 ounces	0.3
Turkey (roasted)	3 ounces	0.3
Egg (poached)	1 large	0.6
Milk (skim)	8 ounces	0.9
Brie (cheese)	1 ounce	0.5

*A three-ounce serving of meat or fish is about the size of a deck of cards.

Table USDA Food Database

Those foods marked in gray are not recommended unless they are derived from whole organic sources and are not pasteurized, homogenized, contain no gluten, or are not processed with sugars.

Studies vary, but almost all the relevant studies only show active response above the forty micrograms per day dosage, which is where you should start. Healthy children should get up to two micrograms per day, healthy adult men and women should get four to five micrograms per day, and those who are looking to improve health should start at fifty micrograms. For those who are pregnant, start at one hundred micrograms, and those who are over fifty should start at one hundred to four hundred micrograms. There is no toxicity with this vitamin, and response appears to improve at the dose increases. This does not work without folate.

Most vitamin B12 supplements are derived from GMO sources, which are not recommended. That is a good reason to use whole organic source vitamins.

Requirements for B Vitamins

1 Gm (gram) = 1000mg (milligrams) 1mg (milligram) = 1000 mcg (micrograms)

Adults Daily	RDA Minimum	Over 50 Years	Integrative Usage	RDA Pregnancy	RDA Maximum
B1 Thiamin	1.2 mg	1.5mg	1.5 –25mg	1.4mg	none
B2 Riboflavin	1.3 mg	1.7mg	1.5- 20mg	1.6 mg	none
B3 Niacin	14mg	20mg	20mg	18mg	35mg
B5Panothinic Acid	5mg	5mg	5 -100mg	6-7mg	none
B6	1.5mg	2mg	25 -100mg	2mg	100mg
Boitin	30mcg	30mcg	30 – 100mcg	30 mcg	none
Folic Acid	400mcg	400mcg	400 – 1000 mcg	600mcg	1000mcg
Vitamin B12	2.4 mcg	500mcg	500 – 1000 mcg	2.8mcg	none

For patients with vitamin B12 malabsorption problems, the injectable form of B12 can be used at one milligram monthly. Oral or sublingual absorption (under-the-tongue tablets or liquid) is also available in five hundred-microgram and thousand-microgram doses. **These products should have no corn or soy in their ingredients.**

Vitamin A

When it comes to vitamin A, this is very important. Please note that the body has its own control mechanisms when it comes to the function and usability of this vitamin.

Plants contain carotenoids, some of which are precursors for vitamin A (alpha-carotene, beta-carotene, and beta-kryptoxanthin). Yellow and orange vegetables contain significant quantities of carotenoids. Green vegetables also contain carotenoids with the pigment masked by the green of chlorophyll.

Eggs and dairy also contain animal converted carotenoids in the form of retinol: cod liver oil, eggs, butter, and whole milk. Beta-carotene and other carotenoids, can be converted in the body to retinol and its related compounds (retinoids) are seen in potatoes, pumpkin, carrots, cantaloupe, mango, spinach, broccoli, kale, collards, and butternut squash.

Food	Serving	Vitamin A, RAE	Vitamin A, IU	Vitamin A, mcg	Retinol,IU
Cod liver oil	1 teaspoon	1,350 mcg	4,500 IU	1,350 mcg	4,500 IU
Fortified breakfast cereals	1 serving	150-230 mcg	500-767 IU	150-230 mcg	500-767 IU
Egg	1 large	91 mcg	303 IU	89 mcg	296 IU
Butter	1 tablespoon	97 mcg	323 IU	95 mcg	317 IU
Whole milk	1 cup (8 fl oz)	68 mcg	227 IU	68 mcg	227 IU
2% fat milk (vitamin A added)	1 cup(8fl oz)	134 mcg	447 IU	134 mcg	447 IU
Nonfat milk (vitamin A added)	1 cup(8fl oz)	149 mcg	497 IU	149 mcg	497 IU
Sweet potato mashed	1/2 cup mashed	555 mcg	1,848 IU	0	0
Sweet potato baked	1/2 cup	961 mcg	3,203 IU	0	0
Pumpkin, canned	1/2 cup	953 mcg	3,177 IU	0	0
Carrot (raw)	1/2 cup, chopped	538 mcg	1,793 IU	0	0
Cantaloupe	1/2 medium melon	467 mcg	1,555 IU	0	0
Mango	1 fruit	79 mcg	1,263 IU	0	0
Spinach	1/2 cup, cooked	472 mcg	1,572 IU	0	0
Broccoli	1/2 cup, cooked	60 mcg	200 IU	0	0
Kale	1/2 cup, cooked	443 mcg	1,475 IU	0	0
Collards	1/2 cup, cooked	386 mcg	1,285 IU	0	0
Squash, butternut	1/2 cup, cooked	572 mcg	1,907 IU	0	0

Table USDA Food Database

Those foods marked in gray, are not recommended forms of vitamin A since these are fortified foods with synthetic (previtamin A) and not recommended. Dairy foods should be organic (without fortification).

To date, no toxic results or damage, has been found from the use of vitamin A as beta-carotene. The only recommended form of vitamin A is provitamin A. It, has been shown that you can eat carrots until you turn orange, and you will still have no signs or symptoms of adverse effects. So, use provitamin A (beta-carotene) and not preformed vitamin A (in forms mentioned in chapter 18). Again, we see the difference between a synthetic and the real deal.

Due to multiple problems associated with the use of preformed vitamin A, many vitamin companies have reduced their preformed vitamin A in their supplements to 750 micrograms (2,500 IU) to prevent detectable side effects. The research suggests that this form of vitamin A is too destructive to the human body—and any form of preformed vitamin A, should be strictly avoided. The use of preformed vitamin A only causes damage. Be aware—and eat your colorful veggies!

Vitamin D- The Sunshine Vitamin

There are few vitamins, that are recommended in supplemental form, but this is one of them. All people (young and old) should have their vitamin D (25 hydroxyvitamin D) level tested, and know their vitamin D levels. First at birth, then every three months until the proper level is achieved with supplementation (including sunshine), and every two to three years after appropriate levels have been established in the body. **Vitamin D during pregnancy is very important, and all pregnant women should be tested.** Their vitamin D levels, should be adjusted to meet or exceed fifty nanograms per milliliter so that the infant can be born with at least thirty nanograms per milliliter. This is not optimum, but is at least minimum for healthy birth and development. **This is the sunshine vitamin—so sun exposure first and supplementation second.**

The skin can produce vitamin D with exposure to UV rays from the sun. Some doctors are now using safe tanning beds for the treatment of multiple skin conditions, with noted positive effects, new cell growth, and elevated levels of vitamin D. Please remember when using the sun, avoid the use of sun-block or other chemical preparations on the skin since these can alter skin cell growth and result in skin cancer. Limit sun exposure to thirty to forty minutes at a time and then cover up or get out of the sun.

The current recommendation for supplementation is thirty-five international units of vitamin D3 (natural vitamin D) per pound of body weight.

25- Hydroxy Vitamin D

<u>New Values</u> **For All Ages**

Deficient Levels	< 50 ng/ml
* Optimal Levels	50 to 70 ng/ml
** Required During Illness	70 to 100 ng/ml
Excess	> 100 ng/ml

Research reflects the belief that vitamin D, beta-carotene, vitamin C, and vitamin K all work together in a symbiotic relationship, much like the B vitamins. They each function with the aid of the other. It takes a community.

The Pathway of Vitamin D

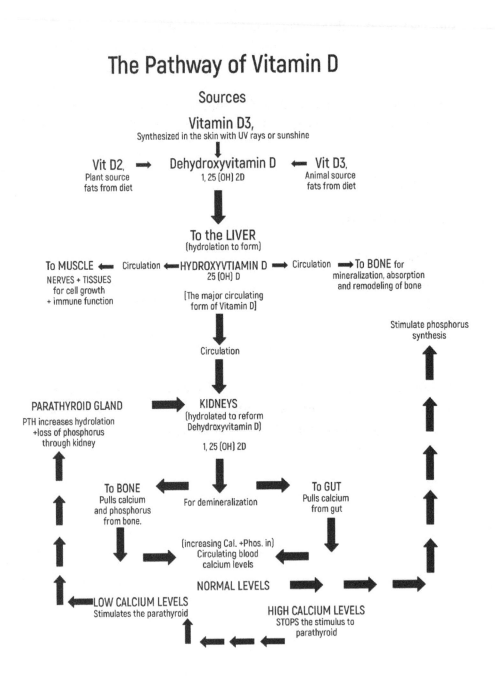

Sources

Vitamin D3,
Synthesized in the skin with UV rays or sunshine

Vit D2, → **Dehydroxyvitamin D** ← **Vit D3,**
Plant source   1, 25 (OH) 2D   Animal source
fats from diet   fats from diet

To the LIVER
(hydrolation to form)

To MUSCLE ← Circulation ← **HYDROXYVTIAMIN D** → Circulation → **To BONE** for
NERVES + TISSUES   25 (OH) D   mineralization, absorption
for cell growth   and remodeling of bone
+ immune function   [The major circulating
                        form of Vitamin D]

Circulation

Stimulate phosphorus
synthesis

PARATHYROID GLAND → **KIDNEYS**
PTH increases hydrolation   (hydrolated to reform
+loss of phosphorus   Dehydroxyvitamin D)
through kidney
                              1, 25 (OH) 2D

To BONE ← For demineralization → **To GUT**
Pulls calcium   Pulls calcium
and phosphorus   from gut
from bone.

(increasing Cal. +Phos. in)
Circulating blood
calcium levels

NORMAL LEVELS → →

LOW CALCIUM LEVELS ←   **HIGH CALCIUM LEVELS**
Stimulates the parathyroid   STOPS the stimulus to
                                    parathyroid

See chapter 18 for additional understanding of vitamin D and its effect on the function of the body—and remember it works better with vitamins A, C, and K.

Glycemic Index

Earlier in the book, we made mention to the glycemic index. Below, you will find the numeric values, that have been placed on non-bondable as well as bondable fuels. These values are a direct indicator of the production of insulin, or how much insulin is produced within the <u>first hour </u>of eating (insulin response). **These values will not tell you how much insulin response occurs after that first hour, and you already know that the ability of that sugar to bond with insulin is the all-important factor here. Since excess insulin and insulin spikes occur two to four hours after eating, these are the culprits we need to control.** This chart might give you a better understanding of bondable versus non-bondable. Remember that the use of chemicals and high-heat processing literally destroys the outer shell of electrons in the sugar and it can no longer bond with insulin.

Sugars

Crystalline Fructose 173   Does Not Bond—Heat Processed
(Fruit sugar concentrate, made from corn)

Invert Sugar 120   Does Not Bond—Heat Processed
(Patented chemical sweetener)

High-Fructose Corn Syrup 120   Does Not Bond—Heat Processed
(Fruit sugar concentrate, made from corn)

Sucrose 100   50 percent Does Not Bond   Commonly known as table sugar
(50 percent fructose and 50 percent glucose) and with heat exposure 100 percent does not bond

Xylitol 100   Does Not Bond
(Chemically patented Sweetener—poisonous to animals)

Tagatose 92   Does Not Bond
(Heat processed, chemically patented sweetener)

Glucose 74   Bonds with minimal (low) heat exposure
(Vegetable sugar)

High DE Corn Syrup 70   Does Not Bond
(Fructose, derived from corn through heat process)

Sorbitol 55   Does Not Bond
(Patented Sweetener made from Genetically Altered Foods)

Mannitol 50   Does Not Bond
(Patented Sweetener made from Genetically Altered foods)

Any sugars below the 50 marker are recommended by the Glycemic index for diabetics or those attempting to reduce type 2 diabetes.

Trehalose 45   Does Not Bond
(Mushroom sugar, only metabolized by intestinal bacteria in humans)

Regular Corn Syrup 40   Does Not Bond
(Heat-processed sweetener, Fructose made from Genetically Altered Foods)

Galactose 32   Bonds if RAW, No Heat Processing
(Milk Sugar, also found in Mother's Milk)

Maltose 32   Bonds if Raw, No Heat Processing
(Grain Sugar—All processed grains Do Not Bond)

Lactose 15   Bonds if Raw, No Heat Processing
(Milk Sugar—All commercial processed milk Does Not Bond)

Now you can see why it makes sense to eat lots of raw vegetables and drink raw milk. And mother's milk is the best.

Fermentation 101

For those who are interested in increasing their biologics (beneficial gut bacteria) and achieving a much higher number of absorbable vitamins, remember that some vitamins can only come from your biologics, like B vitamins, then these websites are for you:

- Mercola.com, mercola library: Fermented Foods—How to Culture Your Way to Optimal Health
- Dr. Campbell-McBride, Gut and Psychology Syndrome (the GAPS Diet)
- Immunonutrition, Cultured and Fermented Foods
- Caroline Barringer, Fermented Foods, www.culturedvegetables.net

For those who are interested in juicing their vegetables for a stronger vitamin and mineral content in your overall diet, these websites are for you.

- Juiceladycherie.com for juicing 101, including starter recipes
- Mercola.com, Mercola Library: Surprising Health Benefits of Vegetables, or just type in the word "Juicing"
- Mercola library: Benefits of Juicing, Your Keys to Radiant Health

People who want to increase their fat intake can add raw butter, organic eggs, coconut cream, coconut oil, avocado, coconut butter, or cream to your juice.

Several diet experts suggest never juicing the peel of oranges or grapefruit since they contain toxic oils. Aviod fruit when juicing. Lemon, lime, and spices are great flavor additives in very small amounts. If you add fats, then add chocolate (100 percent organic cocoa powder). Yum! If you want fruit, eat the whole fruit without the skin or peel.

Other Recommended Websites for Healthy Foods and Organics

- Institute for Responsible Technology or Alliance for Natural Health
- www.nongmoshoppingguide.com
- www.eathealthier.org

For Ketosis and the ketogenic diet

- "Tripping over the truth: The return of the metabolic theory of cancer illuminates a new hopeful path to a cure"
- Dietary Therapies.com
- "Keto Clarity" and Livin La Vita Low-carb website
- Single Cause, Single Cure Foundation
- Metabolic optimization.com
- The Charlie Foundation for Ketogenic Therapies
- TheTruthAboutCancer.com—and watch the global quest.

For Mineral Balance

- Natural Sea Salt, Celtic Sea Salt: www.realsalt.com
- For Trace Minerals, www.traceminerals.com
- www.mineralresourcesint.com
- Magnesium Maltate, Source Naturals
- www.sourcenaturals.com

For Hair Mineral analysis

- Trace Elements Inc. (Laboratory)
- www.aurorahealthandnutrition.com

For Probiotics

- www.nutricology.com

Remember that probiotics must be refrigerated—any high-count, high-quality probiotic will be found in the refrigerator section.

For Whole Food Vitamins

- Daily Complete Liquid Vitamins, www.puretrim.com
- Raw Vitamin C, www.rawvitamins.com
- Whole food vitamins and supplements, www.Mercolaproducts.com

For Other Supplements

- Super DHA, Carlson www.carlsonlabs.com
- Omega-3 fatty acids, www.purealaskaomega.com
- Pure Alaska omega: Available at Costco and Sam's Clubs
- Vitamin D3, 5,000 IU, Nature's Way Products (contains no toxins or soy)
- MSM or Organic Sulfur, The West Coast Organic Sulfur Project, www.organicsulfur-msm.ca
- MSM Pure Powder, www.herbstoreusa.com
- Nature's Way Products, MSM capsules (less bioavailability)

Glossary of Terms

Acetylcholine: Brain neurotransmitter that has a wide variety of applications, but it is primarily known for its ability to stimulate muscle contractions. It not only travels in the brain but the vagus nerve as well. Chapters 8, 18.

Adenosine triphosphate (ATP): The term for the formation of energy, which is made in the mitochondria (power plants) found in all cells. Chapters 9, 12, 14, 17.

Albumin: A family of globular proteins that maintains osmotic pressure in the circulating blood and acts as transport for calcium, sodium, potassium, hormones, bilirubin, T4 (thyroid hormone), and some organic-based pharmaceuticals. Chapter 13.

Amino acids: Organic compound containing carbon, hydrogen, oxygen, and nitrogen (five hundred known amino acids) found in peptides, polypeptides, and proteins. Chapter 10.

Antibodies: Element formed in B cells and killer cells, by copying the DNA of the invading organism, which, when needed, it can recognize again. Chapter 18.

Antigen: An invading microbe (foreign toxic non-self-invaders), can be bacterial, viral, or fungal in nature. Chapter 18.

Antioxidant: That element found in food, which can formulate to limit oxidation reactions in the body by neutralizing the extra oxygen component (ROS) as seen in glutathione. Chapters 12, 18.

Arrhythmias: Irregular heartbeats, seen in normal cardiac function, may be increased by neuro-stimulants and toxins and can lead to heart problems, including heart attack. Chapter 8.

Aseptic necrosis: Bone death without the presence of infection. Chapter 17.

Aspartame (NutraSweet): A chemically derived form of sugar proven to cause direct brain damage (a non-bondable). Chapters 2, 7.

Avidin: An enzyme found in egg white that binds to biotin (a sulfur-bonded protein) preventing absorption of sulfur. Chapter 18.

Bacteroides (enterotype): Bacterial colonies that ferment protein and fats. Chapter 8.

Beneficial bacteria (probiotic bacteria): Bacteria that live in the small and large intestine and benefit the body by breaking down and fermenting foods, producing the nutrients available for absorption by the body. Chapters 4, 18.

Bile: The term used for digestive enzymes, salts, and waste materials, stored in the gallbladder, that break down and emulsify fats passing through the duodenum for continued digestion. Chapters 4, 13.

Biocytin: A form of sulfur-bonded protein, found in foods containing protein. Chapter 18.

Brittle diabetic: The diabetic unable to control blood sugars due to false elevation in blood sugars from non-bondable food use. Chapter 2.

Candida: Pathogenic or destructive yeast-like growth, fungal in nature, that can occur throughout the digestive tract and tends to become abundant (overgrowth) after repeated use of antibiotics. Chapter 15.

Carcinogens: Known agents (chemical, environmental, and food-source), that cause cancer in the human body. Chapters 13, 20.

Carotenoids: Plant source precursors to vitamin A. Chapter 18.

Casein: Phosphoproteins; commonly seen in the milk of mammals. When unprocessed, it provides healthy amino acids along with calcium and phosphorous to the nutritional supply. Chapters 9, 15.

Cholesterol: A lipid or fat molecular structure that is made by the liver, an essential structural component of all cell membranes. Chapters 13, 15, 20.

Cirrhosis: The result of, development of scar tissue in the liver, due to loss of liver function or toxic damage, and usually seen in the final stage of liver disease. Chapter 18.

Coenzymes: A non-protein chemical compound, that activates enzymes and assists in molecular structure transformation and/or function, as seen in vitamins. Chapter 18.

Corium sensing: A form of signaling, or group communications used by bacteria. Chapter 4.

Creatinine phosphokinase: A blood test used to detect liver damage. Chapter 20.

Crystalline fructose: Fructose (fruit sugar can be derived from corn or soy). This form is three to four times the concentration of high-fructose corn syrup, "fructose on speed," a non-bondable. Chapters 2, 7.

Cysteine: Animal- and plant-sourced sulfur-bonded protein; not made by the human body. Chapters 13, 15.

Cytokines: A form of protein; seen as interleukins or lymphocytes, that act, as intracellular mediators (inflammatory response signals—enzymes) in the immune response, for the purpose of self-defense. Chapter 18.

Deamonization: The breakdown of nitrogen found in excess protein, by the kidneys, resulting in kidney damage. Chapter 9.

Decidua reflexia: A barrier between the circulation of the mother and the fetus, formed by epithelial cells tightly bonded together, allowing only nutrients to pass. Chapter 15.

Dehydration: The result of, excessive loss of body water, with an accompanying disruption of electrolyte (mineral) balance of the body. Chapters 8, 12.

Dehydroepiandosterone (DHEA): A minor hormone in the human growth hormone complex that acts as a counterbalance for stress by decreasing cortisol. Chapters 11, 12.

Dementia: Functional mental instability, usually seen with severe memory loss and loss of physical function. Chapter 18.

Demyelination: A result of cellular inflammation with ammonia production, caused by the free radical glutamine, with loss of the myelin sheath that coats and protects nerve cells. Chapter 15.

Deoxyribonucleic acid (DNA): A chain of molecules, that forms our genetic blueprint, for structure and function of each individual human body. Chapters 1, 9, 17, 20.

Dermatitis: A skin reaction; usually seen in vitamin deficiencies and allergic reactions, characterized by skin flushing and rash. Chapter 18.

Duodenum: The first ten inches of the small intestine, which contains an entry port from the gallbladder, called the common bile duct. Chapters 4, 9, 10.

Endothelial nitric oxide synthesis (ENOS): A process in the skin, that produces a sulfur anion and oxygen, from sunlight exposure (the human body solar battery). Chapter 13.

Enterotype: A category of biologics (bacteria) determined by the types of foods that the bacteria ferment. Chapter 8.

Esterification: The removal of water-containing oxygen from any element; this can be done by the body, as seen in the eyes. It, can also be chemically produced in the production of fat-soluble supplements. Chapters 11, 17.

Exocytosis: The induced- rapid movement of ions, across cell walls of neurons. Chapter 17.

Fetal tubes: Also known as neuro tubes, the basic cellular components for the original formation of the human nervous system during fetal development. Chapter 18.

Free radical: An element that is unbalanced, missing electrons in its outer shell, but instead of bonding, it steals electrons from other elements, causing damage and destruction to those elements from which it steals. Chapters 2, 11, 13, 14, 15.

Fibrinogen: Classified as a glycoprotein in animals, that participates in the formation of blood clots. Chapter 13.

Fructooligosaccharides (FOS): A sugar-based medium in which bacteria can grow, used in some probiotic products. Chapter 4.

Fructose: A fruit sugar, found in fruit, also found in table sugar (one glucose and one fructose molecule), classified as a non-bondable sugar. Chapters 2, 7.

Gallbladder: A sack-like organ that stores digestive enzymes, toxins, and waste products, derived from the liver, to be deposited, into the small intestine via the common bile duct. Chapters 4, 16.

Ghrelin: A hormone produced by the hypothalamus, which travels the vagus nerve and stimulates the stomach to stop digestive secretions. Chapters 2, 8.

Glutathione: An enzyme used by the body to control the aggressive nature of powerful antioxidants like hydrogen peroxide, the master controller. Chapters 13, 14, 15.

Gluten: A protein derived from grains (wheat, rye, and barley) that can cause inflammatory response (intestinal wall irritant) in the intestinal tract. Chapters 7, 15.

Glycemic index: An index used to measure insulin response within the first hour, to sugar content in foods. Chapters 5, 7.

Genetically modified (GM): Made by man, found in both plant and animal sources, not found in nature. Chapter 19.

Genetically modified organism (GMO): The combining of genes of different organisms outside of their species, and not found in nature, with no proven safety. Chapter 19.

Helicobacter pylori (H. pylori): A form of pathogenic bacteria, that lives in the stomach and small intestine. Overgrowth of this bacteria, can cause gastritis and inflammatory response. Chapters 4, 15.

Heme: An element found in iron that binds to oxygen, seen in the hemoglobin of red blood cells. Chapter 18.

High-fructose corn syrup: "Fructose on steroids," a sugar product derived from corn, depending on concentration, can be two to three times the potency of table sugar and five times the value of simple glucose. Chapters 2, 7.

Histamine: Immune response enzyme, that signals to the immune system, the presence of injury in a specific area, attracting white blood cells and platelets to the area in response. Chapter 18.

Horizontal gene transfer: The lateral movement, of foreign genetic material, into other genetic structures. This movement, is seen in intestinal bacteria. Chapters 8, 9, 19.

Hydrogen peroxide: "Our internal sweeper," a chemical formation at the cellular level, derived from CoQ-10, or vitamin C, which can act as an antioxidant, preventing free radical damage, this action will destroy and/or remove bacteria, viruses, and toxins from the tissues. Chapters 14, 16, 17.

Hydrogenation (also partial hydrogenation): The process used in food processing to change a liquid fat to a solid fat, usually seen in processed vegetable oils. Chapter 13.

Hydrotherapy: A form of therapy or detox- treatment of the body using water. Chapter 16.

Hyperbaric: A form of therapy, using oxygen under pressure, raising the atmospheric pressure outside the body. Chapter 16.

Hypertension: The elevation of the blood pressure above that of acceptable levels, characterized by a diastolic (bottom number of pressure reading) remaining consistently above 100 mm/Hg (millimeters of mercury). Chapters 2, 17.

Hyperthermia: Elevated body temperature, usually seen as a high fever. Also, can be seen in the detoxification of the body, the removal of toxins using heat, as in use of a sauna or steam bath. Chapter 16.

Hypocholesteremia: The severe loss of cholesterol in the circulation, leading to death. Chapter 20

Hypothalamus: A chamber under the brain, an organ that produces six different hormones for regulation of function of other organs throughout the body. Most of these hormones travel the vagus nerve. Chapter 12.

Ileus or intestinal colic: Loss of peristalsis or functional movement of the muscles that line colon, which can be seen as constipation or bowel blockage. Chapters 4, 17.

Immunology: The study of the human immune system, our natural defense system. Chapter 3.

Inflammatory response: The end result of tissue irritation, causing swelling in cells and separation of bonds between cells, allowing gaps between cellular structures and entry of unwanted elements. Chapters 9, 15.

Insulin: A hormone produced by the pancreas that binds to glucose and carries it to the cells for utilization as fuel. Chapter 2.

Interferon: A type of cytokine, released by host cells (inflammatory response), in response to the presence of pathogens, viruses, bacteria, parasites, and tumor cells. Chapter 18.

Intravenous: The installation or placement of solid or liquid materials through a vein in the human body. Chapters 16, 18.

Ionic minerals: Water-soluble minerals that can carry an electric charge. Chapter 17.

Ketosis: The formation of ketone bodies from fatty acids found in fat cells and dietary fats, usually seen in starvation mode, but also can be seen as a form of high-fat diet and fat-burning mode. Chapters 5, 9, 11, 13.

Ketonuria: The excessive loss of ketone bodies via the kidneys. Chapters 5, 11.

Krebs cycle: The process by which protein and the lipid droplet are combined to form the early stages of cholesterol. Chapter 13.

Leptin: A hormone produced by fat cells to signal satiety to the hypothalamus in the brain. Chapters 2, 8.

Lipid bilayer: A thin polar membrane made of two layers of lipid (fat) molecules held in place by a sulfur bond in the middle. This forms a sheet that makes a continuous barrier around cells (the 'Oreo cookie structure'). Chapters 11, 13.

Liposuction: Surgical - removal of fat from the body via a long hallow tube. Chapter 11.

Macrophages: Formed from white blood cells, Greek for big eaters, *macros* for large and *phagen* for eat). An amoeboid (self-movement) like a blood cell that can respond to infection and engulf or eat foreign cells. Chapter 18.

Megaloblastic anemia: The result of, the formation of abnormal- enlarged red blood cells, usually- seen as a folate deficiency. This can also be seen as a hydrochloric acid (stomach acid) deficiency. Chapter 18.

Metabolic ketoacidosis: The result of formation or accumulation of extremely large amounts of ketone bodies, that cannot be rapidly consumed or disposed of by the body, usually the result of artificial stimulus. Chapter 5.

Metabolic syndrome: A classification of a group of health problems, which appear to be related, but with no common associated disease cause. Chapters 2, 11.

Methionine: An animal- and plant-sourced sulfur-bonded protein- not made by the human body. Chapters 13, 15, 18.

Meucin lining: A layer of epithelial cells, that bond tightly together and coat the interior lining of the intestinal wall, preventing passage of unwanted elements into the body. Chapter 15.

Myelin sheath: A coating found on nerve cells made from Schwann cells and oligodendrocytes (specialty cells), this coating is used for both peripheral cell and brain cell protection from damage caused by electrical charge traveling the nerve cells surface. Chapters 13, 18.

Myopathy: Loss of muscle tissue function, characterized, by muscle pain and weakness. Chapter 20.

Necrobiosis: The act of natural cell death – normal life span. Chapter1

Necrosis: The early death of cells through injury or disease. Chapter 20, 13

Neuro-excitotoxin: An element formed from protein fragments called glutamine, which creates damage to brain cells with increased formation of ammonia in the brain, resulting in neuron death. Chapters 15, 17.

Neurotransmitters (dopamine, epinephrine, and norepinephrine): A class of hormones and enzymes, that act as electrical conductors in the nervous system, affecting functional activity as well as mood. Chapter 15, 18.

Nicotinamide: A coenzyme derived from niacin (one of the B vitamins) in the body. This element is not related to nicotine found in tobacco. Chapter 18.

Nitric oxide: An enzyme produced by epithelial cells that line the walls of the arteries of the body. This enzyme is necessary for muscle relaxation in the arteries, which lowers blood pressure. Chapter 2.

Non-rapid eye movement (NREM). A stage of sleep, that is intermittent in length and recognized as a decrease in all body systems activities. This is the closest the body gets to total body rest and is vital for good health. Chapter 12.

Opsin: A protein that forms the visual pigment of the eye when combined with retinol and exposed to light. Chapter 18.

Osmosis. The diffusion or movement, of a fluid (molecules), through a semi-permeable membrane, to a region of higher-solute concentration, from a lower-solute concentration, until concentrations are equalized on both sides of the membrane. This is an attempt to equalize concentrations. Chapter 16.

Osmotic pressure: The minimum pressure needed to nullify osmosis or the passage of fluids across a membrane (no net movement of molecules). Chapter 16.

Osteomalacia: Adult rickets; also seen as severe vitamin D deficiency. Chapter 18.

Oosteoporosis: Weak or soft bones, due to a loss of mineral density or gap in bone formation, generally resulting in fractures or broken bones. Chapters 15, 18.

Oxidation: A change in a chemical compound structure, due to a loss of atom or atoms from its outer shell. This change is often- referred to as oxidative damage, changing structure, changes its ability to function. Chapters 13, 18.

Oxidative stress: A form of free radical oxidation in the body, indicated by elevated levels of homocysteine. Chapter 18.

Oxysterols:. Cholesterol, that has been oxidized or used (broken down or changed). Some can be beneficial, while others can be damaging. These same oxysterols help the liver control cholesterol production. Chapter 13.

Peptide: A compound formed by two or more amino acids. In the intestinal tract, these are seen as protein fragments and usually are derived from unhealthy sources. Chapter 15.

Peripheral neuropathy: Loss of nerve sensation or numbness in extremities, usually caused by free radical damage or vitamin deficiencies. Chapters 2, 18.

Peristalsis. The rhythmic - contractions of the intestinal wall, this causes the movement of fecal material through the intestine. Chapters 4, 8.

Phylic acid: Damaging element found in soy that blocks intestinal absorption of critical minerals needed for body function. Chapter 7.

Phytoestrogens: Elements that mimic the function of estrogen hormones and can cause abnormal elevations in estrogen levels. This element is found in soy. Chapter 7.

Phytonutrient or Phytochemical: A plant-derived organic compound that contains nutrient properties that assist or induce the functions associated with vitamins and minerals. Chapter 18.

Phytosterols: Plant-sourced sterols that act as vitamin adjuncts and become a part of human cholesterol, found in vitamin D2. Chapters 11, 18.

Platelet aggregation: The ability of platelets to clump, due to stickiness, for the formation of clots. Chapter 15.

Platelet (thrombocyte): Blood cells formed in bone marrow that circulate in the blood and form clots to stop bleeding. They also act as a carrier for nitric oxide and a stimulus in immune response. Chapter 18.

Polyneuropathy (peripheral neuropathy): A symptom characterized by numbness, tingling, and weakness in the extremities (arms and legs) due to the loss of protective coating of nerves (myelin sheaths). Chapter 18.

Polypeptide chain: A long, continuous peptide chain composed of amino acids, generally distinguished from proteins on the basis of size with polypeptides containing fewer than fifty amino acids. Chapter 10.

Preeclampsia and Eclampsia: A toxemia of pregnancy; characterized by uncontrolled hypertension, headaches, and albumin (excess protein) in the urine and edema or swelling in the lower extremities. Chapter 17.

Prostacyclin: A natural form of blood thinner seen as an enzyme, that maintains active blood flow and prevents excessive clot formation. Chapters 11, 13.

Prevotella: An enterotype, bacterial colonies that ferment sugars. Chapters 4, 8.

Quercetin: A bonding agent found in fruit that binds to fructose and limits its absorption. Chapter 2.

Recombinant DNA technology: The technology, that combines genes from different organisms (outside of their species) to create a new modified gene, not found in nature. Chapter 19.

Rapid eye movement (REM): A cyclic pattern of sleep, characterized by dreaming, and necessary for the maintenance of memory and learning patterns. Chapter 12.

Reticular beds: A network of strands of protein-coated connective tissue that is found in the skin and also supports structures throughout the body. Chapter 14.

Retinoid: Element converted in the body from carotenoids and stored in the eye. Chapter 18.

Retinol (preformed vitamin A): A synthetic compound designed to mimic retenoids in the body. Have been found to be toxic and form birth defects. Not a recommended form of vitamin A. Chapter 18.

Rhabdomyolysis: The end result of muscle-cell necrosis and death with the release of intracellular contents, resulting in **myoglobinurea** (blood in the urine) with renal damage and renal failure, a life-threatening condition. Chapter 20.

Rickets: The term used for severe vitamin D deficiency. It is described as a lack of phosphorous to create balance to form bone matrix, usually described as soft bone. Vitamin D is the main influence in this balance. Chapter 18.

Reactive oxygen species (ROS): Are chemically reactive molecules containing oxygen. This includes ions and peroxides, which are necessary for immune response and protection from pathogens, but they can become free radical molecules without the natural controls found in such elements as glutathione, the body's master controller. Chapter 18.

Schwann cells: Cells that wrap around neurons to form the myelin sheath for protection of the nerve cell and conduction of nerve impulses. Without the sheath, nerve impulses cannot travel. Chapter 13.

Semiubiquinone: Partially oxidized CoQ-10, that coats and protects cell walls and produces hydrogen peroxide. Chapter 14.

Sodium pump: The movement of positive-to-negative ions of potassium and sodium across the cell wall (lipid bilayer), causing the transfer of elements in and out of the cell. Chapter 1.

Stem cells: Specialized biological cells, that can divide and produce more cells (duplicates of itself) for each different or specialized area or tissue in the body. These are the first layer of cells that form in early stages of embryo formation throughout the human body. Chapter 9.

Steroid hormones: Hormones produced by the adrenal glands (testosterone, estrogen, progesterone, and cortisol). This production is regulated by the hypothalamus in the brain. These hormones regulate stress response and sexual function of the human body. Chapters 12, 13.

Sterols: Plant- and animal-sourced cholesterol, also act as a fat-soluble vitamin adjunct, as seen in vitamin D2. Chapter 11.

Stevia: A natural plant sweetener, contains no absorbable glucose, does not bond with insulin, does not cause insulin spikes, and causes no known health damage. This is not a bondable or non-bondable. It is a natural, organic substance, recognized by the body as only a sweetener, that stimulates salivation and appetite. Chapter 2.

Sucralose (Splenda): A chemical (artificial) sugar known to kill intestinal biologics, a non-bondable. Chapter 2.

Sulfotryosine: A non-sulfated protein (Tryosine - amino acid) that is bonded to sulfur within the liver. Chapters 13, 15.

Thromboxane: An enzyme found in blood that stimulates increased blood clot formation. Chapters 11, 13.

Trans fats: A form of oxidized fat that alters cholesterol formation and function. There are two forms: trans fats that come from the saturated fat of animals, which is natural in nature and recognized by the body, and trans fats that are formed from the artificial hydrogenation of vegetable oils, which oxidize easily, are not recognized by the human body, and are classified as lethal oxysterols. Chapters 13, 11.

Type 2 diabetes: The end result of pancreatic failure, caused by the excessive use of non-bondable fuels, with loss of insulin production in the body. Chapter 2.

Ubiquinol: Fully reduced CoQ-10, that coats and protects cell walls and attracts more CoQ-10. Chapter 14.

Ubiquinone: Fully oxidized CoQ-10, that forms the electron transport chain. Chapter 14.

Uric acid: An enzyme created as a by-product of the breakdown of toxins in the liver. This enzyme can become damaging to health in large quantities. Chapters 2, 9.

Ventricle: A vessel that is a part of management of fluid pressures, found in the brain, heart, and other organs, seen as a hollow organ through which fluid can flow. Chapter 8.

Visual purple: The pigment found in the rods and cones of the eye that activates visual reception. Chapter 18.

Very small dense lipoprotein (VSLDL): A particle or fat and protein fragment, produced by the liver from unhealthy or non-bondable foods. Chapters 2, 13.

Walzen factor: A compound made by the body using sterols, which inhibits inflammation in cartilage of joints (arthritis). Chapter 11.

White blood cells (WBCs) (leukocytes): Blood cells, that function as part of the immune system in response to inflammation to control infection. Chapter 18.

Whey: The liquid remaining after milk has been curdled and strained. There are two distinctive types of whey: one comes from whole raw milk and can be made into cheese (a healthy form) and one that comes from pasteurized, homogenized milk that contains dead bacteria and toxins (a toxic form). Chapter 7.

Zoosterol: Animal-sourced sterol that becomes part of human cholesterol formation. Chapter 11.

Test Questions

Chapters 1–2 - How our body uses fuel

1. Name three bondable natural dietary fuels.
   A. green peas, bean sprouts, agave syrup
   B. broccoli, kale, pasteurized milk
   C. black beans, spinach, red peppers
   D. corn, soy, organic honey

2. The hormone insulin is formed from what elements?
   A. LDL cholesterol bonded to calcium
   B. heparin with a vitamin C complex chain
   C. two digestive enzymes bonded to sulfa
   D. two polypeptides (proteins) bonded by sulfa

3. Leptin is a hormone produced by fat cells. What stimulates the fat cell to produce this hormone?
   A. the consumption of toxins by the fat cell
   B. the consumption of excess fuel
   C. the consumption of extracellular fluid
   D. the presence of sodium ions

4. Ghrelin stimulates what nerve to signal the stomach to shut down?
   A. the hypothalamus nerve
   B. the vagus nerve
   C. the pharyngeal nerve
   D. the facial nerve

5. How are all non-bondable sugars, toxins (including chemicals used in food processing), and alcohols processed in the body?
   A. They are processed through the liver through separate pathways.
   B. They are processed through the liver through the same pathways.
   C. They are broken down before they reach the liver and use the same pathway.
   D. They enter the liver as complex molecular chains but use separate pathways.

6. Name three non-bondable fuels.
   A. freshly brewed coffee, orange juice, 100 percent maple syrup
   B. wild brown rice, white rice, table sugar
   C. bran muffin, breakfast cereal, barley malt sweetener
   D. unprocessed organic honey, soft drinks, blackstrap molasses

7. What are the three end-products of processing non-bondable fuels?
   A. fat, glycogen (closed molecule), nitric oxide
   B. lactic acid, LDLs, glycogen
   C. glycogen, uric acid, nitric oxide
   D. VSLDLs, glycogen (closed molecule), lactic acid

8. Accumulations of lactic acid in the circulating blood causes _____, which can cause damage to the _____.
   A. swollen blood vessels, arteries
   B. swelling in fingers and toes, thyroid
   C. gout, kidneys
   D. stiff arteries, heart

9. Excessive lactic acid can also affect the blood pressure by blocking _____. This causes arteries to _____ and _____ blood pressure results.
   A. nitric oxide, stiffen, elevated
   B. uric acid, soften, decreased
   C. crystals, swelling, elevated
   D. cholesterol, stiffen, high

10. LDL cholesterol is a vital component of all cells. Large buoyant LDLs are necessary for what activities in the bloodstream?
    A. keeping arteries clean
    B. absorbing cellular debris
    C. transport of nutrients (CoQ-10 and vitamins)
    D. making plaque

11. Plaque is derived from dead dry cells on the inner lining of the arteries. Small amounts are a necessary part of what?
    A. sulfa formation
    B. heparin formation
    C. nutrient transport
    D. clot formation

12. A closed molecule is?
    A. a molecule that can't open
    B. a bondable molecule
    C. a molecule with balanced electrons in its outer shell
    D. a molecule bonded to sulfa

13. Peripheral arterial disease or hardening of the arteries, is a result of high volumes of what by-product?
    A. LDLs
    B. VSLDLs
    C. HDLs
    D. cholesterol

14. High volumes of non-bondable glycogen (the closed molecule), are the direct cause of what?
    A. hypertension
    B. belly fat
    C. kidney failure
    D. liver failure

15. The long-term consumption of an 80 percent non-bondable diet, will cause what?
    A. obesity

B. diabetes

C. metabolic syndrome

D. all of the above

16. What are the two main problems that result from increased pressure from belly fat and decreased function of the liver?
    A. kidney dysfunction, dilated blood vessels
    B. decreased blood flow, increased toxins
    C. continued circulating toxins in bloodstream, multiple (almost continuous) insulin spikes
    D. increased free insulin, increased blood pressure

17. Continuous multiple insulin spikes can be traced to what disease?
    A. Alzheimer's
    B. hypertension
    C. kidney failure
    D. heart disease
    E. diabetes

18. Diabetes is
    A. the end result of excess sugar intake
    B. the end result of pancreatic failure
    C. the end result of insulin increases
    D. A and C

19. Excessive, multiple insulin spikes cause
    A. brain fog
    B. pancreatic fatigue
    C. increased ghrelin production
    D. A and B

20. The loss of leptin and ghrelin signaling will cause
    A. continued hunger
    B. decreased insulin production
    C. an increase to the tumbleweed affect causing pancreatic fatigue
    D. A and C

21. Free-floating bondable glucose
    A. acts like a free radical
    B. causes oxidation (cellular destruction)
    C. is prevented with the presence of insulin
    D. all of the above

22. A false positive blood sugar reading can be caused by
    A. low insulin
    B. free-roaming non-bondable glucose (glycogen)
    C. high insulin
    D. free-roaming bondable glucose (poly-glucose)

23. The exterior protective coating of all cells throughout the body is composed of _____.
    A. protein (amino acids)
    B. nitric oxide
    C. cholesterol
    D. sulfa

24. The lipid bi-layer supports electrical activity, which is seen in _____ cells.
    A. bone
    B. skin
    C. muscle
    D. nerve

25. Sodium and potassium create electrical charges that facilitate nutrient movement in and out of the cell. With a positive electrical charge, _____ the cell and a negative electrical charge _____ the cell.
    A. inside, outside
    B. through, around
    C. outside, inside
    D. around, through

26. A healthy BMI for the average adult is?
    A. 22–24
    B. 19–23
    C. 24–28
    D. 25–30

27. For the bodybuilder, the BMI should be?
    A. 18–22
    B. 22–24
    C. 23–28
    D. 23–30

28. Morbid obesity affects all vital organs and may not occur until after signs of metabolic syndrome have arrived. Name two early signs of metabolic syndrome.
    A. elevated blood pressure
    B. renal failure
    C. prediabetes diagnosis
    D. A and C

29. The fat index is?
    A. the waist measurement of the smallest area around the abdomen, below the rib cage and above the belly button while standing
    B. the most important measurement for indicating level of health
    C. this number, when elevated, indicates increased pressure on internal organs
    D. all of the above

30. What will satisfy the appetite and prevent insulin spikes better than portion control?
    A. eating raw vegetables as snacks
    B. drinking water before meals
    C. increasing protein intake
    D. eating very small amounts of snack foods

E. A and B

F. C and D

31. What is the maximum fat index for adult women?
    A. 37 inches
    B. 34 inches
    C. 34.6 inches
    D. 36 inches

32. What is the maximum fat index for adult men?
    A. 38 inches
    B. 40 inches
    C. 41 inches
    D. 39 inches

33. The Mediterranean diet is a vegetable-based diet using a wide variety of vegetables daily. How many grams of protein should be the maximum consumed in any one meal (this includes vegetable proteins like beans, green peas, and brown rice).
    A. 15 grams
    B. 25 grams
    C. 30 grams
    D. 40 grams

34. Non-bondable fuels consist of?
    A. most high-glycemic index foods (generally above an index of 45)
    B. artificial sugars and fructose
    C. raw organic vegetables
    D. A and B

35. USDA organic is the label to look for to avoid genetically altered foods. Genetically altered foods include?
    A. vegetable oils, canola oil
    B. sugar beets, corn, and sweet corn
    C. tomatoes, honey, and soybeans
    D. all of the above

Chapter 4 and 5 - Getting from Point A to Point B And Cellular Metabolism

36. Hydrochloric acid is necessary for the breakdown of what element?
    A. fat
    B. cholesterol
    C. protein
    D. carbohydrates

37. The main components of stomach acid are found in what minerals?
    A. sodium, chloride
    B. sodium, potassium, and chloride
    C. potassium, chloride, and iron
    D. zinc and sodium

38. The breakdown of protein provides a wide variety of amino acids, which are necessary for the formation of _____ and _____ throughout the body.
    A. enzymes and hormones
    B. hormones and blood cells
    C. fatty acids and enzymes
    D. mineral compounds and hormones

39. Each crystal in whole crystal sea salt contains?
    A. 85 percent sodium and 15 percent trace minerals
    B. only sulfa
    C. the minerals that are in direct proportion to the minerals found in the human body
    D. all of the above

40. "Digestion problems," heartburn, and GERD are indicators of
    A. too much stomach acid
    B. mineral deficiencies
    C. not enough stomach acid
    D. B and C

41. The gallbladder stores waste products from the body, along with bile and digestive enzymes. What is the stimulus for the gallbladder to contract?
   A. protein
   B. carbohydrates
   C. fats
   D. none of the above

42. Bacteria work together in large functional groups (colonies) and communicate with each other. For every cell in the human body, there are _____ bacterial cells helping to keep it alive.
   A. 100
   B. 10
   C. 1 trillion
   D. 1,000

43. Bacteria found in your small intestine are microscopic, yet they fill the twenty feet of small intestine with how many pounds of bacteria?
   A. 8–10 pounds
   B. 3–5 pounds
   C. 2 pounds
   D. 1–3 pounds

44. Bacteria become active grow and multiply at _____degrees and will die at _____ degrees.
   A. 60–85
   B. 72–85
   C. 50–65
   D. 55–72

45. Normal digestion should take?
   A. 72–80 hours
   B. 14–44 hours
   C. 15–24 hours
   D. 24–36 hours

46. At what time of day does the body have the lowest amount of glycogen floating around its cells?
    A. 6–10 p.m.
    B. 1–2 a.m.
    C. 6–10 a.m.
    D. 2–4 a.m.

47. Fatty acids that are stored in the fat cell are expelled when stimulated and become _____ in the extracellular spaces (floating around the cells).
    A. glucose
    B. ketone bodies
    C. poly-glucose
    D. glycogen

48. We lose fat when we burn _____.
    A. glucose
    B. glycogen
    C. ketone bodies
    D. ketosis

49. Burning _____ as _____ is known as starvation mode.
    A. glucose, fatty acids
    B. glycogen, ketone bodies
    C. fatty acids, glycogen
    D. ketone bodies, secondary form of fuel

50. Using a continuous form of mild ketosis in the body will kill unhealthy cells.
    A. true
    B. false

51. Burning ketone bodies for fuel is a normal form of metabolism, but stimulating ketone bodies without exercise can cause what?
    A. metabolic ketoacidosis
    B. a flood of ketones into the body that muscles cannot use

C. elevated blood pressure and damage to the heart

D. all of the above

52. If we eat 80 percent bondable fuels, we can

A. automatically utilize "calories in, calories out"

B. allow leptin and ghrelin signals to complete

C. decrease fat cell size with simple cardio exercise each morning

D. all of the above

Chapter 6 – It Takes a Community

53. The liver is of primary importance in the function of all other organs in the body. It

A. performs five hundred different functions daily

B. is our toxic waste disposal plant

C. is the largest gland in the human body

D. all of the above

54. The liver will attempt to break down and utilize anything you eat that manages to get past your intestinal tract (immune defense system).

A. true

B. false

55. What is the best personal indicator (with or without lab tests) for liver damage?

A. height and weight

B. waist size

C. BMI

D. A and C

56. What are some of the typical problems we fail to associate with liver function?

A. osteoporosis

B. hormone imbalance and depression

C. thyroid problems

D. all of the above

57. The true way to treat a medical problem is to find the cause and correct it.
    A. true
    B. false

58. Liver chemistries are a good indicator of early metabolic syndrome.
    A. true
    B. false

59. *Complete* liver failure is fully reversible.
    A. true
    B. false

Chapter 7 – What's Wrong With These Foods

60. The first step in health improvement through nutrition is
    A. eliminating processed grains from the diet
    B. eliminating all sugars from the diet
    C. eliminating all chemicals and toxins from the diet
    D. eliminating all GMOs (genetically altered foods) from the diet

61. Processed grains contain
    A. chemical preservatives
    B. natural vitamins and minerals
    C. no nutrition
    D. A and C

62. Celiac disease is an allergic response in the intestinal tract to
    A. fat
    B. sugars
    C. artificial sugars
    D. gluten

63. Celiac disease affects _____ Americans.
    A. 1 out of every 1,000
    B. 1 out of every 500

C. 1 out of every 133

D. 1 out of every 5,000

64. Diseases related to gluten reactions (inflammatory-autoimmune response)

A. irritable bowel

B. malabsorption syndrome with multiple vitamin deficiencies

C. intestinal lymphoma (cancer)

D. all of the above

65. Whey consists of

A. dead red and white blood cells, serum albumin, dead bacteria, and mucus

B. residues of pharmaceuticals and hormones, including IGF (insulin growth factor—a GMO)

C. A and B

D. none of the above

66. What is the maximum protein load for the liver in any one meal?

A. 30 grams

B. 20 grams

C. 25 grams

D. 50 grams

67. Pasteurized, homogenized milk from commercial farms also contains toxic waste in the form of pharmaceuticals (pain medications, antibiotics, hormones, and steroids). To date, we have found no way to remove these toxins from the milk supply.

A. true

B. false

68. The main dangers of whey *do not include*

A. allergies

B. toxic destruction of bacteria in the intestinal tract

C. malabsorption syndrome

D. multiple forms of cancer

69. Soy, in any form, organic or not, is not a health food and contains no intrinsic value.
    A. true
    B. false

70. Baby formula containing soy will give an infant female hormones equivalent to _____ birth control pills a day.
    A. 1–2
    B. 3–5
    C. 4–6
    D. 8–10

71. As of January 2012, how many products (including vitamins and supplements) in this country contain soy?
    A. 10,000
    B. 25,000
    C. 30,000
    D. 34,000

72. 98 percent of the soy and corn produced in this country is genetically altered and should not be part of a healthy diet.
    A. true
    B. false

Chapter 8 – Bits and Pieces

73. What nerves in the human body *are connected* to the body through the spinal cord?
    A. sensory and motor nerves for muscle movement and skin response
    B. the nerves to the kidneys and the heart
    C. the sensory and motor nerves of the face and neck
    D. the nerves of the small intestine and bladder

74. Pressure stimulation applied to either end of the vagus nerve will do what?
    A. speed up the nearest organ

B. slow down the organs it branches directly to

C. speed up all the organs it branches to

D. slow down all the organs it branches to

75. Can the vagus nerve be controlled by mental action or thought?

A. yes

B. no

76. Can the vagus nerve be affected by foods?

A. yes

B. no

77. It is safe to assume you are okay after passing out from vaso-vagal syncope or stimulation of the vagus nerve if

A. you have no injuries and you are not dehydrated

B. you have no cardiac problems

C. your pulse returns to normal (60–70 beats per minute) within 20–30 minutes

D. all of the above

E. A and C only

78. Chemical messages between organs in the body move via the vagus nerve.

A. must go through the brain first

B. are all controlled by brain function

C. stimulate each other directly

D. are produced by food

E. A and B

F. C and D

79. Increasing the stimulus to the vagus nerve with caffeine will increase metabolism?

A. yes

B. no

Chapter 9 - Tissue Regeneration

80. Every cell in the human body is replaced every
    A. 3–5 years
    B. 5–7 years
    C. 7–10 years
    D. 15–20 years

81. Cells in the human body generate from a base layer of cells found in each and every organ called
    A. branch cells
    B. base cells
    C. sickle cells
    D. stem cells

82. New liver cells grow or replicate every _____, while brain cells grow or replicate every _____.
    A. 8 months, 1 month
    B. 10 months, 50 days
    C. 5 months, 4 days
    D. 2 months, 120 days

83. When we look at health improvement, we look at the function of the _____ first.
    A. heart
    B. liver
    C. brain
    D. muscles

84. Regeneration of healthy tissue is different for every person.
    A. true
    B. false

Chapters 10 and 11 – Protein and Fat

85. Peptides, enzymes, and hormones are derived from?
    A. proteins

B. vitamins

C. fats

D. minerals

86. Methionine and cysteine are?

    A. plant- and animal-based proteins

    B. can be synthesized by the human body

    C. are generally sulfur-bonded

    D. must be acquired from food

    E. A, C, and D

    F. B and C

87. In acute starvation or extreme bodybuilding,

    A. the body burns glucose

    B. the body burns fats

    C. the body burns protein

    D. the body burns ketones

88. The minimum daily requirement for protein in women is

    A. 45–55 Grams

    B. 60–70 Grams

    C. 70–80 Grams

89. The minimum daily requirement for protein in men is

    A. 55–60 Grams

    B. 65–70 Grams

    C. 75–80 Grams

90. Healthy proteins are not found in these foods

    A. red and black beans, green peas, walnuts

    B. sunflower seeds, brown rice, almonds

    C. corn, wheat, soybeans

91. Wild-caught is the statement to look for when purchasing fish. What state does not allow commercial-farmed fishing?

    A. Maine

    B. Texas

C. Alaska

D. California

92. Chemically bonded, or genetically altered proteins are not recognized by the body. These proteins are found in

A. corn

B. whey

C. soy

D. all of the above

93. Each meal with 3–4 ounces of healthy meat protein will result in

A. hundreds of protein molecules for chemical formations

B. new digestive enzymes, peptides, and hormones

C. the basic elements of ketosis

D. A and B

E. A and C

F. B and C

94. Excess protein can cause

A. elevated uric acid and hypertension

B. peripheral neuropathy (damage to nerves in hands and feet)

C. renal failure

D. decreased nitric oxide formation with increased platelet formation

E. all of the above

95. Excess protein (glutamine) from unhealthy sources

A. are found in some non-bondable food sources

B. are found in soy, whey, corn, wheat, rye, and processed milk

C. A and B

D. none of the above

96. Inflammatory response in the blood-brain barrier

A. is caused by unhealthy proteins that cross into the brain

B. is caused by unhealthy proteins that cross the gut wall barrier

C. can result in brain damage and brain disease

D. is also seen as leaky gut syndrome

E. all of the above

97. In most cases, modern medicine (doctors) do not associate brain damage or brain disease with any dietary causes

A. true

B. false

98. Loss of both vitamin D and sulfur can be caused by

A. excess fat consumption

B. excess vitamin consumption

C. excess protein consumption

D. excess sugar consumption

99. The number of fat cells your body has and the amount of fat you consume are directly related.

A. true

B. false

100. What is the balance needed for healthy fats in the diet animal to plant fat in teaspoons to tablespoons

A. 2:4

B. 1:7

C. 1:4

D. 1:1

101. Belly fat (the spare tire) comes from

A. consumption of bondable fuels

B. consumption of non-bondable fuels

C. consumption of fats

D. consumption of sugars (fructose), including artificial sugars

E. A and C

F. B and D

102. Omega-3 fatty acids are found in

A. organic butter

B. chicken and eggs

C. fish

D. coconut oil

E. A and D

F. all of the above

103. Healthy monounsaturated and polyunsaturated fatty acids come from

    A. olive oil, avocado, safflower oil

    B. palm oil, corn oil

    C. soy oil, canola oil

    D. all of the above

104. The human body will convert

    A. unsaturated fats to saturated fats LA to ALA

    B. ALA to EPA to DHA

    C. all healthy fats to saturated fats

    D. A and B

    E. all of the above

105. Healthy saturated fats are used by the liver to produce

    A. insulin

    B. triglycerides

    C. thyroid hormones

    D. free fatty acids

    E. all of the above

    F. B and D

    G. A and C

106. Free radicals are

    A. unbound bondable elements floating free in the system

    B. missing electrons in the outer shell to form balance

    C. the cause of oxidation

    D. steal electrons from other elements

    E. all of the above

107. In an element, when the outer shell of electrons is out of balance, as seen in free-floating glucose or glutamine (free floating protein), they become free radicals and
    A. cause cellular bonding
    B. cause cellular damage
    C. bond to other elements
    D. steal electrons from other elements
    E. B and D
    F. A and C

108. Oxidation can become damage to cellular tissue and occurs when bondable elements are allowed to float freely in the circulation without a chemical bond.
    A. true
    B. false

109. The damage caused by diabetes is from
    A. glucose becoming a free radical
    B. oxidation of tissues from glucose
    C. loss of sufficient insulin to bond with glucose
    D. all of the above

110. In the body, elevated serum cholesterol levels occur during
    A. weight gain
    B. illness or injury
    C. lack of exercise
    D. chronic inflammatory response
    E. A and C
    F. B and D

111. Excess healthy fat in the diet
    A. becomes free fatty acids
    B. will make you fat
    C. is disposed of through the kidneys and the lungs
    D. will raise your cholesterol

E. is burned by ketosis
F. will cause brain damage
G. C, B, and D
H. B, F, and A
I. A, C, and E

112. Healthy fat in the diet should
    A. consist of 40–60 percent of the total daily intake
    B. consist of healthy fuels only
    C. be balanced, plant to animal fats
    D. create ketosis
    E. all of the above
    F. A, B, and C

113. The ketotic diet requires strict monitoring and can kill cancer
    A. true
    B. false

114. The protein found in whey, and casein are not
    A. genetically altered
    B. form free-floating glutamine
    C. become free radicals in the body
    D. will cause brain damage
    E. will cause inflammatory response

Chapter 12 – The Overlooked Elements; Water Sleep and Exercise

115. The common, usually unnoticed symptom of dehydration is
    A. sweating
    B. hunger
    C. increased heart rate
    D. shortness of breath

116. Water is
    A. 2 hydrogen molecules and 1 oxygen molecule
    B. H_2O
    C. A and B

117. Lack of water in the body will
    A. create dehydration
    B. decrease oxygen reactions
    C. decrease CoQ-10 function
    D. aggravate and increase any incidence of illness
    E. depress cellular response
    F. all of the above
    G. A and B

118. To maintain proper fluid balance in the body, one should drink
    A. 2/3 their weight in ounces of water daily
    B. 1/3 their weight in ounces of water daily
    C. 1/2 their weight in ounces of water daily
    D. 3/4 their weight in ounces of water daily

119. Dehydration will not increase with
    A. coffee
    B. heavy exercise
    C. alcohol
    D. soda

120. Reverse osmosis removes most heavy metals and toxins from water
    A. true
    B. false

121. The brain moves back and forth through two realms of sleep every 1–2 hours throughout the night
    A. REM and NREM
    B. rapid eye movement and non-rapid eye movement
    C. active electrical rewiring and flushing out dead cells and debris
    D. A and B
    E. all of the above

122. Both REM and NREM sleep are critical for proper brain function.
    A. true
    B. false

123. Sleep deprivation *will not cause*
    A. momentary to lengthy lapses in consciousness
    B. depression that may progress or worsen
    C. loss of cognitive function
    D. weight loss

124. Sleep deprivation (loss of quality as well as quantity) in young adults is not aggravated by
    A. consumption of non-bondable fuels
    B. inappropriate sleep guidelines set in childhood
    C. exercise
    D. excessive light and noise during the evening hours

125. Improved sleep can be enhanced by
    A. prescription sleeping medications
    B. psychiatric or mood-enhancing drugs
    C. exercise and the use of bondable fuels only
    D. minimal night hour stimulus
    E. C and D
    F. A and B

126. Excessive exercise as seen in overtraining can do more damage than good.
    A. true
    B. false

127. Weight loss can result from ketosis
    A. exercise to burn fat as fuel
    B. exercise to burn poly-glucose as fuel
    C. exercise to burn protein as fuel
    D. A and B
    E. B and C

128. Ketosis can be created after fasting (7 PM–7 AM) with exercise
    A. after all poly-glucose has been utilized
    B. after excess poly-glucose is stored in fat
    C. after a meal

D. after a protein load

E. A and B

F. C and D

129. Adenosine triphosphate is

A. metabolism inside the cell for energy

B. the chemical formed outside the cell for energy

C. the waste product of ketosis

D. the chemical extracted from non-bondable fuels

E. burning healthy protein for fuel

130. Burning protein only occurs after all poly-glucose and fats are completely burned and

A. can be accomplished with protein loading

B. is the end result of starvation or extreme exercising

C. is required for bodybuilding

D. B and D

E. A and B

131. Exercise does not have to be overt and aggressive in order to be effective.

A. true

B. false

132. Exercise will not

A. increase endorphins and improve circulation

B. affect leptin and ghrelin signaling

C. increase production of growth hormones and testosterone

D. increase mental clarity and decrease depression

E. decrease fat stores, help fight illness and disease

Chapter 13 – The Missing Elements: Cholesterol

133. The liver combines fatty acids (the lipid droplet) and sulfur-bonded proteins from Acetyl-CoA, to make

A. a lipid droplet coated in proteins

B. healthy cholesterol

C. a bonded fatty acid

D. all of the above

134. Cholesterol produces

   A. longer-lasting cells
   B. stronger cell walls
   C. improved cell wall permeability
   D. stronger cells
   E. A and D
   F. all of the above

135. The dry weight of the brain is _____ cholesterol

   A. 40 percent
   B. 50 percent
   C. 60 percent
   D. 80 percent

136. All scar tissue, both inside and outside the body, is composed of

   A. fats
   B. cholesterol
   C. proteins
   D. white blood cells

137. To date, how many oxysterols have been identified?

   A. 20
   B. 50
   C. 30
   D. 40

138. But only _____ oxysterols are considered to be "lethal."

   A. 7
   B. 5
   C. 3
   D. 6

139. Methionine, cysteine, and sulfotyrosine are all _____ that contain sulfur.
   A. fats
   B. vitamins
   C. enzymes
   D. proteins

140. The production an oxygen and a sulfur ion from sunlight on the skin is the
   A. conversion of nitric oxide or ENOS
   B. conversion of protein to vitamin D
   C. conversion of fat to ENOS
   D. conversion of sodium to ENOS

141. The sulfur-bonded protein wrapped around the lipid will create a strong bond to
   A. cell walls
   B. platelets
   C. other sulfated proteins
   D. connective tissue

142. Damage to cholesterol (oxidation) comes from
   A. trans fats
   B. oxysterols
   C. free radicals
   D. A and B
   E. A and C

143. Active cholesterol sulfate as fully formed cholesterol can travel freely through _____ due to their sulfur content
   A. cell walls
   B. bone
   C. brain tissue
   D. any tissue

144. Active cholesterol sulfate can become the new cell wall for "any cell" throughout the body.
   A. true
   B. false

145. Removing fried foods, margarines, soft spreads, hydrogenated and partially hydrogenated vegetable oils, and powdered eggs from the diet will
   A. prevent trans-fat damage
   B. prevent free radical damage
   C. A and B

146. What are the basic healthy household cooking oils? 1. Peanut oil 2. Olive oil. 3. Palm oil. 4. Coconut oil. 5. Butter
   A. 1, 3, and 5
   B. 2, 4, and 5
   C. 1, 2, and 3
   D. 2, 3, and 5

147. HDL returns to the liver and becomes
   A. new triglycerides
   B. fatty deposits
   C. bile
   D. cofactors
   E. A and C
   F. B and D

148. Poorly formed and unstable cholesterol that can be easily oxidized and come from unhealthy foods like
   A. grains
   B. beans
   C. wheat
   D. fish
   E. soy
   F. peas
   G. peanuts

H. corn
I. B, C, F, and G
J. E, B, H, and F
K. A, E, H, and C

149. Natural body antioxidants are found in vitamins C, E, B6, and CoQ-10. Food sources of these antioxidants are
A. healthy proteins
B. whole vitamins
C. healthy fats
D. fermented vegetables
E. A, B, and D
F. C and D

150. The delicate balance between prostacyclin and thromboxane that maintains blood flow and controls blood clot formation is broken by
A. oxysterols
B. trans fats
C. vitamin C
D. CoQ-10
E. all of the above

151. The main determining factor in reading the NMR lipo profile test is
A. number of LDLs
B. number of triglycerides
C. size of LDL particles
D. number of small LDL particles

152. The need for healthy cholesterol sulfate depends on the foods consumed and
A. the presence of illness
B. the presence of injury
C. the presence of chronic illness
D. the size of the cholesterol produced

E. A and B

F. all of the above

153. Another measurement of cholesterol for healthy function is the ratio of

A. triglycerides to LDLs

B. LDLs to HDLs

C. triglycerides to HDLs

154. The only "bad" cholesterol is an _____ one, and the best cholesterol is a _____ one, 1. poorly formed 2. fluffy. 3. oxidized. 4. sulfated. 5. damaged. 6. phosphorated

A. 1 and 2

B. 2 and 4

C. 3 and 4

D. 5 and 6

Chapter 14 – The Missing Elements: COQ-10

155. CoQ-10 is produced by all cells from

A. fats

B. minerals

C. proteins

D. sugars

156. The production of hydrogen peroxide from CoQ-10 is a by-product of

A. oxidation

B. bonding

C. reduction

D. fusion

157. As an antioxidant, hydrogen peroxide will

A. protect CoQ -10

B. protect the inside of the cell

C. protect the outside of the cell

D. prevent damage from bacteria, viruses, and heavy metals

E. B, C, and D

F. A and D

158. CoQ-10 bonds with and protects
    A. fats
    B. proteins
    C. cell walls

159. The use of statin drugs causes drug-induced CoQ-10 deficiency.
    A. true
    B. false

160. There are no set levels for CoQ-10 in the body.
    A. true
    B. false

Chapter 15 – The Missing Elements: Sulfur

161. Minerals found in areas where volcanic activity has occurred contain high levels of
    A. sodium
    B. potassium
    C. sulfur
    D. chloride
    E. calcium

162. We acquire sulfur in _____ ways?
    A. 2
    B. 3
    C. 5
    D. 4

163. In farming, the use of pesticides and herbicides
    A. damages plant formation
    B. blocks the plants from absorbing sulfur
    C. makes sulfur more available to plants
    D. kills plant roots

164. The one element the body uses in abundance for bonds between elements is
    A. potassium
    B. protein
    C. sulfur
    D. sugars

165. The sulfur-to-sulfur bond is the _____ of all the bonds in the body.
    A. strongest
    B. shortest-lasting
    C. weakest
    D. most erratic

166. Sulfotyrosine is made in
    A. the skin
    B. the brain
    C. the liver
    D. the bones

167. Sulfotyrosine is a major component in
    A. enzyme formation
    B. bone formation
    C. brain hormones
    D. energy formation

168. The master controller of oxygen oriented reactions (hydrogen peroxide) is?
    A. glutathione
    B. glutamine
    C. poly-glucose
    D. sulfur

169. The sulfur-to-sulfur (protein-to-protein) bond between cells is extremely strong, and it can be found in
    A. the lining of the intestinal wall
    B. the surface of the skin

C. the lining of the heart wall

D. the lining of arteries and veins

E. all of the above

F. C and D

170. The sulfur-to-sulfur bond creates a seal between cells that

A. is watertight

B. will prevent passage of bacteria and viruses

C. absorbs platelets from arterial walls

D. will allow open intestinal absorption

E. A and B

F. C and D

171. The presence of sulfur in the body assists and is essential for many functions. Sulfur can be formed in the skin. 1_____ from platelets is released into the 2_____, for deposit in the tissues, and with exposure to UV light this creates 3_____.

A. nitric oxide

B. reticular bed

C. ENOS

D. platelet aggregation

172. The presence of sulfur compounds in the circulating blood maintains

A. sulfation

B. a negative charge on most elements

C. aggregation

D. pH balance

173. Sulfated ions or sulfation is

A. the conversion of other molecules with sulfur

B. the binding of protein to protein

C. the breakdown of sulfur-bonded elements

D. the movement of oxygen through the tissue

174. The lack of sulfur in the body may be a result of cascaded losses due to
    A. clumping
    B. oxidation
    C. stealing
    D. urinary loss

175. Free-floating amino acids known as glutamine can create 1_____ in a structure's barrier and squeeze between the leaky gaps to enter the 2_____ and cause 3_____.
    A. damage
    B. action
    C. brain
    D. bone
    E. neurological damage
    F. free radical function
    G. irritation and swelling

176. Pathogenic bacteria (anaerobic, without oxygen) in the intestinal tract will 1_____ sulfur in foods so it 2_____ be absorbed by the body.
    A. bond
    B. break down
    C. can
    D. cannot

177. An increase in unhealthy source proteins will, 1 _____ absorption of sulfur in the 2_____.
    A. bond
    B. block
    C. intestinal tract
    D. brain

178. The increase of sulfation and the utilization of sulfur in the intestinal tract has a direct relation to
    A. the amount of hydration

B. the number of probiotics

C. the types of fats consumed

D. the presence of anaerobic bacteria

179. Without sulfur, oxygen cannot be carried throughout the body in hemoglobin, and it cannot be carried from hemoglobin to the tissues.

A. true

B. false

180. In fetal development, growth of the fetus depends on nutrients being able to pass the 1_____ or barrier, which keeps the maternal circulation 2 _____ the fetal circulation.

A. maturna reflexa

B. decidua reflexa

C. blood-brain barrier

D. completely separate from

E. connected to

181. The need for sufficient sulfur levels in the body by today's medical standards can only be determined by

A. the presence of healthy cholesterol sulfate levels

B. the presence of illness or disease

C. the measurement of circulating oxygen

D. the presence of increased sulfur or vitamin D in the urine

Chapter 16 - Detoxification

182. There are four ways the body disposes of toxic or waste materials. The organs of the intestinal tract, _____, _____, and _____.

A. the liver, the skin, the kidneys

B. the spleen, the kidneys, the gallbladder

C. the skin, the kidneys, the gallbladder

D. the sweat glands, the kidneys, the liver

183. There are several areas the lymphatic system dumps into for disposal of wastes:
   A. the skin, the kidneys, the gallbladder
   B. the circulation, the tonsils, the sweat glands
   C. the kidneys, the liver, the gallbladder
   D. the spleen, the colon, the tonsils

184. When we lose weight, we force fat cells (via ketosis) to empty, we burn the fat (ketone bodies) as fuel, and we shuttle the toxins to the _____ for neutralization and disposal.
   A. circulation
   B. liver
   C. lymphatic system
   D. kidneys

185. Dead red blood cells, dead white blood cells along with macrophages, dead cancer cells, heavy metals, and toxic chemicals all enter the lymphatic system. The main component that keeps this system functioning is
   A. minerals
   B. macrophages
   C. water
   D. fats

186. The solid waste (dead cells) is disposed via
   A. the kidneys
   B. the skin
   C. the gallbladder
   D. the colon

187. Detox should not be attempted until the _____ is functioning at a normal level.
   A. liver
   B. kidneys
   C. skin
   D. intestinal tract

188. _____ is a major contributor to abnormal intestinal function.
   A. Use of laxatives
   B. Constipation
   C. Inflammatory response
   D. Decreased biologics

189. What is not a form of skin detox?
   A. hypothermia
   B. baking soda baths
   C. Epsom salt baths
   D. hyperthermia

190. Aggressive weight loss (30 pounds or more) requires more intense forms of detox. A safe and effective form involves
   A. liver cleansing
   B. gallbladder stimulation
   C. kidney flushes
   D. colon cleansing

191. The toxic solid waste disposal plant in the human body is
   A. the skin
   B. the liver
   C. the kidneys
   D. the gallbladder

192. High levels of calcium, cadmium, aluminum, and mercury can be removed from the body via
   A. hyperthermia
   B. colon cleansing
   C. chelation therapy
   D. gallbladder stimulation

193. _____treatments have been found to be extremely effective in removing toxins, treating trauma and even stroke patients. But

this kind of therapy in the United States is expensive and difficult to obtain.

A. Hyperthermia therapy
B. Hydrotherapy
C. Hypothermia therapy
D. Hyperbaric therapy

194. Most over-the-counter herbal mixes that do not contain laxatives are safe for gentle cleansing of the colon. But _____should not be attempted without the presence of a trained professional, certified in the field.

A. coffee enemas
B. mechanical colon cleansing
C. herbal therapy
D. hyperthermia

195. Starvation or fasting for extended periods of time will result in low blood sugar levels. The fasting blood sugar level must be kept above 1_____ as a blood sugar below 2_____ can result in coma and death.

A. 70
B. 50
C. 60
D. 40
E. 30

Chapter 17 - Minerals

196. The body's minerals are divided into two groups, 1 _____ which is needed in 2_____, and 3_____which is needed in 4_____.

A. macro
B. in small amounts (micrograms)
C. in small amounts (milligrams)
D. substantial amounts (milligrams)

E. trace

F. in substantial amounts (micrograms)

197. What percent of calcium becomes a part of bone structure?
A. 50
B. 87
C. 98
D. 75

198. Exocytosis is?
A. increased hormone formation
B. increased irritability of nerves
C. increased electrical activity in nerves and muscles
D. increased mineral formations

199. The _____ gland controls or regulates the calcium level in the blood.
A. parathyroid
B. thyroid
C. adrenal
D. pituitary

200. The parathyroid gland 1_____ via the kidneys, and 2_____ via the intestinal tract.
A. increases calcium loss
B. stimulates increased absorption of calcium
C. decreases absorption of calcium
D. prevents calcium loss

201. Overconsumption of calcium in the diet can
A. increase parathyroid function
B. create an imbalance with multiple minerals
C. increase kidney function
D. improve bone

202. Supplementation with calcium as a whole natural food should not exceed _____ milligrams per day.
   A. 2,000
   B. 1,500
   C. 1,000
   D. 500

203. Calcium and phosphorous will bind together in the body to form?
   A. adenosine triphosphate (ATP)
   B. the matrix for bone formation
   C. glutathione
   D. CoQ-10

204. Every cell produces phosphorous from
   A. electrical activity
   B. ATP (energy production)
   C. coenzymes
   D. cholesterol sulfate

205. Phosphorous is found in foods that contain protein—but not bonded to protein.
   A. true
   B. false

206. Phosphorous is bonded to fats and is released from its bond during fat metabolism or ATP.
   A. true
   B. false

207. How should you gauge phosphorous intake?
   A. If you are eating enough veggies, you are getting enough phosphorous.
   B. If you are eating enough fat, you are getting enough phosphorous.
   C. If you are eating enough protein, you are getting enough phosphorous.
   D. If you are eating enough bondable fuels, you are getting enough phosphorous.

208. Potassium is the third most abundant mineral in the body. It plays a direct role in
    A. nerve stimulation
    B. muscle contraction
    C. nerve transmission
    D. muscle relaxation
    E. C and D
    F. A and B

209. Too much potassium (elevated potassium levels) can result from
    A. overuse of supplementation
    B. renal failure, tissue trauma, and burns
    C. use of diuretics and vomiting
    D. A and B
    E. A and C

210. Too much potassium is known as hyperkalemia. Too little potassium is known as _____.
    A. hyponatremia
    B. hypokalemia
    C. hypovolemia
    D. hypothermia

211. Too little or low potassium levels can come from
    A. overuse of diuretics, licorice and coffee
    B. use of potassium sparing diuretics
    C. prolonged vomiting and diarrhea
    D. A and C
    E. B and D

212. Supplementation with sulfur in the form of MSM, biotin, or organic sulfur should be guided by
    A. blood levels
    B. the presence of illness or disease
    C. urinary sulfur loss (levels in urine)

213. Healthy food sources of sulfur include
    A. organic eggs
    B. organic meats and poultry
    C. wild caught fish and seafood
    D. unprocessed milk and some legumes
    E. A and B
    F. all of the above

214. We are very salty people—sodium comprises 0.2 percent of the total body sodium. What is table salt comprised of?
    A. sodium and chloride
    B. sodium and potassium
    C. sodium, potassium, and chloride

215. Table salt
    A. can be found in almost all processed foods
    B. will not create balance to our body chemistry
    C. is not recommended in any diet
    D. A and C
    E. all of the above

216. Unprocessed sea salt crystals contain a combination of major and trace elements, in equal balance to the human body. Use liberally.
    A. true
    B. false

217. Magnesium is found in foods containing high levels of chlorophyll, unfiltered hard water,
    A. meat, and poultry
    B. chocolate, and green, leafy vegetables
    C. seafood, artichokes
    D. A and C
    E. B and C

218. Magnesium is attracted to _____, and they will deplete each other when either is in excess.
    A. sodium

B. phosphorous

C. calcium

D. potassium

219. Magnesium is readily balanced by kidney filtration, and it is difficult to develop a magnesium excess.

A. true

B. false

220. Loss of magnesium in the tissues causes

A. muscle cramps and migraine headaches

B. numbness and muscle twitching

C. nerve tingling and muscle spasms

D. A and B

E. all of the above

221. Excess calcium and the presence of calcium in tissues throughout the body is an indication of magnesium deficiency.

A. true

B. false

222. Iron is a necessary micronutrient for the

A. transport of sulfur in the blood

B. transport of red blood cells

C. transport of oxygen in red blood cells

223. The mineral content of our foods determines

A. the vitamin content

B. the absorption rate

C. the function of biologics

Chapter 18 - Vitamins

224. The average adult intake of organic vegetables (servings, ½ cup) to meet the present RDA in the United States daily is

A. 4–6

B. 5–7

C. 8–10

D. 2–4

225. Vitamins can be absorbed and utilized without the presence of balanced minerals.
   A. true
   B. false

226. Besides balanced minerals, what else is necessary for absorption and utilization of vitamins?
   A. increased fluid intake
   B. healthy function of the digestive tract
   C. the presence of vitamin cofactors
   D. A and C
   E. all of the above

227. The best forms of vitamins are found in whole food source or whole vitamins derived from
   A. fermented foods
   B. whole organic foods
   C. chemically extracted foods
   D. A and B
   E. A and C

228. Esterification is
   A. the removal of oxygen from a compound or element
   B. the combining of an alcohol and an acid to yield water and an ester
   C. a form of fat-soluble preservation
   D. all of the above

229. To create ketosis, we must move the ketone bodies from the tissues into the cell. This is facilitated by a carrier seen in
   A. vitamin A
   B. vitamin C
   C. vitamin B
   D. protein

230. This element is regulated by the kidneys, increases CoQ-10 action, acts as an antioxidant protecting RNA and DNA and can be utilized directly by bone and muscle tissue:
    A. protein
    B. oxygen
    C. vitamin C
    D. vitamin D

231. Swelling in a wound (inflammatory response)
    A. increases histamine formation
    B. isolates a wound
    C. signals white blood cells and platelets for detoxification and stabilization
    D. all of the above

232. Continued inflammatory response over time signals
    A. specialized white blood cells to the wound area
    B. the release of cholesterol sulfate from the reticular bed
    C. the increase of platelets to the area
    D. A and B
    E. A and C

233. Macrophages are
    A. specialized white blood cells
    B. our trash compactors
    C. cells that consume or eat dead cellular material
    D. B and C
    E. all of the above

234. Cytokines and interferon are enzymes that signal
    A. T cells
    B. B cells
    C. red blood cells
    D. ROS
    E. specialized white blood cells

F. A, B, D, and E

G. all of the above

235. ROS (reactive oxygen species) is seen as
    A. oxidation of toxins and foreign material (bacteria and viruses)
    B. enzymes that are activated by vitamin C
    C. hydrogen peroxide
    D. all of the above

236. What cell produces antibodies?
    A. T cells
    B. B cells
    C. killer cells
    D. ROS
    E. A and D
    F. B and C

237. Antibodies are cells that contain
    A. coded copies of foreign DNA
    B. coded copies of the bodies DNA
    C. pieces of the antigen
    D. oxygen

238. T cells destroy foreign material by?
    A. consuming them
    B. targeting their DNA
    C. attaching to the antigen for destruction
    D. oxidizing the antigen

239. Killer cells
    A. carry a carbon code of the body's DNA
    B. consumes foreign material
    C. can distinguish between self (the body's DNA) and foreign DNA
    D. B and C
    E. A, B, and C

240. Specialized white blood cells are formed in
    A. the marrow of long bones
    B. the reticular bed
    C. the spleen
    D. A and B
    E. A, B, and C

241. High-dose therapy with vitamin C has been used as an adjunct to cancer therapy by alternative medicine with noted success.
    A. true
    B. false

242. Studies have found that disease prevention with the use of vitamin C begins at _____ and ranges upward.
    A. 200 milligrams daily
    B. 400 milligrams daily
    C. 800 milligrams daily
    D. 1,000 milligrams daily

243. All B vitamins are
    A. fat-soluble
    B. water-soluble
    C. bonded to sulfur
    D. interactive with each other
    E. B and D
    F. A and C

244. When you think B vitamins, think
    A. liver
    B. muscles
    C. brain
    D. bones

245. B vitamins work together, this cooperative and interdependent effort is best seen in
    A. fetal neuro tube development .
    B. bone formation

C. steroid hormone and neurotransmitter formation

D. muscle strength

E. A and C

F. B and D

246. Throughout the rest of the body, this interdependent relationship of B vitamins is directly connected to

A. prevention of liver damage from toxins

B. formation of strength of DNA and RNA

C. formation and strength of red and white blood cells

D. increased strength and function of the immune system

E. A and C

F. all of the above

247. Vitamin B1 (thiamine) is necessary for

A. detox of the liver

B. breakdown of fatty acids for brain hormone formation

C. formation of red blood cells

D. neuromuscular function

248. Vitamin B2 or riboflavin is necessary as a cofactor for the absorption of

A. B6

B. folate

C. niacin

D. iron

E. none of the above

F. all of the above

249. Vitamin B2 or riboflavin has been found to have a direct relation to

A. lowering preeclampsia and eclampsia (uncontrolled hypertension) in pregnancy

B. reduction of cataract formation in the eyes

C. reduction of migraine headaches

D. activation of folate in the body

E. A and C

F. all of the above

250. Classified as an antioxidant, riboflavin is necessary for the formation of
    A. CoQ-10
    B. glutathione
    C. glutamine
    D. ENOS

251. The coenzyme formed by niacin is necessary for the transfer of electrons during oxidation and requires _____ to become active.
    A. B1 and B2
    B. B6, B2, and iron
    C. pantothenic acid
    D. biotin

252. Niacin is derived from the breakdown of tryptophan, found in meat, which yields the hormone _____.
    A. epinephrine
    B. thyroid
    C. melatonin
    D. testosterone

253. Niacin and its derivatives (nicotinamide) are related to nicotine found in tobacco.
    A. true
    B. false

254. Vitamin B5 or pantothenic acid is essential for the formation of _____ within the cell.
    A. steroid hormones
    B. coenzyme-A
    C. ENOS
    D. energy from fats and sugars
    E. A and C
    F. A, B, and D

255. Pantothenic acid is necessary for the formation of _____ and _____.
    A. endorphins (neurotransmitters), melatonin (sleep hormone)
    B. acetylcholine (neurotransmitter), melatonin (sleep hormone)
    C. steroid hormones, thyroid hormones
256. Pantothenic acid is also necessary for
    A. the formation of lipids in the liver for cholesterol
    B. the formation of digestive enzymes
    C. the synthesis of hemoglobin from iron
    D. the formation of white blood cells
    E. A and C
    F. B and D

257. Vitamin B6 or pyridoxine can be synthesized by the human body.
    A. true
    B. false

258. Pyridoxine is classified as a coenzyme, found in protein foods, that play a direct role in
    A. 100 different chemical reactions inside and outside of the cell
    B. production of neurotransmitters
    C. formation of heme from iron for hemoglobin
    D. all of the above

259. Dosage of vitamin B6 can be directly-correlated to 1_____intake, making 2_____the basis for adequate intake.
    A. fat
    B. protein
    C. minimum protein intake
    D. minimum fat intake

260. Vitamin B7 or biotin is
    A. bonded to a protein with a sulfur bond
    B. bonded to sugars with a sulfur bond
    C. bonded to fats with a sulfur bond
    D. a vitamin bonded to sulfur

261. What is biotin necessary for?
    A. the synthesis of fatty acids
    B. the breakdown of proteins
    C. the turning of ketone bodies back to glucose in the cell
    D. ketosis
    E. A and B
    F. A, C, and D

262. The highest source of biotin is found in 1_____ or minimally cooked 2_____.
    A. raw milk
    B. raw egg yolk
    C. salmon
    D. whole eggs

263. 1. The requirement for biotin increases during pregnancy.
    A. true
    B. false

    2. Biotin deficiency during pregnancy goes largely unrecognized.
    A. true
    B. false

264. Biotin is
    A. produced from proteins by intestinal bacteria
    B. is extracted from fats within the cell
    C. is extracted from proteins within the liver
    D. is absorbed still containing its sulfur bond
    E. A and D
    F. B and C

265. Deficiency in biotin can be seen in
    A. hair loss and scaly, red rash around eyes, nose, mouth, and genital area
    B. numbness and tingling in extremities
    C. depression, lethargy, and hallucinations
    D. all of the above

266. Deficiency in biotin can be connected to deficiency in healthy bacterial count in the intestinal tract.
    A. true
    B. false

267. Most synthetic forms of folate are referred to as folic acid. The true chemical name of this vitamin is folate or folates.
    A. true
    B. false

268. The main source of folate is from
    A. green, leafy vegetables
    B. fruit
    C. root vegetables
    D. beans and legumes
    E. A and D
    F. B and C

269. Folate is necessary for?
    A. breakdown and bonding of methionine to sulfur (SAM)
    B. proper DNA replication inside the cell
    C. formation of healthy red blood cells in bone marrow
    D. formation of neuro tube structures in pregnancy
    E. prevention of premature birth in pregnancy
    F. B and D
    G. all of the above

270. SAM (S-Adenosylmethionine) is a sulfur-bonded protein that
    A. is a product of breakdown and bonding of methionine
    B. produces neurotransmitters, epinephrine, and norepinephrine
    C. requires only folate to produce
    D. A and B
    E. A and C

271. Homocysteine is
    A. a by-product of ATP production
    B. can be recycled back to methionine

C. requires only folate to be converted back

D. A and B

E. A and C

272. Blood levels of homocysteine are used to measure

A. inflammatory response or immune function

B. renal function

C. steroid hormone function

D. liver function

273. Oxidative stress is the result of

A. uncontrolled homocysteine acting as a free radical

B. a result of B12, B6, and folate deficiencies

C. a result of any or all B12, B6, or folate deficiencies

D. A and C

E. A and B

274. B vitamins are a form of master controller of

A. homocysteine levels

B. renal function

C. bone function

D. oxidative stress

E. A and D

F. B and C

275. Folate is directly connected to healthy red blood cell production in bone marrow. A deficiency in folate is seen as

A. small, malformed red blood cells

B. enlarged, abnormal red blood cells

C. deficiency in number of red blood cells

D. loss of oxygen carrying capacity of red blood cells

E. A and C

F. B and D

276. Megaloblastic anemia

A. causes breakdown in the kidneys

B. stems from enlarged, abnormal red blood cells

C. is the same anemia caused by B12 malabsorption

D. B and C

E. A and C

277. B12 and folate have an interlinked relationship, one cannot work without the other.

A. true

B. false

278. Vitamin B12 is the _____ structure chemically of all the vitamins.

A. smallest

B. largest

C. most active

D. least active

279. The essential cofactor found in B12 is _____.

A. iron

B. cobalt

C. cesium

D. sulfur

280. Along with B12, this cofactor must be present to produce methionine from homocysteine.

A. folate

B. B1

C. B6

D. B7

281. The human body is capable of synthesizing vitamin B12, it is also present in _____.

A. vegetables

B. fruits

C. nuts and legumes

D. animal sources

282. Vitamin B12
    A. is a heat-sensitive vitamin
    B. is a cold-sensitive vitamin
    C. is necessary for fat metabolism (energy from fat)
    D. is necessary for glucose metabolism
    E. A and C
    F. B and D

283. The end result of protein breakdown and metabolism with B12 is
    the formation of
    A. muscle tissue
    B. myelin sheaths
    C. neurotransmitters
    D. liver enzymes
    E. A and D
    F. B and C

284. Vegetarian and vegan diets lack _____ for adequate B12
    absorption.
    A. fats
    B. healthy animal protein
    C. sufficient minerals
    D. vegetable protein

285. B12 deficiency can be seen as
    A. iron deficiency anemia
    B. tingling in arms and legs
    C. elevated homocysteine levels
    D. memory loss, dementia
    E. A and C
    F. all of the above

286. We cannot form myelin sheaths without vitamin B12. Diseases
    involved in this area of damage include
    A. Alzheimer's disease
    B. autism

C. depression and cognitive disorders

D. birth defects

E. all of the above

F. A and C

287. When we think of B vitamins we must think of the

A. liver

B. bone

C. brain

D. heart

288. Vitamin A is a _____-soluble vitamin.

A. fat

B. water

289. Significant precursors to vitamin A are found in

A. carotenoids

B. fats

C. yellow, orange, and green vegetables

D. pre-vitamin A

E. A and C

F. B and D

290. The difference between pro-vitamin A and pre-vitamin A is significant, as all pre-vitamin A compounds

A. are synthetic

B. cause birth defects

C. have been found to be toxic

D. block the absorption and function of vitamin D in the body

E. A and C

F. all of the above

291. Retinol is

A. the base compound necessary for vision

B. the compound needed for vitamin A breakdown

C. will combine with opsin to form visual purple

D. A and C

E. all of the above

292. Retinol is stored in the surface layers inside the eye. It is activated and binds with opsin when stimulated by repeated exposure to _____.

   A. heat

   B. light

   C. cold

   D. pressure

293. Vitamin A is also known to affect 1_____ formation and 2_____ production.

   A. DNA and RNA

   B. neurotransmitters

   C. growth hormones

   D. steroid hormones

294. The most important factor in the use of vitamin A as pro-vitamin A is in

   A. liver health

   B. brain health

   C. fetal development

   D. skin health

295. Pro-vitamin A is essential for the development of 1_____ from 2_____in the fetus.

   A. white blood cells

   B. red blood cells

   C. reticular bed

   D. stem cells

296. Pro-vitamin A is essential for the formation of 1_____ from 2_____ in adults as well as the fetus.

   A. hemoglobin

   B. cholesterol sulfate

C. reticular bed

D. iron

297. Impaired dark adaptation is known as

    A. astigmatism

    B. night blindness

    C. glaucoma

    D. cataracts

298. Severe vitamin A deficiency over a prolonged period of time can result in

    A. glaucoma

    B. cataracts

    C. dry eye

    D. stigmatism

299. Progressive changes seen in vitamin A deficiency can result in

    A. corneal scars

    B. glaucoma

    C. eventual blindness

    D. corneal ulcers

    E. A, C, and D

    F. all of the above

300. Provitamin A deficiency (carotenoid deficiency) during pregnancy can result in

    A. bone disturbances

    B. birth defects

    C. kidney failure

    D. liver disease

301. Iron deficiency, anemia, and frequent, prolonged infections are an indication of

    A. liver disease

    B. vitamin a deficiency

    C. iron and zinc deficiency

    D. kidney failure

E. B and C

F. A and D

302. The only recommended form of vitamin A supplementation is
    A. Pre-vitamin A
    B. Pro-vitamin A
    C. beta-carotene
    D. retinol acetate or palmate
    E. A and D
    F. B and C

303. The breakdown and absorption of vitamin D can only occur with
    A. Pro-vitamin A
    B. Pre-vitamin A
    C. beta-carotene
    D. retinol acetate or palmate
    E. A and C
    F. B and D

304. Vitamin D affects
    A. bones
    B. cell structure
    C. immune function
    D. all of the above

305. Vitamin D has been found in white blood cells, and at acceptable levels, it can
    A. prevent multiple forms of cancer
    B. improve muscle function
    C. improve neurological function
    D. improve bone structure
    E. all of the above
    F. A and D

306. 1_____ is the term used for vitamin D deficiency. In adults, it is called 2_____.
    A. osteoporosis

B. osteomalacia

C. rickets

D. osteoarthritis

307. Rickets is described as a lack of phosphorous. Vitamin D
    A. influences the calcium to phosphorous ratio (2:1)
    B. increases the absorption of the matrix into bone
    C. increases re-absorption into the bone
    D. A and B
    E. all of the above

308. Newborn pediatric rickets is rare in the United States.
    A. true
    B. false

309. Adult rickets (osteomalacia or soft bone) is rare in the United
    States.
    A. true
    B. false

310. Which form of vitamin D has the positive effects on bone, muscle
    and brain health?
    A. Dehydroxy vitamin D (1, 25(OH)2D)
    B. Hydroxy vitamin D (25 (OH) D)

311. The 1_____ gland controls the tight loop that can increase the
    2_____ levels.
    A. thyroid
    B. parathyroid
    C. blood calcium
    D. bone calcium

312. 1_____ will pull calcium and phosphorous from bone. 2
    _____ will force calcium and phosphorous back into bone.
    A. Dehydroxy vitamin D
    B. Hydroxyl vitamin D

313. This absorption and re-absorption pattern or pathway cannot occur without
    A. healthy liver function
    B. healthy kidney function
    C. healthy parathyroid gland
    D. all of the above

314. The parathyroid gland is stimulated by low levels of 1_____ in the blood. It then causes increased production of 2_____ in the kidneys, which increases the calcium and phosphorous absorption from 3 _____ and pulls calcium and phosphorous from bone, increasing the 4 _____ levels.
    A. Hydroxy vitamin D
    B. Dehydroxy vitamin D
    C. calcium
    D. intestinal tract
    E. blood calcium

315. Healthy vitamin D blood levels start at
    A. 40 ng/ml
    B. 50 ng/ml
    C. 60 ng/ml
    D. 70 ng/ml

316. The high levels of 1_____ in the body will offset the destructive effects of _____.
    A. Hydroxy vitamin D
    B. liver enzymes
    C. dehydroxy vitamin D
    D. uric acid

317. Excess dehydroxy vitamin D is seen in
    A. Liver failure
    B. Parathyroid disease
    C. Excessive use of calcium carbonate preparations
    D. Renal disease

E. A and C

F. All of the above

318. Since the average vitamin D level of the adult female in the United States is 18 to 20 nanograms per milliliter or (severe deficiency), then we can say that
A. most infants are born with rickets
B. infants are not affected by the mother's level
C. vitamin D at adequate levels are necessary to prevent infantile rickets.
D. A and C
E. B and C

319. The only known symptom of rickets in children is
A. fever
B. skin rash
C. head sweating
D. muscle twitching

320. Adult rickets (osteomalacia) appears to be associated in severe cases of
A. gastric reflux
B. migraine headaches
C. muscle weakness
D. abdominal pains

321. Vitamin D levels should be tested
A. once a year
B. at birth and every three months until a healthy level is achieved
C. every two years
D. every two to three years after healthy levels have been established
E. A and C
F. B and D

322. During pregnancy, vitamin D levels should be followed, and pregnant or not, all women
    A. should avoid any calcium carbonate preparations
    B. should avoid bottle feeding if at all possible
    C. know and adjust their own vitamin D levels
    D. all of the above

323. Two ingredients found in infant formula that should be completely avoided since they block absorption of vitamin D and many minerals in an infant's intestinal tract are
    A. sugars
    B. palm olein
    C. soy
    D. whey
    E. A and D
    F. B and C

324. To calculate the body's average (maintenance dose) needed dose of vitamin D3 for oral supplementation (for any age),
    A. multiply 35 IU times the body weight in pounds
    B. multiply 25 IU times the body weight in pounds
    C. multiply 42 IU times the body weight in pounds
    D. multiply 32 IU times the body weight in pounds

325. Like the B vitamins, these vitamins also work together in a symbiotic relationship
    A. vitamin D
    B. beta carotene
    C. vitamin C
    D. vitamin K
    E. all of the above
    F. A and D

326. People deficient in vitamin D who have rickets (osteomalacia) tend to have elevated levels of clot formation (vitamin K deficiency). This explains
   A. traumatic injuries at birth
   B. ruptured arteries and bleeding in the brains of infants
   C. unexplained bruising or bleeding under the skin
   D. A and B
   E. All of the above

327. Vitamin K2 is necessary for
   A. maintenance of stable matrix formation in bone
   B. breakdown of bone during remodeling
   C. clotting of blood
   D. prevention of clots in blood

328. Vitamin K2 is recommended for supplementation in those people with osteomalacia or osteoporosis and is a good reason to ferment your own vegetables.
   A. true
   B. false

329. Sterols are
   A. healthy plant fats
   B. healthy animal fats
   C. elements that support the immune system, increasing disease resistance
   D. found in vitamin D2
   E. B and C
   F. A, C, and D

330. Sterols are found in
   A. all vegetables
   B. some fruit
   C. all seeds, nuts, and beans
   D. kelp and other seaweeds

E. all of the above

F. A and C

331. Sterols are highly sensitive to
    A. heat
    B. mechanical grinding
    C. cold (freezing)
    D. chemical processing
    E. A, C, and D
    F. all of the above

332. Sterols enhance
    A. vitamin D absorption and utilization
    B. all B vitamin absorption and utilization
    C. the production of DHEA and reduced stress
    D. all of the above
    E. A and B

333. Increased production of DHEA will
    A. enhance estrogen production
    B. enhance progesterone production
    C. enhance testosterone production
    D. drive down cortisol levels for stress balance
    E. A and D
    F. all of the above

334. To date, _____ different sterols have been identified.
    A. 100
    B. 250
    C. 300
    D. 500

335. Each individual sterol performs a different action, including hormone and vitamin precursors, increased cell membrane

strength, synthesis of progesterone and vitamin D, and formation of anti-inflammatory compounds.
   A. true
   B. false

336. What do the Paleo diet, the Mediterranean diet, and vegan and vegetarian diets have in common that benefits the use of sterols?
   A. consumption of vegetables
   B. consumption of fats
   C. high consumption of raw vegetables
   D. low consumption of fats

337. What is missing in vegan or vegetarian diets?
   A. healthy animal protein
   B. a balance of plant-to-animal source fats
   C. a balance of plant-to-animal source proteins
   D. B and C
   E. all of the above

338. Crude fat oils—otherwise known as vegetable oils (canola or rapeseed, cottonseed, and corn)
   A. are genetically altered foods
   B. are refined vegetable oils with destroyed sterols
   C. contain synthetic agents and chemicals
   D. are not recognized by the body as useable
   E. are hydrogenated and become trans fats when heated
   F. all of the above

339. Sterols (plant fats) have no antioxidant properties.
   A. true
   B. false

340. Grains and wheat contain sterols
   A. which, once processed, are replaced with synthetic vitamins
   B. which are destroyed in processing
   C. which enhance iron absorption
   D. which controls DHEA reduction

E.   A and B

F.   C and D

341. The minimum amount of plant-based foods needed for a healthy diet should consist of
  A. 20 percent raw and 20 percent lightly cooked
  B. 50 percent raw and 20 percent lightly cooked
  C. 60 percent raw and 20 percent lightly cooked
  D. 40 percent raw and 20 percent lightly cooked

342. The total plant-to-animal source-based food balance should be approximately
  A. 50 percent plant source, 50 percent animal source
  B. 80 percent plant source, 20 percent animal source
  C. 60 percent plant source, 40 percent animal source
  D. 70 percent plant source, 30 percent animal source

343. Primary animal source omega-3 fatty acids are found in
  A. beef
  B. eggs and poultry
  C. fish
  D. pork

344. When it comes to supplementation, omega-3 fatty acids should be measured by _____ content.
  A. EPA
  B. DHA
  C. ALA
  D. LA

345. In supplements, the balance of EPA to DHA should be 1_____EPA to 2_____ DHA.
  A. 40 percent
  B. 50 percent
  C. 20 percent
  D. 10 percent

346. It has been recommended that every diet (with or without supplementation) should contain
    A. 12 ounces of fish per week
    B. 6 ounces of fish per week
    C. 1 serving of fish per week
    D. 3 servings of fish per week

347. The requirement for plant-to-animal source-fats should remain
    A. 2:1 tablespoons to teaspoons
    B. 1:1 tablespoons to teaspoons
    C. 4:1 tablespoons to teaspoons
    D. 3:1 tablespoons to teaspoons

348. Carbohydrate is
    A. a term not used in this book
    B. an overused term to describe sugars, non-bondable and nonessential nutrients in foods that are simply not healthy
    C. a necessary part of a healthy diet
    D. a term used to describe a wide variety of foods that contribute to healthy body function
    E. A and B
    F. C and D

349. Fructose is
    A. a natural sugar found in fruit
    B. an artificial sugar
    C. classified as a non-bondable
    D. A and C
    E. B and C

Chapter 19 – GMO's The Nightmare Come True

350. Recombinant DNA technology is
    A. the combining of genes from different organisms
    B. the combining of genes from the same organisms
    C. the reduction of genes in an organism
    D. the splicing of genes within a species

351. Genetically modified, genetically engineered, and transgenic organisms are found in
A. medicines
B. vaccines
C. food
D. food ingredients
E. feeds
F. fibers
G. A, C, and D
H. all of the above

352. By genetic manipulation, the biotech industry has literally changed the structure of foods genetically.
A. true
B. false

353. Foods that are genetically modified or GM include
A. corn, soy, and sugar beets
B. sweet corn, rice, and canola
C. tomatoes, potatoes, and squash
D. papaya and cotton oil
E. A and B
F. All of the above

354. The introduction of a gene pesticide or herbicide into plant genes will create a living pesticide or herbicide. This process is reversible.
A. true
B. false

355. Today there is independent testing required by the USDA and FDA to prove safety of these crops.
A. true
B. false

356. The initial failure of these GM crops prompted
A. new research
B. the USDA's attention

C. an increase in the number of gene traits used

D. the use of bacteria, viruses, and even human genes in plants

E. A and B

F. C and D

357. The United States does not require any toxicological studies to determine the adverse effects or safety of GM crops.

A. true

B. false

358. The 'comparative study' is the only requirement for safety of GM foods. This compares

A. the GM crop structure to non-GM crop structure

B. the GM crop chemistry and feeding response to non-GM chemistry and feeding response

C. the GM crop effect on the environment to the non-GM crop effect on that same environment

359. The comparison testing is done by the GM industry and is

A. checked or overseen by the USDA and FDA

B. not overseen by any organization

C. proprietary (owned by the company) and not revealed to any sources

D. accepted by the USDA and FDA with a declaration of safe

E. B, C, and D

F. All of the above

360. If it looks like a duck, then it will quack the same; therefore it is safe. And no further testing is necessary.

A. This is the only form of testing in the United States.

B. This has nothing to do with science or safety.

C. This is tinkering with genetics without any knowledge of what it could produce.

D. This is perfectly safe for human health

E. A, B, and C

F. all of the above

361. Today, the United States requires toxicological studies on genetically altered crops.
    A. true
    B. false

362. Europe requires ninety-day studies by the GM industry on single-trait crops only.
    A. true
    B. false

363. Horizontal gene transfer involves
    A. the transfer of genes into the digestive tract
    B. the transfer of DNA from GM plants into the DNA of human gut bacteria
    C. the creation of a living pesticide in human intestines
    D. the development of antibiotic-resistant mega bacteria (super bugs) in the human intestinal tract.
    E. B, C, and D
    F. All of the above

364. The Shroder independent study on GM rice found
    A. toxic or disruptive bacteria in the digestive tracts
    B. the GM rice did not pass the comparative study test
    C. overall "possible toxicological findings"
    D. A and B
    E. all of the above

365. The Kroghslo study of 2008 found inhaled particles from the powdered Bt toxin in the feed to create allergic reactions.
    A. true
    B. false

366. The Austria 2008 rat feeding study found
    A. GM corn caused small liters with a high death rate
    B. GM corn caused no unexpected deaths from cancer
    C. the death rate in the GM fed rats was twice the rate of the control or non-GM fed group

D. GM corn and soy mixed caused a mortality rate of 55.3 percent in infant rats
E. all of the above
F. A, C, and D

367. The Russia 2010 study on GM soy roundup ready, increased infant mortality rates, increased birth defects, and third-generation sterility.
    A. true
    B. false

368. In the Russian study, Dr. Surov called the test results
    A. "lost forever"
    B. "reproductive disasters"

369. In GM crops, the Bt toxin is
    A. designed to tolerate large amounts of herbicide and pesticide spray
    B. bacillus thuringiensis
    C. found in corn and soy roundup ready
    D. all of the above

370. In Quebec in 2011, the discovery of significant levels of insecticidal protein, Cry 1Ab, present in Bt crops, in the blood of sixty-nine women, both pregnant and non-pregnant, and their fetuses.
    A. true
    B. false

371. GMOs (genetically modified organisms) are in our food today and have been there for the past seventeen years. This is not a contributing factor to the rise of metabolic syndrome or syndrome X in the United States.
    A. true
    B. false

372. Is it possible that, in eighty years, the uncontrolled use of GMOs or GM products in our foods could be the cause of our own demise?
   A. yes
   B. no

373. Rapeseed, when first developed, was toxic. A second stack of genes was added to form double-zero rapeseed, which
   A. was then found edible
   B. was renamed canola
   C. was originally used only as animal feed
   D. was produced into cooking oils
   E. A, B, and D
   F. all of the above

374. The use of GM crops in Canada to feed honeybees to make honey has resulted in a ban of all Canadian honey to Europe.
   A. true
   B. false

375. GM soy is
   A. found in 40,000 products across the US
   B. found in nutritional supplements
   C. found in infant formulas
   D. all of the above

376. GM corn and sweet corn in the United States comprises 98 percent of all produced corn.
   A. true
   B. false

377. Quest cigarettes, are produced from GMO tobacco.
   A. true
   B. false

378. Almost all vegetable oils and margarines made in the United States are made from
   A. soy

B. corn

C. canola

D. cottonseed

E. A and B

F. all of the above

379. Unless the oil is marked non-GMO or certified organic, it is genetically modified.

A. true

B. false

380. Unless the supplement label reads certified organic or non-GMO, then

A. vitamin C comes from GM corn

B. vitamin E comes from soy

C. vitamin A, B2, B6, and B12 are derived from GMOs

D. vitamin D and K are derived from carriers of GM sources

E. all of the above

F. B and C

381. The recommendation from this book is to

A. eat only certified organic foods (look for the USDA-certified organic label)

B. put corn in your gas tank—not in your mouth

C. avoid all products containing corn, soy, canola, cottonseed, and sugar beets

D. all of the above

Chapter 20 – A Question of Personal Choice

382. Who actually set the normal cholesterol blood levels in the US?

A. FDA

B. USDA

C. pharmaceutical industry

D. American Heart Association

383. Our brain is by dry weight
    A. 50 - 60 percent cholesterol
    B. 20 - 30 percent cholesterol
    C. 35 - 40 percent cholesterol
    D. 15 – 20 percent cholesterol

384. Cholesterol is the main element in lipid rafts, the outer shell or protective coating of
    A. all cells
    B. nerve cells
    C. muscle cells
    D. liver cells

385. What is the best way to maintain healthy cholesterol in the body?
    A. bondable versus non-bondable diet
    B. the use of healthy fats in the diet
    C. the use of healthy protein in the diet
    D. A and C
    E. all of the above

386. The three substances produced from acetyl-Co-A are
    A. cholesterol, uric acid, and ubiquinone
    B. ubiquinone, dolichol, and cholesterol
    C. nitric oxide, cholesterol, and dolichol

387. Dolichol
    A. is essential for the formation of DNA proteins
    B. must be present to replicate DNA from one cell to the next
    C. is necessary to maintain genetic programming in both egg and sperm
    D. all of the above

388. Given the information above, should men of childbearing age take statins?
    A. yes
    B. no

389. Ubiquinone or CoQ-10 is
    A. vital for cell function throughout all cells
    B. increases oxygen use inside as well as outside the cell
    C. is vital for protection from viruses and bacteria
    D. acts as an antioxidant for cell wall protection
    E. all of the above
    F. A and B

390. The lack of CoQ-10 to protect the cell membrane and the diminished capacity of the body to replace damaged cell walls, with the steadily growing death of cell walls, is called
    A. necrobiosis
    B. cellular necrosis
    C. natural cell death
    D. death of cells through injury or disease
    E. A and C
    F. B and D

391. All statins work the same way
    A. by blocking the formation of HMG-Co-A reductase enzyme
    B. by blocking only cholesterol formation
    C. by blocking cholesterol release in the liver
    D. A and C

392. If HMG-Co-A reductase cannot form, then
    A. cholesterol cannot form
    B. ubiquinone cannot form
    C. dolichol cannot form
    D. all of the above
    E. A and B

393. When the normal blood cholesterol remains low,
    A. the body is unable to repair rapidly increasing cellular damage
    B. cell wall structures are weakened
    C. eventual necrosis and cell death occurs
    D. cell death can occur anywhere in the body

E. A, C, and D

F. All of the above

394. To date, there is no independent research that proves that the presence of elevated cholesterol is a direct cause of heart attacks.
   A. true
   B. false

395. Along with headaches, nausea, unexplained fevers, and insomnia, which may be the result of microscopic tissue death, we can add
   A. myopathy, rhabdomyolysis, and renal failure
   B. liver damage, polyneuropathy, and retinal hemorrhage
   C. brain hemorrhages and infertility
   D. all of the above
   E. A and B

396. The CARE study of the year 2000 addressed the problem of cancer and found that the risk of breast cancer increased by _____ percent in women using statin drugs.
   A. 50
   B. 110
   C. 500
   D. 1,500

397. According to the research presented, what population needs to take statin drugs for cholesterol reduction.
   A. 10–20
   B. 20–50
   C. 50 and over
   D. B and C
   E. none of the above

398. In the over-fifty population, are diseases and multiple diagnosis ever associated with the use of statin drugs?
   A. yes
   B. no

399. To date, no studies have ever been conducted that can show any decrease in the risk of heart disease for _____ — no matter their age.
  A. men
  B. women
  C. the elderly
  D. children

400. What is the best way to maintain healthy cholesterol?
  A. the use of bondable versus non-bondable foods teaching
  B. the use of cholesterol-lowering drugs
  C. the maintenance of a healthy liver
  D. the use of a low-fat diet
  E. B and D
  F. A and C

Test Answers

Chapters 1 and 2 – How Our Body Uses fuel

1. C.
Agave syrup contains fructose (a non-bondable), pasteurized milk contains lactose that has been exposed to high heat and the outer shell of electrons can no longer bond (a non-bondable). Corn and soy are now genetically altered foods, their molecules are either too big, or they are not recognized by the body as food, thus; they are also non-bondable.

2. D.
The hormone insulin, is formed by two polypeptides that are derived from protein and bonded together by sulfur.

3. B.
All fat cells produce leptin upon consumption of excess poly-glucose, including the consumption of the 'closed molecule' of glycogen that is produced by the liver.

4. B.

Ghrelin, is formed in the hypothalamus stimulates the vagus nerve, which slows down the production of hydrochloric acid, and satiety results.

5. B.

Non-bondable sugars, once they cross the intestinal wall, become simple and complex chains of molecules. The body does not recognize the complex toxins as food and the closed molecules as well as the very large chain structures cannot bond with insulin. All these molecules are sent directly to the liver and are processed through the same pathways, producing the same by-products.

6. C.

100 percent maple syrup, wild brown rice, and unprocessed organic honey will all bond with insulin. Barley malt sweetener contains, hydrolyzed soy and is processed.

7. D.

The end products of non-bondable processing by the liver are lactic acid (which blocks the formation of nitric oxide in the blood), VSLDLs (very small dense lipoproteins) necessary in small amounts but cause heart disease in large amounts, and glycogen the closed molecule, which cannot bond with the insulin that it stimulates.

8. C.

Small amounts of lactic acid remain diluted and cause no problems. Large amounts produce crystals that block tiny arteries, causing swelling and pain and eventual damage to the arteries (gout). This damage, can also be seen in the kidneys, blocking the tiny renal tubules and resulting in renal failure (kidney failure).

9. A.

Nitric oxide, which is formed in the bloodstream, keeps the arteries soft and elastic so blood pressure can rise and fall naturally. Lactic acid blocks nitric oxide formation, which causes arteries to stiffen, and elevated or high blood pressure results.

10. C.
CoQ-10 and vitamins utilize LDLs for transport in the bloodstream. In fact, the presence of CoQ-10 keeps the LDLs large, fluffy, and buoyant. Without CoQ-10, the LDL molecule shrinks and becomes damaged and unusable.

11. D.
The body needs small amounts of plaque to form clots. Without it, we would not stop bleeding after an injury.

12. C.
A molecule with balanced electrons in its outer shell is called; a 'closed molecule', and it cannot bond.

13. B.
Very small dense lipoproteins (VSLDLs) tend to lodge in the arterial wall and increase the eventual formation of plaque to unnecessarily large amounts (peripheral artery disease).

14. B
High volumes of non-bondable glycogen (the closed molecule) cannot bond with the insulin that it actually stimulates. As a result, it is slowly - consumed by fat cells in and around the vital organs, forming **belly fat**.

15. D.
The continued consumption of large amounts of non-bondable fuels over a long period of time (years) will result in accumulation of by-products that result in obesity, diabetes, hypertension, renal failure, and eventual hepatic failure (metabolic syndrome).

16. C.
The increase in belly fat causes adverse pressure on the liver, which decreases the size of the blood vessels and reduces the amount of toxins that can be filtered- readily. This causes the toxins to remain circulating in the bloodstream, allowing them to cause damage to other organs— and even cause cancer. At the same time, the reduced function of the liver causes slower production of by-products from the liver. This means the slow, almost continuous production of glycogen (the closed molecule), which in

turn, causes multiple, almost continuous stimulation of insulin spikes and resulting brain damage and hunger.

17. A.

Multiple, almost continuous stimulation of insulin spikes cause a continuous elevated level of free insulin in the brain, which blocks the absorption of bondable poly-glucose (brain food), which starves the brain cells. More cells die than can be replaced with new growth. The resulting damage and shrinkage of the brain is seen in Alzheimer's.

18. B.

The pancreas becomes forcefully fatigued, with multiple aggressive stimulation (insulin spikes) cause it to fail (the 'light bulb effect').

19. D.

Excess free insulin causes pancreatic fatigue and tends to accumulate in the brain, causing brain fog (confusion, inability to concentrate 'attention deficit syndrome'). This accumulation of insulin blocks the leptin/ghrelin signals, and ghrelin cannot be formed.

20. D.

In this scenario, the production of insulin continues to increase.

21. D.

Free-floating, bondable glucose is damaging to all tissues and is found in diabetes.

22. B.

Free-roaming non-bondable glucose (glycogen) causes a false increase in the blood sugar reading (false positive). False positive blood sugars can result in overmedication with insulin and possible death. Wide-ranging blood sugars are the classic sign of a 'brittle diabetic'.

23. C.

The exterior protective coating of all cells is composed of a bi-layer of cholesterol (two layers held together by protein).

24. D.
The lipid bi-layer also supports electrical activity. An electrical charge can run smoothly across its surface without damaging the cell's interior. This is seen in all nerve cells.

25. C.
A positive electrical charge, is created outside the cell by increasing numbers of positively charged ions facilitated by potassium. And a negative charge is created by increasing numbers of negative ions inside the cell, facilitated by sodium. Just remember P+ (potassium positive) Na- (sodium negative). The cell pushes out the negative to draw in the positive.

Chapter 3 – The BMI and Why

26. B.

27. C.

28. D.
Renal failure is usually a late sign of metabolic syndrome.

29. D.
All of the above

30. E.
Drinking water before meals will slow down digestion, and ice water will drive up metabolism (the thermal affect) but not affect insulin spikes. Increased protein intake (above 25 grams) will only damage liver function and also affects insulin spikes. Eating small amounts of snack foods (non-bondable) will actually stimulate insulin spikes. Eating small amounts of raw vegetables (bondable fuel) will not affect insulin spikes.

31. C.
For most women, 31.5" to 34.6" is overweight, and more than 34.6 inches is obese.

32. B.

For Men, 37" to 40" is overweight, and more than 40" is obese.

33. B.

The liver can only process 25 grams of protein in any one sitting. It is allowable for bodybuilders to increase their protein intake slightly with healthy source proteins only—and only during heavy resistance training or muscle building.

34. D.

All organic raw vegetables are bondable.

35. D.

The list of GMOs is long. Soy and corn should not be a part of your diet simply because 98 percent of all soy and corn, is genetically altered in this country. And soy is not a food, soy is a weed.

Chapter 4 and 5 – Getting From Point A to Point B and Cellular Metabolism

36. C.

Hydrochloric acid breaks down protein bonds, along with digestive enzymes provided by the gallbladder, reducing that protein molecule to a size readily used by bacteria, which continues to break down protein to base amino acids for absorption into the intestinal wall.

37. B.

Sodium, chloride, and potassium are, only found in sea salt, in proper proportion to the balanced minerals found in the human body. Potassium is not found in table salt.

38. A.

A vast majority of the enzymes and hormones that are formed in the human body, are protein-bound structures derived from base amino acids.

39. C.
The mineral balance found in each crystal of sea salt is essentially the same as that found in the human body's mineral balance.

40. D.
When balanced minerals are not present, sufficient hydrochloric acid cannot be produced and protein cannot be broken down. The use of antacids, depletes normal levels of stomach acid and will force the stomach to work harder to produce sufficient stomach acid to break down proteins. This can result in sudden high flow of acid and 'reflux' with the acid splashing into the esophagus, resulting in tissue burns and pain. These burns result in scarring of the esophagus.

41. C.
Fats need to be present in the diet. This is the stimulus for the gallbladder to contract, producing the digestive enzymes to break down these fats.

42. B.
There are one trillion human cells to ten trillion bacterial cells: "our invisible body armor."

43. B.
Although this figure may vary slightly with individuals, a low bacteria count in the intestinal tract can result in incomplete digestion, malabsorption syndrome, and a host of other diseases.

44. B.
Anything over eighty-five degrees will kill bacteria, including high body fevers.

45. C.
Any length of time over twenty-four hours; allows risk of dehydration, constipation, and accumulated dry products of digestion to form on the wall the colon.

46. C.

This gives slow-moving fat cells ten to twelve hours to consume excess glycogen in the extracellular spaces.

47. B.

Ketone bodies, are formed from amino acids released from fat cells. This is an alternative form of fuel.

48. C.

Not just weight loss but fat loss—with decrease in fat cell size.

49. D.

The muscles have no poly-glucose to produce energy. They must use 'ketone bodies', converting them back to glucose inside the healthy cell.

50. A.

True—only healthy cells can use this process.

51. D.

Not a safe form of weight loss and will not affect metabolic syndrome. Gradual increases in ketosis can be achieved without damage and will affect metabolic syndrome.

52. D.

Some people actually need up to 95 percent bondable fuels to achieve their goals.

Chapter 6 – It Takes A Community

53. D.

It truly is the most important organ in the human body.

54. A.

Once past your first line of defense (the intestinal tract and the immune system), the liver must come into play as a second line of defense.

55. B.

The waist size will tell you how much compressive pressure is on your liver. As the size increases, the pressure also increases, leading to markedly decreased liver function.

56. D.

Osteoporosis and thyroid problems are generally a result of mineral deficiency, but the liver provides the levels of vitamin D that regulate bone formation.

57. A.

Treat the cause—not the symptom.

58. B.

Most blood chemistries, of the liver, will not become elevated until after diabetes, hypertension, and heart disease have already arrived.

59. B.

Liver cells grow very slowly. Once failure is complete, it takes too long to recover (approximately one to three years).

Chapter 7 – What's Wrong With These Foods

60. B.

Followed by; elimination of grains, along with processed foods and GMOs.

61. D.

They are no longer a part of a healthy diet

62. D.

This is an autoimmune type of inflammatory response in the intestinal wall. This intestinal wall response is similar to 'leaky gut syndrome'. See Chapter15

63. C.

And this number could be much smaller since routine testing is not done.

64. D.

All of the symptoms related to each of these diseases stem directly from inflammatory response.

65. C.

Whey is not a health food.

66. C.

The liver cannot process more than twenty-five grams of protein in a six-hour period (excess free protein causes kidney damage).

67. A.

To date, we have found no way to remove the chemicals from the milk.

68. C.

Malabsorption syndrome is the end- result of mineral deficiencies. Whey does not block mineral absorption through the intestine, but soy does.

69. A.

Soy is a **toxic weed**—not a health food.

70. C.

Please read your labels—no soy. If it is not fermented, don't put it in your mouth.

71. D.

This number continues to climb—please read your labels.

72. A.

GMOs or genetically altered foods have never been proven safe for human consumption. And those independent studies that have been done, lead us to believe that these 'Franken-foods' are frighteningly dangerous. Until they have been proven safe for human consumption, they should be avoided completely, especially soy and corn. **Opt for 100 percent USDA organic.**

Chapter 8 – Bits and Pieces

73. A.

Those nerves that run through the spinal cord give us muscle movement, skin and muscle sensation and response. These nerves are under our control.

74. D.

It does not matter, which end of this nerve is stimulated, the (pressure) stimulation will travel the length of the nerve, slowing organ function.

75. B.

The vagus nerve is completely independent of brain control. **You can't think yourself thin.**

76. A.

Neuro-stimulants such as caffeine, ginseng, and neuro-depressants such as narcotics can increase or decrease organ function through chemical stimulation.

77. D.

Vaso-vagal syncope (passing out)will result in a pulse rate of approximately forty beats per minute. The body should return to normal (60–70 beats per minute) within twenty to thirty minutes.

78. F.

You cannot think yourself thin—but you can influence the vagus nerve with foods.

79. B.

Metabolism requires fuel, and excessive stimulation will drive ketosis into ketoacidosis.

Chapter 9 – Tissue Regeneration

80. C.

You are not the person you were ten years ago.

81. D.

Stem cells contain the original genetic code or DNA that keeps us who we are for the rest of our lives.

82. C.

Liver cells grow or replicate very slowly, every five months, whereas brain cells grow or replicate very rapidly, every four days.

83. B.

The liver is the most important organ in the human body. Without it, nothing else works.

84. A.

True

All humans process food, regenerate cells, and maintain body function the same. But every person has a different rate of tissue regeneration that is dependent on food (nutrition), activity, and level of internal health.

Chapters 10 and 11 – Proteins and Fats

85. A.

The base structure for all peptides, enzymes, and hormones is protein.

86. E.

Methionine and cysteine, cannot be synthesized by the human body.

87. C.

The body will burn glucose first and then fats (ketosis), and it will not burn protein unless it absolutely has to.

88. A.

89. A.

Extreme exercisers and bodybuilders should never exceed eighty to one hundred grams of healthy protein a day and under twenty-five grams per meal.

90. C.

Unhealthy proteins promote inflammatory response and damage to vital organs.

91. C.

The only state in the United States that has laws prohibiting commercial farm fishing is Alaska.

92. D.

Whey is the by-product of milk pasteurization, containing bovine growth hormones derived from GMOs. Unhealthy proteins, are usually chemically bonded due to processing (use of chemicals and heat) or genetic alteration.

93. D.

The basic elements of ketosis are provided by fatty acids stored in fat cells or fats converted to ketones in the liver. Once released, they become 'ketone bodies' (a clean-burning fuel)—not protein.

94. E.

Keep in mind that the breakdown of excess protein is processed through the same pathway as non-bondable fuels. As a result the same byproducts are produced. 'Demonization' or the passage of excess nitrogen through the kidneys causes destruction to very small blood vessels (also seen in hands and feet). The main reasons why, proteins should be limited.

95. C.

Proteins do not bond with insulin, but these unhealthy sources also contain sugars that are processed in the liver, which do not bond with insulin. Some non-bondable food sources, are usually seen as processed foods. The key word here is **unhealthy**.

96. E.

Unhealthy proteins are the key words here, and protein should be limited.

97. A.

In most cases, the diet is usually the last item to be looked at when making a diagnosis or treatment.

98. C.

Excess protein consumption will cause increased filtration by the kidneys and loss of vitamin D and sulfur in the urine.

99. B.

Fat does not make you fat—sugar does.

100. D.

In grams, the ratio is wider. In tablespoons, fourteen grams of plant fat equals one tablespoon, and 2.6 grams of animal fat equals one teaspoon.

101. F.

One of the main by-products of non-bondable foods is glycogen (the closed molecule). It stimulates the production of insulin, but it will not bond to that insulin.

102. F.

Also found in cocoa, nuts, and some seeds.

103. A.

Found in plant-source healthy fats. Palm oil is processed and hydrogenated. Corn, soy, and canola oils are all genetically altered.

104. E.

All **healthy fats** become healthy saturated fats, which the liver can use.

105. F.

Insulin and thyroid hormones are protein-based hormones.

106. E.

Oxidation is caused by free radicals, that steal electrons from other elements to balance their own structure.

107. E.

Free radicals are missing electrons (unbalanced) and steal from other elements rather than bonding, resulting in damage.

108. A.
Free radicals are unbounded elements, most elements in the body are bonded. Oxidation can be the process of oxygen combining with other elements (CoQ-10) or an increase in positive valance (needs electrons) due to loss of electrons. An element that has been 'oxidized' has lost its electrons to other elements (usually an oxygen reaction or free radicals). The body cannot easily control free radicals, but it can control oxygen reactions with glutathione.

109. D.
Loss of insulin (the 'light bulb effect') is the end- process of pancreatic failure.

110. F.
Inflammatory response is one of the triggers for increase in release of LDLs. The other trigger is human growth hormone. When children are growing, they will naturally have a higher LDL.

111. I.
Healthy fat does not make you fat. Healthy fat does not raise your cholesterol. Healthy fat does not cause brain damage.

112. E.
Excess healthy fat is burned as ketosis. Unused ketones are disposed of through the lungs and the kidneys without tissue damage.

113. A.
This requires both blood and urine monitoring to keep the urine acidity and blood sugars at acceptable levels.

114. A.
Whey and casein are not GMOs, but they may contain GMOs due to animal feeding and processing. They also cause free - floating glutamine and free radical damage, also seen in the use of corn, soy and wheat.

Chapter 12 – The Overlooked Elements; Water, Sleep and Exercise

115. C.
Sweating and shortness of breath are the result of excessive exercise, which results in dehydration. Rapid heart rate without exercise usually goes unnoticed.

116. C.

117. F.
The lack of water and its oxygen component will reduce reactions that remove toxins, thus decreasing cell function.

118. C.

119. D.
Soda will not increase dehydration, but it will increase your weight and keep you addicted to foods through the loss of the leptin and ghrelin connection.

120. A.
The removal of fluorides and chlorines, can only be accomplished with reverse osmosis.

121. E.
Inhibiting this pattern can result in loss of neuro-patterns (re-wiring) or memory and an increase the amount of spinal fluid debris as seen in Alzheimer's disease.

122. A.

123. D.
Leptin and ghrelin signals appear to be affected by sleep deprivation with loss of satity.

124. C.
Healthy daily exercise will enhance both the quality and quantity of sleep. Non-bondable fuels (sugars) prevent REM and NREM sleep.

125. E.
Prescription sleeping medications and psychiatric mood-enhancing drugs block REM sleep by slowing electrical function and NREM sleep by preventing brain shrinkage. Drug-induced sleep or coma can limit or destroy both REM and NREM sleep.

126. A.
Too much exercise or overtraining can result in ketoacidosis, rhabdomyolysis (excessive protein breakdown), and multiple forms of tissue damage, which is life threatening.

127. A.
Once poly-glucose has burned, 'ketone bodies' can be released and burned. Ketosis is the burning of fat (ketone bodies) for fuel.

128. E.
Eating a meal will reintroduce poly-glucose, which is burned first. A protein load can cause tissue damage, should only be used for tissue building and is burned last (starvation mode).

129. A.
ATP (energy) is formed in the mitochondria, the power plant inside the cell.

130. B
Healthy protein loading is never necessary. More than seventy-five to one hundred grams a day, may be used by power athletes and bodybuilders—but only after they have burned all available fats in the body. This is a form of deliberate body starvation and can be dangerous.

131. A.

132. B.
Leptin-to-ghrelin signaling **is only affected by what you eat.**

Chapter 13 – The Missing Elements; Cholesterol

133. D.
Cholesterol, all forms of bonded fatty acids, and a lipid droplet coated in proteins are called healthy cholesterol.

134. F.

135. A.

136. B

137. D.

138. A.

139. D.

Methionine and cysteine contain sulfur, and the liver adds sulfur to tyrosine to form sulfotyrosine. These are all proteins.

140. A.
Nitric oxide and UV rays from sunlight will produce oxygen and a sulfur anion, otherwise known as ENOS.

141. C.
All proteins bond readily to sulfur.

142. E.
Damage to cholesterol comes from trans- fats that become free radicals. These, are classified as lethal oxysterols.

143. D.
Sulfur acts as a bonder and a carrier. It can move through any tissue in the body.

144. A.
The neat little package provides strength and structure (the 'Oreo cookie structure' or lipid bi-layer) to all cells in the body.

145. C.
Hydrogenated and partially hydrogenated vegetable oils, rancid oils, fried foods, and powdered eggs become trans- fats that oxidize cholesterol, changing its structure.

146. B.

147. E.

148. K.

Organic beans, peanuts, and fish are all healthy proteins and fats.

149. E.
Healthy probiotics are necessary for the production of vitamins for the body, especially the B vitamins.

150. B.

151. C.
The NMR particle test, was designed to distinguish **size**. We need those fat, fluffy LDLs that keep us healthy.

152. F.
When considering healthy function, all these factors must be considered.

153. C.

154. C.
The only "bad" cholesterol is an oxidized one, and the best cholesterol is a sulfated one.

Chapter 14 – The Missing Elements; COQ-10

155. C.
CoQ-10 is; formed from and is attracted to proteins.

156. A.
As CoQ-10 oxidizes, changing its states; it forms ubiquinone and hydrogen peroxide.

157. E.

158. B.

159. A.

Statin drugs directly block the formation of CoQ-10.

160. A.

161. C.

Chapter 15 – The Missing Elements; Sulfur

162. D
We can get sulfur through skin, food, water, and supplements.

163. B
Pesticides and herbicides block the roots from absorbing minerals.

164. C
Sulfur bonds to almost all other elements, but it has an affinity for proteins.

165. A.

166. C
Once, this bond is created it cannot be broken.

167. C

This bond gives the brain hormones strength and mobility for crossing the blood-brain barrier.

168. A.

Glutathione will prevent hydrogen peroxide from getting out of control and causing tissue damage.

169. E.

This bond is the most important in the prevention of inflammatory response.

170. E.

Preventing the absorption of unwanted elements past the wall or barrier.

171. 1. A 2. B 3. C

ENOS equals oxygen and a sulfur ion, formed in the reticular beds of the skin.

172. B.

This prevents elements from sticking together or clumping.

173. A.

Adding sulfur to change compound structures—not necessarily a protein bond.

174. C.

The liver requires large amounts of sulfur to function and is the first in line to steal.

175. 1. G 2. C 3. E

This is inflammatory response, also seen in the intestinal tract.

176. 1. B 2. D

Converting needed SO_4 (-2) sulfate to $S(2)$ a sulfide, which the body cannot absorb.

177. 1. B 2. C

Amino acid fragments (Glutamine) blocks sulfur use.

178. B.

Fermented foods improve the biologic or probiotic count and decrease anaerobic growth or presence.

179. A.

Iron sulfate and sulfur oxide.

180. 1. B 2. D

Both the circulation of the fetus and mother are completely separate.

181. D.

This test, is only used in scientific studies. This leaves us with the presence of illness or disease as only a guideline for the need for sulfur.

Chapter 16 - Detoxification

182. C.

These are the exit ports for toxins and solid waste

183. B.

The lymphatic system 'dumps' into the circulation for disposal through the gallbladder and kidneys, the tonsils that deposit back into the digestive system, and the sweat glands on the surface of the skin.

184. C.

185. C.

Fluid movement influenced by muscular action or massage is the only form of movement in this system. This fluid movement, can also be influenced by heat in soaking or saunas.

186. C.

The gallbladder is our solid waste disposal plant, which empties into the small intestine.

187. D.

If the intestinal tract is slow or constipation occurs, toxins can accumulate and reabsorb into the body.

188. C.

It's not how you eat, it's what you eat.

189. A.

Severe cold will not allow toxins to pass through the skin.

190. B.
Safe and easily done by anyone.

191. D.
The gallbladder is the only organ that handles solid waste.

192. C.
Under alternative medicine supervision.

193. D.
There are three hundred chambers in the United States, and more than two thousand in Russia.

194. B.
Mechanical colon cleansing, must be done under trained supervision.

195. 1. C 2. E

Chapter 17 - Minerals

196. 1. A   2. D   3. E   4. B

197. C.
Only 2 percent of calcium remains circulating. The bones are for structure, not storage.

198. C.
This can be seen inside as well as outside the cell. Hormones and some minerals can cause increased electrical activity.

199. A.
Located on both sides of the thyroid gland—and completely separate from thyroid function.

200. 1. D   2. B
This gland increases calcium in the bloodstream when the calcium level is low, it can be lovingly be called 'our squirrel'.

201. B.
This cascading effect can eventually result in multiple disease problems, including bone and mineral loss.

202. C.
The parathyroid can only adjust for low levels of calcium—not high.

203. B.
Calcium and phosphorous combination supplements are already bound to each other and go straight to blood and soft tissues, causing hardening of the tissues (often mistaken for tendonitis). This type of supplement is not recommended. Calcium and phosphorous must be bonded to the proper ratios **inside the body by vitamin D—not outside.**

204. B.
All cells produce ATP, and one of its by-products is phosphorous.

205. A.

206. A.
Usually found in protein, but it bonds to fats. In the liver, these are seen as phospholipids.

207. C.

208. E.
The other side of the sodium pump, sodium is pushed out (muscle contraction) with ATP to draw in the potassium, causing muscle relaxation.

209. D.
Diuretics and vomiting will increase potassium loss.

210. B.
Hypo means below level.

211. D.
Potassium-sparing diuretics will raise the potassium.

212. B.
There are no medical guidelines or levels for sulfur in the body.

213. F.

214. A.
You can't make stomach acid out of it.

215. E.
Excess sodium is responsible for fluid retention and elevated blood pressure, and it is found in high levels in most processed foods.

216. A.
Using unprocessed natural sea salt liberally in the diet will not cause an imbalance.

217. E.

Magnesium is not found in meats.

218. C.

Too much calcium will pull magnesium from muscles.

219. A.

It is difficult if not impossible to create an excess of magnesium due to efficient kidney filtration. Excess is often seen in the use of concentrated magnesium preparations, like laxatives.

220. E.

Neuro-stimulation in the tissues increases when the magnesium decreases—commonly seen as exocytosis.

221. B.

Excess calcium or calcium deposits throughout the body are not necessarily an indication of a magnesium deficiency, but studies have found that calcium deposits (bone spurs), can be reduced by increasing magnesium intake.

222. C.

223. A.

Vitamins cannot be utilized by the body without the presence of balanced minerals.

Chapter 18 - Vitamins

224. C.

We need eight to ten servings of a variety of vegetables to meet the RDA since vegetables in the United States have such low vitamin and mineral content.

225. B.

226. E.
Cofactors are a part of whole vitamins and are necessary for many vitamins to be utilized in the body.

227. D.
Fermented foods create high numbers of biologics (probiotics), which produce many vitamins from food, and those vitamins rely on those cofactors to function.

228. D.
Fats and fat-soluble vitamins, are esterified when processed, removing oxygen, a necessary cofactor, and extending shelf life (preservation).

229. B.
Vitamin C serves as a ketone carrier for fat metabolism in the cell.

230. C.
This vitamin has been studied for years and is still not fully understood.

231. D.

232. D.
Platelets are a part of the initial response.

233. E.

234. F.
T cells and B cells are specialized white blood cells. Red blood cells are not part of this response.

235. D.
ROS is activated by vitamin C (the end- product is oxygen and hydrogen peroxide).

236. F.
Antibodies, are formed by copying the DNA of the antigen inside the B cell or killer cell.

237. A.

B cells and killer cells carry a code of body DNA and can recognize self from others.

238. C.

T cells are like little bombs with suction cups.

239. E.

Killer cells engulf and consume (eat) foreign material, while B cells break down foreign cell walls.

240. D.

The spleen is used for storage of white blood cells, specialized cells, and extra blood.

241. A.

Debate still exists between conventional and alternative therapies in regard to the dosage used in high-dose therapies.

242. B.

All studies to date show little or no effect below the four hundred milligrams daily dose.

243. E.

B vitamins appear to be interdependent on each other for absorption as well as function.

244. C.

The complement of B vitamins has more effect on brain health than any other organ.

245. E.

B vitamins play a key role in fetal growth and proper development.

246. F.

247. B.

Vitamin B1 has a direct relationship with fatty acids that contribute to brain hormones, but this relationship is only complete with the presence of niacin.

248. F.

B6, folate, niacin, and iron, cannot be absorbed into the body without the presence of B2.

249. F

This significant vitamin is necessary during pregnancy

250. B.

Glutathione, our master controller of ROS, must have B2 present to form.

251. B.

This coenzyme is necessary for all oxidation and reduction (CoQ-10) reactions.

252. C.

Sixty milligrams of tryptophan will yield one milligram of niacin.

253. B.

254. F.

Vitamin B5 is essential for forming red blood cells and iron—but not ENOS.

255. B.

Pantothenic acid is necessary to form acetylcholine (a neurotransmitter) and melatonin (a brain hormone that controls sleep patterns).

256. E.

Pantothenic acid is necessary for lipid formation for cholesterol and is also seen in myelin sheaths of nerves and in the synthesis of hemoglobin from iron.

257. B.
Vitamin B6 is a necessary element found in healthy proteins from both plant and animal sources.

258. D.
Vitamin B6 is essential in multiple chemical reactions throughout the body, and along with vitamin B5, pantothenic acid (vitamin B6) is a necessary coenzyme in neurotransmitter formation and formation of hemoglobin.

259. 1. B   2 C
The minimum healthy protein intake will supply the minimum B6 intake or need from both plant and animal sources.

260. A.
Biotin is bonded to proteins using a sulfur bond.

261. F.
The breakdown and synthesis of fatty acids (ketosis), in ketosis fats burn—not proteins.

262. 1. B   2. D
Raw egg yolk contains the highest form of biotin (sulfur-bonded protein) found in foods.

263. 1. A   2. A
This may be due to decreased intestinal function due to insufficient bacteria to allow absorption of biotin.

264. E.
This is one of the strongest sulfur bonds.

265. D.
Scattered symptoms make it difficult to diagnose and treat.

266. A.
Biologics (probiotics) have a direct effect on the availability of biotin for absorption.

267. A.

Folic acid is the term used for the chemical derivative.

268. E.

Healthy sources are organic green, leafy vegetables, beans, and legumes.

269. G.

Studies have found that folate deficiency during pregnancy is linked to premature births.

270. D.

This requires both vitamin B6 and B12 to produce break down for methionine bonding.

271. D.

Requires both, folate and B12 to, convert back to methionine.

272. A.

Elevated levels of homocysteine, are seen in many chronic diseases and are treated with B vitamins.

273. D.

A deficiency in any one of these vitamins (B6, B12, or folate) will result in increased oxidative stress and elevated homocysteine levels.

274. E.

Oxidative stress is seen with elevated homocysteine levels.

275. F.

Enlarged, abnormally shaped red blood cells are seen in normal numbers, but they lack the capacity to carry oxygen.

276. D.

Loss of iron (found in protein) from digestion, results in enlarged, abnormal red blood cells (megaloblastic anemia).

277. A.

278. B.
This molecular structure contains a metal ion—cobalt.

279. B.

280. A.
B6 is necessary for homocysteine formation, but folate and B12 are needed for conversion back to methionine. The two; B12 and folate, activate each other.

281. D.
Healthy food sources of vitamin B12 are unprocessed, organic animal products.

282. E.
This vitamin is derived from proteins and is sensitive to heat, which means minimal low-temperature cooking and no pasteurization.

283. F.
Think brain!

284. B.
Healthy animal protein only!

285. F.
Iron-deficiency anemia comes from B12 malabsorption syndrome. Elevated homocysteine may be due to B6, B12, or folate deficiencies.

286. E.
These problems, are all connected to brain development and function. Again—think brain.

287. C.

288. A.
Fat-soluble vitamins means there must be fat in the diet for breakdown and absorption.

289. E.
Brightly colored vegetables contain carotenoids.

290. F.
Pro-vitamin A's are carotenoids and good for you. Pre-vitamin As are all synthetic compounds and can cause substantial health damage.

291. D.
Synthetic retinol is **not the same** as the retinol formed by the eye and will cause damage. Retinol formed by the eye does not break down vitamin A.

292. B.
Retinol is stored in the inner lining of the eye and can only be stimulated and activated by light exposure. It is not affected by heat, cold, or pressure.

293. 1. A 2. C
This vitamin has a direct effect on growth hormones, but it does not appear to affect neurotransmitters.

294. C.
Pro-vitamin A, carotenoids, are vital to the proper growth and development of the fetus.

295. 1. B 2. D
Without healthy stem cell development, birth defects and cancer can occur.

296. 1. A 2. D
Formation of hemoglobin from iron requires both A and B vitamins.

297. B.
Stigmatism is inappropriate light refraction, glaucoma is increased inner-eye pressure, and cataracts are opacity in the lens of the eye.

298. C.

299. E.
Vitamin A deficiency does not affect internal eye pressure.

300. B.

301. E.
Vitamin A, zinc, and iron work together at the cellular level and appear to reduce the length and severity of illness and disease.

302. F.
Keep in mind the difference between pre-vitamin A and pro-vitamin A, and you will know that **pre-vitamin A is not recommended.**

303. E.

304. D.
Vitamin D has been studied at length recently, and it has been found to have effects involving not just bone, but cell structure (cholesterol sulfate), and immune health.

305. E.
Acceptable blood levels must be above 50 nanograms per milliliter (by blood analysis) of Hydroxy vitamin D or (25 (OH) D.

306. 1. C 2. B
These are both structural terms for soft bone or bone demineralization, rickets in children, and osteomalacia in adults.

307. E.

308. B.
The average vitamin D level of most women in the United States is eighteen to twenty nanograms per milliliter, which is classified as severe deficiency. Infants are born with 60–70 percent of the mother's levels, this is rickets.

309. B.
The average adult in the United States has a vitamin D level of twenty to thirty-five nanograms per milliliter, which is classified as deficiency and osteomalacia.

310. B.

Dehydroxyvitamin D will pull calcium from bone, which is a negative effect.

311. 1. B 2. C

The parathyroid is stimulated by low blood calcium levels.

312. 1. A 2. B

313. D.

Each organ plays a specific role in this pathway. Without healthy liver function, hydroxy vitamin D is lost and balance is lost. Without parathyroid and kidney function, the calcium and phosphorous balance is lost.

314. 1. C 2. B 3. D 4. E

This is the parathyroid loop that controls availability of calcium in the body.

315. B.

Fifty nanograms per milliliter, to one hundred nanograms per milliliter, depending on your health status.

316. 1. A 2. C

The end- result is remodeled bone structure.

317. A.

In renal disease, the kidneys are unable to convert hydroxy vitamin D back to dehydroxy vitamin D, and loss of calcium availability results (low calcium levels). In parathyroid disease, not enough dehydroxy-vitamin D is made, and the end- result is low blood calcium levels. The use of calcium carbonate preparations blocks the use of phosphorus in the matrix formation, but it does not affect the formation of hydroxy vitamin D. In liver disease, the loss of hydroxy vitamin D formation will result in excess dehydroxy vitamin D and loss of bone formation. Without healthy liver function, we can't make bone.

318. D.

Infants are born with 60–70 percent of the mother's vitamin D level.

319. C.

This symptom, is not- generally used by modern medicine, but it was discovered in research from very old medical literature.

320. A.

It is not- generally recognized by modern medicine, but studies show a direct association to vitamin D deficiency.

321. F.

Everyone should know their vitamin D levels.

322. D.

Calcium carbonate preparations, should not be used as bone-strengthening agents (Tums and Rolaids) and should especially be avoided during pregnancy.

323. F.

Palm olean (synthetic supplement that mimics palmic acid) will block vitamin D absorption and soy will block the absorption of calcium, zinc, and iron in the intestinal tract. Whey protein does not block absorption of minerals or vitamin D but it should also be avoided as it contributes to large amounts of hormones, antibiotics and pain killers, causing distructive changes in infant development.

324. A.

325. E.

It takes a community: vitamin D, beta-carotene, vitamin C, and vitamin K all work together.

326. D.

Unexplained bruising or bleeding under the skin is the result of clotting deficiency or high levels of vitamin K1.

327. A.

Clot prevention in blood requires vitamin K1—not K2.

328. A.

Vitamin K, is formed by bacteria in the intestinal tract. Fermentation of foods will create the needed bacteria as well as vitamin K.

329. F.

Healthy plant fats work as adjuncts to vitamins and minerals

330. E.
331. E.

Mechanical grinding, macerating, or juicing fresh plants, does not affect sterols.

332. D.

333. F.

It will also improve the production of thyroid growth hormones and is used by the liver for the production of cholesterol.

334. B.

335. A.

The action of these different sterols is wide and encompasses hundreds of different functions in the body. It is even seen in studies to affect arthritis.

336. C.

Sterols, must be consumed raw in order to be beneficial to the body.

337. E.

Vegetarians are missing a balance of plant to animal source fats, and plant-to-animal-source proteins due to a lack of healthy animal source foods.

338. F.

339. A.

Their actions as cofactors for vitamins and minerals is invaluable.

340. E.

Once processed, grains and wheat have no sterols.

341. B. or C.

This would form a minimum base for a healthy diet.

342. B.

Fats come from both plant and animal sources.

343. C.

344. B.

Avoiding the blood-thinning increase provided by EPA.

345. 1. D   2. B

Too much EPA can actually prevent DHA from crossing the blood-brain barrier.

346. A.

This is the recommendation of the US Department of Health and Human Services.

347. B.
348. E.

The word carbohydrate does not belong in nutrition related to body function. Outside of the indirect cause of belly fat, **there is no specific body function for a carbohydrate**. Just think of carbohydrates as non-bondables and vegetables that contain natural sugars as bondable.

349. D.

Fructose is a sugar naturally found in fruit. It is classified as a non-bondable, and it needs to be limited to one fresh whole piece of fruit daily.

Chapter 19 – GMO's The Nightmare Come True

350. A.
The genes used are taken from different organisms, unrelated to the plant's genealogy.

351. H.
This includes food ingredients such as high-fructose corn syrup, vitamins, and clothing fibers.

352. A.
When genetic structure changes we have a 'new organism'—with unknown actions or potential.

353. F.
White rice contains human genes. Corn and sweet corn contain a 'living pesticide'.

354. B.
Once these new structural organisms are created, they cannot be reversed. If not controlled, cross-pollination of plants will literally change **all of that specific plant species.**

355. B.
No independent tests are required.

356. F.
Stacked traits were introduced (multiple crossing of organisms in one plant) when single traits failed. This was followed by the use of bacteria, viruses, and even human genes.

357. A.

358. A.
If it looks like a duck, then it should quack the same; therefore, it is 'safe'.

359. E.

These comparison studies have never been revealed to the public (can only be revealed under court order) and are accepted as 'safe' by the USDA and FDA.

360. E.

Safety has nothing to do with this form of testing.

361. B.

Toxicology studies are not necessary according to the United States government.

362. A.

Most of Europe's GM crops are stacked traits.

363. E.

364. E.

365. A.

366. F.

The corn used caused unexpected deaths from cancer.

367. A.

Unable to finance or reproduce the study, it was lost.

368. B

369. D.

This toxin can cross-pollinate with non-GM crops, changing their genetic structure as well.

370. A.

371. B.
It, may in fact be a contributing cause to metabolic syndrome in the United States.

372. A.

373. F.
It was moved from animal feed to human food.

374. A.
Most of Europe has banned genetically altered foods for human consumption.

375. D.
Soy is **'not a food'**, converting it to GM just makes it that much worse.

376. A.
Corn should go into the gas tanks of our cars—and not our mouths.

377. A.
It still causes cancer.

378. F.
Blended oils or vegetable oils, are made from any or all these.

379. A.
No labeling is required.

380. E.
If it labeled non-GMO or certified organic, then the vitamin is whole and organic. Most vitamins on the market today come from GM products.

381. D.

Chapter 20 – A Question of Personal Choice

382. C.
It, was recommended by the pharmaceutical industry, which was agreed to by the FDA.

383. C
Refer to chapter 13.

384. A.
Lipid rafts (the 'Oreo cookie' structure), a layer of sulfated protein coated on each side with a layer of fat.

385. E.
Bondable versus non-bondable will reduce the production of unhealthy triglycerides. Healthy fats and proteins will produce healthy triglycerides.

386. B.
This is the HMG-Co-A reductase enzyme pathway.

387. D.
388. B.
Sperm also contains DNA, which needs dolichol for replication and healthy reproduction.

389. E.
Statins block the formation of CoQ-10 in the body.

390. F.
Necrobiosis is, by definition, natural cell death (normal life span). Necrosis is, by definition, the early death of cells through injury or disease.

391. A.
It blocks all formation of ubiquinone, dolichol, and cholesterol in the liver.

392. D.
Statins block more than just cholesterol formation in the liver.

393. F.

When cholesterol remains low, weakening of cell walls comes from other factors such as free radical damage or uncontrolled oxidation reactions. The inability to replace and maintain cholesterol in cells results in necrosis and eventual cell death and is a secondary statin affect.

394. A.

Care must be taken to recognize the source and validity of the research provided.

395. D.

The reports and research involving the damage from these so-called 'side effects' are repeatedly verified in multiple independent studies from the past eighteen years.

396. D.

When the immune system and its ability to repair, is depleted or even destroyed by a lack of healthy cholesterol sulfate, then disease can take over and flourish.

397. E.

The use of statin durgs is not supported by science, nor is its use advocated for any population—not even those suffering from familial hypercholesterolemia (inherited high cholesterol – a theory not yet proven). **Change the way you look at food—and change your life!**

398. B.

Degenerative disease is an 'accepted norm' in medical science, and 'side effects' or 'problems' that may arise from statin use, are generally treated with more pharmaceuticals.

399. B.

There has never been an independent study to show benefits for any population, especially women.

400. F.

Change the way you look at food—and change your life!

References

Chapter 1

1. Hall, John E., Guyton, Arthur C. (2006). *Textbook of Medical Physiology*. St. Louis, Mo: Elsevier Saunders. ISBN 0-7216-0240-1.
2. Forrest MD, Wall MJ, Press DA, Feng J (December 2012). "The Sodium-Potassium Pump Controls the Intrinsic Firing of the Cerebellar Purkinje Neuron." PLoS ONE 7 (12): e51169. doi:10.1371/journal.pone.0051169. PMC 3527461. PMID 23284664.
3. Cannon, C (July 2004). "Paying the Price at the Pump: Dystonia from Mutations in a Na^+/K^+-ATPase." Neuron 43 (2): 153–154. doi:10.1016/j.neuron.2004.07.002. PMID 15260948.
4. Young, EA, Fowler CD, Kidd GJ, Chang A, Rudick R, Fisher E, Trapp BD (April 2008). "Imaging correlates of decreased axonal Na^+/K^+ ATPase in chronic multiple sclerosis lesions." Ann Neurol 63 (4): 428–35. PMID 18438950.
5. Gray, Pikering, and Howden, *Gray's Anatomy: Descriptive and Surgical Anatomy: General Anatomy and Histology: The Animal Cell, and the Nerves.* Lea Brothers & Co. 2003.
6. National Institute for General Medical Science, Science of Biology: www.sciencesource.ca, "ATP and the Sodium Pump."
7. Robert Thompson, MD, Kathleen Barns, *The Calcium Lie: The Sodium Pump and Ion Transport.* In Truth Press 2008.
8. Heymsfield, S, Waki M, Kehayias J, Lichtman S, Dilmanian F, Kamen Y, Wang J, Pierson R (1991). "Chemical and elemental analysis of humans in vivo using improved body composition models." *Am J Physiol* 261 (2 Pt 1): E190–8. PMID 1872381.

9. Sychrová, H (2004). "Yeast as a model organism to study transport and homeostasis of alkali metal cations" (PDF). *Physiol Res.* 53 Suppl. 1: S91–8. PMID 15119939.

Chapter 2

1. Dr. Robert Lusting Dept. of Pediatrics, UCSF Faculty Bio Page, Sugar: The Bitter Truth.
2. Dr. J Mercola, articles. mercola.com, "Agave: A Triumph of Marketing over Truth." Archives/2009.
3. Dr. J Mercola, "Sweet Deception," 2006.
4. Dr. Richard Johnson, "The Sugar Fix," 2008.
5. Jean-Marc Schwarz PhD. UC Berkley, Nutritional Science, Molecular Studies.
6. Cline, Ma, Tintinalli, Kelen Stapczynski, "Emergency Medicine: Acute Hypoglycemia, Diagnosis and Management," 2000.
7. Alliance for Natural Health Feb. 2011, "How Sweet Isn't Cutting Through the Hype and Deception."
8. Dr. Deepak Chopra, *Alternative Medicine, The Definitive Guide: Treating Diabetes and Dietary Guidelines*, 2002.
9. Stephen McPhee, Maxine Papadakis, "Current Medical Diagnosis and Treatment, Metabolic Syndrome, Syndrome X," Insulin Resistance Syndrome. 2010.
10. Fauci, Braunwald, Kasper, Hauser, Longo, Jameson, Loscalzo, *Harrison's Principles of Internal Medicine: Metabolic Syndrome, Diagnosis and Treatments:* 17th ed. 2009.
11. Stephanie Seneff, Ann Lauritzen, Robert Davidson and Laurie Lentz-Marino, "Is Endothelial Nitric Oxide Synthase a Moonlighting Protein Whose Day Job is Cholesterol Sulfate Synthesis? Implications for Cholesterol Transport, Diabetes and Cardiovascular Disease." Entropy 2012, 14, 2492-2530, doi:10.3390/e14122492.
12. Stephanie Seneff, Glyn Wainwright, and Luca Mascitelli, "Is the Metabolic Syndrome Caused by a High Fructose, and Relatively Low Fat, Low Cholesterol Diet?" Archives of Medical Science, 2011, 7, 1: 8-20, doi:10.5114/aoms.2011.20598.

13. Stephanie Seneff, Glyn Wainwright, and Luca Mascitelli, "Nutrition and Alzheimer's Disease: The Detrimental Role of a High Carbohydrate Diet," *European Journal of Internal Medicine* 22 (2011) 134–140, doi:10.1016/j.ejim.2010.12.017.

14. Sulfur: Could This Be the Hidden Factor Behind Obesity, Heart Disease, and Chronic Fatigue? September 17, 2011 Mercola Video Log. Interview with Stephanie Seneff, senior scientist at MIT with an undergraduate degree in biology from MIT, and a minor in food and nutrition and has been conducting research there for over three decades.

15. Phyllis A Balch CNC, Prescription for Dietary Wellness, Sugar by Any Other Name. Copyright Canada, 2003.

16. Cline, Ma, Tintinalli, Kelen and Stapczynski, Emergency Medicine 5th ed., *Diabetic Emergencies/Fluid and Electrolyte Balance.* McGraw Hill, 2000.

17. Deepak Chopra, Trivieri, and Anderson, *Alternative Medicine: The Definitive Guide* 2nd. Ed. More Food, Less Nutrients: Inno Vision Health Media 2002.

18. Pereira MA, Kartashov AI, Ebbeling CB, Van Horn L, Slattery ML, Jacobs DR Jr, Ludwig DS.: Fast-food habits, weight gain, and insulin resistance (the CARDIA study): 15-year prospective analysis. Lancet 2005 Jan 1–7, 365(9453):36–42.

19. Robert H. Lusting MD. UCSF Faculty Bio Page, "Sugar, The Bitter Truth, The Fructose epidemic," *The Bariatrition*, 2009 Vol, 24 No. 1, 10.

20. Ludwig D.S., Peterson, K.E. and Gortmaker, S.L. "Relation between consumption of sugar-sweetened drinks and childhood obesity: a prospective, observational analysis," *The Lancet,* Feb. 17, 2001 Volume 357, issue 9255, 505–508.

21. Wells H. F. and Buzby J. C. "Dietary assessment of major trends in U.S. food consumption, 1970–2005. USDA Economic Research Service, Economic Information Bulletin Number 33, March 2008.

22. Vartanian L.R., Schwartz M. B. and Brownell K. D. "Effects of soft drink consumption on nutrition and health: A systematic review and meta-analysis" AJPH April 2007, vol. 97, No. 41, 667–675.

23. Apovian C. M. "Sugar-sweetened soft drinks, obesity, and type 2 diabetes" JAMA 2004, 292: 978–979

24. Esterbrook J. "Schools that can soda cut obesity," CBS News Health, April 23, 2004.

25. Palmer J.R., Boggs D.A., Krishnan S., Hu F. B., Singer M., and Rosenberg L. "Sugar-sweetened beverages and incidence of type 2 diabetes mellitus in African American women" Arch Intern Med. 2008, 168(14):1487–1492.

26. Stanhope K. L., et al. "Consuming fructose-sweetened, not glucose-sweetened, beverages increases visceral adiposity and lipids and decreases insulin sensitivity in overweight/obese humans" J Clin Invest. 2009 May 1,119(5):1322–1334.

27. Faith M. S., Dennison B. A., Edmunds L. S., Stratton H. H. "Fruit juice intake increased adiposity gain in children from low-income families: weight status by environment interaction" Pediatrics 118:2066-2075.

28. Taubs, G. "Good Calories, Bad Calories: Challenging the Conventional Wisdom on Diet, Weight Control, and Disease," 2007, Knopf, and Medical Grand Rounds presentation, Datmouth-Hitchcock,

29. Lim, J. S., Mietus-Snyder M. L., Valente, A., Schwartz, J. M., and Lustig, R. H. "Fructose, NAFLD, and metabolic syndrome," Dept. of Pediatrics and Medicine, University of California, San Francisco, 2009.

30. Ouyang, X., Cirillo P., Sautin, Y., McCall S., Bruchette, J. L., Diehl, A. M. Johnson, R. J., Abdelmalek, M. F. "Fructose consumption as a risk factor for non-alcoholic fatty liver disease" J. Hepatol. 2008 Jun, 48(6):993–9.

31. Le, K. A., Ilth, M., Kreis, R., Faeh, D., Bortolotti, M., Tran C., Boesch, C., and Tappy, L. "Fructose overconsumption causes dyslipidemia and ectopic lipid deposition in healthy subjects with and without a family history of type 2 diabetes" Am J Clin Nutr. 2009 Jun, 89(6):1760–5.

32. Hillier T.A., Pedula K.L., Schmidt B.A., Mullen J.A., Charles M., Pettitt D. J. "Childhood obesity and metabolic imprinting:

The ongoing effects of maternal hyperglycemia" *Diabetes Care,* September 2007 vol. 30 no. 9, 2287–2292.

33. U.S. Department of Health and Human Services, Administration for Children and Families, Early Childhood Learning and Knowledge Center (ECLKC) "Prevention of overweight and obesity in infants and toddlers."

34. Rosendale, R. MD., Designs for Health Institute's Boulder Fest Seminar, Aug 1999, Insulin and Its Metabolic Effects.

35. Braunwald, Fauci, Hauser, Longo, and Jaameson: Principles of Internal Medicine: Pathologic Consequences of Obesity, Cardiovascular Disease, Exorcise & Cholesterol Management, 15th ed., 2001.

36. Centers for Disease Control and Prevention. National Diabetes Fact Sheet: National Estimates and General Information on Diabetes and Prediabetes in the United States, 2011. Atlanta, GA: U.S. Department of Health and Human Services, Centers for Disease Control and Prevention, 2011.

37. Heinig, M, Johnson, RJ (December 2006). "Role of uric acid in hypertension, renal disease, and metabolic syndrome." Cleveland Clinic Journal of Medicine 73 (12): 1059–64. doi:10.3949/ccjm.73.12.1059. PMID 17190309.

38. Banach, K., Bojarska, E., Kazimierczuk, Z., Magnowska, L., Bzowska, A. Kinetic Model of Oxidation Catalyzed by Xanthine Oxidase—The Final Enzyme in Degradation of Purine Nucleosides and Nucleotides. Nucleosides Nucleotides Nucleic Acids 2005, 24, 465–469.

39. "What is Gout: What Causes Gout?" MedicalBug. 6 January 2012. Retrieved 6 May 2012.

40. Malik VS, Popkin BM, Bray GA, Després JP, Willett WC, Hu FB. (November 2010). Sugar-sweetened beverages and risk of metabolic syndrome and type 2 diabetes: a meta-analysis. Diabetes Care 33 (11): 2477–2483. doi:10.2337/dc10-1079. PubMed 20693348.

41. Cappuccio, F.P., Strazzullo, P, Farinaro, E., Trevisan, M (July 1993). "Uric acid metabolism and tubular sodium handling. Results from a population-based study." *JAMA* 270 (3): 354–9. doi:10.1001/jama.270.3.354. PMID 8315780.

42. Dehghan, A, van Hoek, M, Sijbrands, EJ, Hofman, A, Witteman, JC (February 2008). "High serum uric acid as a novel risk factor for type 2 diabetes." *Diabetes Care* 31 (2): 361–2. doi:10.2337/dc07-1276. PMID 17977935.

43. Nakagawa T, Hu H, Zharikov S, et al. (March 2006). "A causal role for uric acid in fructose-induced metabolic syndrome." *American Journal of Physiology.* Renal Physiology 290 (3): F625–31. doi:10.1152/ajprenal.00140.2005. PMID 16234313.

44. Becker BF (June 1993). "Towards the physiological function of uric acid." *Free Radical Biology & Medicine* 14 (6): 615–31. doi:10.1016/0891-5849(93)90143-I. PMID 8325534.

45. Glantzounis GK, Tsimoyiannis EC, Kappas AM, Galaris DA (2005). "Uric acid and oxidative stress." *Current Pharmaceutical Design* 11 (32): 4145–51. doi:10.2174/138161205774913255. PMID 16375736.

46. Nguyen S, Lustig RH. Just a spoonful of sugar helps the blood pressure go up. Expert Rev Cardiovasc Ther. 2010 Nov, 8(11):1497–9.

47. J. V. Zhang, P. G. Ren, O. Avsian – Kretchmer, C. W. Lus, R. Rauch, A.J.W. Hsueh, "Obestatin, a Peptide Endcoated by Ghrelin gene, Opposes Ghrelin's effects on food intake:" *Food Science,* 11 Nov. 2005: Vol 310. No. 5750 PP996-999. [DOI:10.1126/science.1117255].

48. R. Nogueriras and M. Tschop, Separation of conjoined Hormones Yealds opposite rivals, Science STKE, 15, Nov. 2005, vol. 2005 issue 310: PPtw408 [doi:10.1126/stke.3102005tw408], Dueling Hunger Hormones?

49. Weiss R, Bremer AA, Lustig RH. "What is metabolic syndrome, and why are children getting it?" *Ann N Y Acad. Sci.* 2013 Apr, 1281:123–40.

50. Lustig RH. Fructose: it's "alcohol without the buzz." *Adv Nutr.* 2013 Mar, 4(2):226–35.

51. Tomiyama AJ, Schamarek I, Lustig RH, Kirschbaum C, Puterman E, Havel PJ, Epel ES. "Leptin concentrations in response to acute stress predict subsequent intake of comfort foods." *Physiol Behav.* 2012 Aug 20, 107(1):34–9.

52. Lustig RH, Schmidt LA, Brindis CD. "Public health: The toxic truth about sugar." *Nature.* 2012 Feb 2, 482(7383):27–9.

53. Bremer AA, Lustig RH. Effects of sugar-sweetened beverages on children. Pediatr Ann. 2012 Jan, 41(1):26–30.

54. Belinda S Lennerz, David C Alsop, Laura M Holsen, Emily Stern, Rafael Rojas, Cara B Ebbeling, Jill M Goldstein, and David S Ludwig. Effects of dietary glycemic index on brain regions related to reward and craving in men. Am J Clin Nutr, June 26, 2013 DOI: 10.3945/ajcn.113.064113.

Chapter 3

1. "Who's fat? New definition adopted." CNN. June 17, 1998. Retrieved 2010-04-26.

2. "Physical status: The use and interpretation of anthropometry." WHO Technical Report Series (Geneva, Switzerland: World Health Organization) 854 (854): 1–452. 1995. PMID 8594834.

3. "Executive Summary." Clinical Guidelines on the Identification, Evaluation, and Treatment of Overweight and Obesity in Adults: The Evidence Report. National Heart, Lung, and Blood Institute. September 1998. xi–xxx.

4. Taylor, R. S. (2010). "Use of Body Mass Index for Monitoring Growth and Obesity." Pediatrics & Child Health 15 (5): 258. PMC 2912631. PMID 21532785.

5. Romero-Corral, A, Somers, V K, Sierra-Johnson, J, Thomas, R J, Collazo-Clavell, M L, Korinek, J et al. (2008). "Accuracy of body mass index in diagnosing obesity in the adult general population." *International Journal of Obesity,* 32 (6): 959–66. doi:10.1038/ijo.2008.11. PMC 2877506. PMID 18283284.

6. Kang SM, Yoon JW, Ahn HY, Kim SY, Lee KH, et al. (2011) "Android fat depot is more closely associated with metabolic syndrome than abdominal visceral fat in elderly people." PLoS ONE 6: e27694.

7. Lumeng CN, Saltiel AR (2011) "Inflammatory links between obesity and metabolic disease." *Journal of Clinical Investigation,* 121: 2111–2117.

8. Janssen I, Katzmarzyk PT, Ross R (2005) "Body mass index is inversely related to mortality in older people after adjustment for waist circumference." *Journal of the American Geriatrics Society* 53: 2112–2118.

9. Simpson JA, MacInnis RJ, Peeters A, Hopper JL, Giles GG, et al. (2007) "A comparison of adiposity measures as predictors of all-cause mortality: the Melbourne Collaborative Cohort Study." *Obesity* 15: 994–1003.

10. WHO (2011) Waist Circumference and Waist-Hip Ratio: Report of a WHO Expert Consultation, Geneva, 8–11 December 2008. Technical report, World Health Organization.

11. Klein S, Allison DB, Heymsfield SB, Kelley DE, Leibel RL, et al. (2007) "Waist circumference and cardiometabolic risk: a consensus statement from Shaping America's Health." *Diabetes Care,* 30: 1647–1652.

12. Burton R (2010) "Waist circumference as an indicator of adiposity and the relevance of body height." *Medical Hypotheses,* 75: 115–119.

13. Trunk Fat as a Determinant of Liver Disease, 24 February 2010, Jacquelyn J. Maher *Gastroenterology,* April 2010, vol. 138, issue 4, 1244–1246.

14. Bujalska IJ, Kumar S, Stewart PM (1997). "Does central obesity reflect 'Cushing's disease of the momentum?" *Lancet* 349 (9060): 1210–3. doi:10.1016/S0140-6736(96)11222-8. PMID 9130942.

15. Bacon, Linda, Aphramor, Lucy (January 24, 2011). "Weight Science: Evaluating the Evidence for a Paradigm Shift." Nutr J. 10 (9). doi:10.1186/1475-2891-10-9. PMC 3041737. PMID 21261939.

16. Després, Jean-Pierre, Lemieux (14 December 2006). "Isabelle." Abdominal obesity and metabolic syndrome. *Nature* 444: 881–887. Retrieved March 12, 2012.

17. Poelhlman, E. T. "Abdominal obesity: the metabolic multi-risk factor." *Coronary Heart Disease.* Exp. 9:469-471, 1998.

18. Huffman DM, Barzilai N (2009). "Role of visceral adipose tissue in aging." BIOCHEMICA ET BIOPHYSICA ACTA 1790 (10): 1117–1123. doi:10.1016/j.bbagen.2009.01.008. PMC 2779572. PMID 19364483.

19. Griesemer, Rebecca Lynn (July 25, 2008). "Index of Central Obesity as a Parameter to Evaluate Metabolic Syndrome for White, Black, and Hispanic Adults in the United States," (Master's thesis). Georgia State University.
20. Deepak Chopra, L. Trivieri Jr., John Anderson. "Body Mass Index: Alternative Medicine, the definitive guide." 2nd. Ed. 821–836.
21. The Weston A. Price Foundation, Rs, "Soy in foods."
22. Dr. Kaalylaya Daniel, "The Whole Soy Story."

Chapter 4

1. Reusser, M.E., McCarron, D.A., Nutr Rev., 1994: 52, 367–375.
2. Rosenberg, I.H., Solomons, N.W. "In: Absorption and Malabsorption of Mineral Nutrients." Alan R. Liss, 1984, 2.
3. Alexander G. Schauss, PhD, "Minerals and Human Health, The Rationale for Optimal and Balanced Trace Element Levels," *The Journal of Agriculture and Food Chemistry* 2006.
4. van Kessel JC, Rutherford ST, Shao Y, Utria AF, Bassler BL. (2013) "Individual and combined roles of the master regulators AphA and LuxR in control of the Vibrio harveyi quorum-sensing regulon." *J Bacteriol* 195:436–443.
5. Rutherford ST, Bassler BL. (2012) "Bacterial quorum sensing: its role in virulence and possibilities for its control." In Cold Spring Harbor Perspectives. *Bacterial Pathogens,* Eds Maloy S and Cossart P. Cold Spring Harbor Press.
6. Bassler BL (2010) "Cell-to-Cell Communication." *Proc Am Philos Soc* 154:307–314. Annu Rev Microbiol. 2001,55:165–99. "Quorum sensing in bacteria." Miller MB (1), *Bassler* BL. Author information: (1) Department of Molecular Biology, Princeton University.
7. Kenneth Todar, PhD, "The Normal Bacterial Flora of Humans," *Textbook of Bacteriology,* .net. 201, 3 1–5.
8. Guarner, F, Malagelada, J (2003). "Gut flora in health and disease." *Lancet,* 361 (9356): 512–9.
9. Sears, Cynthia L. (2005). "A dynamic partnership: Celebrating our gut flora." *Anaerobe* 11 (5): 247–51. doi:10.1016/j. anaerobe.2005.05.001. PMID 16701579.

10. Steinhoff, U (2005). "Who controls the crowd? New findings and old questions about the intestinal microflora." *Immunology Letters* 99 (1): 12–6. doi:10.1016/j.imlet.2004.12.013. PMID 15894105.

11. Arumugam, Manimozhiyan, Raes, Jeroen, Pelletier, Eric, Le Paslier, Denis, Yamada, Takuji, Mende, Daniel R., Fernandes, Gabriel R., Tap, Julien, Bruls, Thomas, Batto, Jean-Michel, Bertalan, Marcelo, Borruel, Natalia, Casellas, Francesc, Fernandez, Leyden, Gautier, Laurent, Hansen, Torben, Hattori, Masahira, Hayashi, Tetsuya, Kleerebezem, Michiel, Kurokawa, Ken, Leclerc, Marion, Levenez, Florence, Manichanh, Chaysavanh, Nielsen, H. Bjørn, Nielsen, Trine, Pons, Nicolas, Poulain, Julie, Qin, Junjie, Sicheritz-Ponten, Thomas, Tims, Sebastian (2011). "Enterotypes of the human gut microbiome." *Nature* 473 (7346): 174–80. doi: 10.1038/nature09944. PMC 3728647. PMID 21508958.

12. Wu, G. D., Chen, J., Hoffmann, C., Bittinger, K., Chen, Y.-Y., Keilbaugh, S. A., Bewtra, M., Knights, D., Walters, W. A., Knight, R., Sinha, R., Gilroy, E., Gupta, K., Baldassano, R., Nessel, L., Li, H., Bushman, F. D., Lewis, J. D. (2011). "Linking Long-Term Dietary Patterns with Gut Microbial Enterotypes," *Science* 334 (6052): 105–8. doi:10.1126/science.1208344. PMC 3368382. PMID 21885731.

13. Zimmer, Carl (April 20, 2011). "Bacteria Divide People Into 3 Types, Scientists Say." *New York Times*. Retrieved April 21, 2011. "A group of scientists now report just three distinct ecosystems in the guts of people they have studied."

14. Coppa, Giovanni V, Bruni, Stefano, Morelli, Lorenzo, Soldi, Sara, Gabrielli, Orazio (2004). "The First Prebiotics in Humans." *Journal of Clinical Gastroenterology* 38 (6 Suppl): S80–3. doi:10.1097/01.mcg.0000128926.14285.25. PMID 15220665.

15. Coppa, G.V., Zampini, L., Galeazzi, T., Gabrielli, O. (2006). "Prebiotics in human milk: A review." *Digestive and Liver Disease* 38: S291–4. doi:10.1016/S1590-8658(07)60013-9. PMID 17259094.

16. Wynne, Anthony G, McCartney, Anne L, Brostoff, Jonathan, Hudspith, Barry N, Gibson, Glenn R (2004). "An in vitro assessment of the effects of broad-spectrum antibiotics on the human gut microflora and concomitant isolation of a Lactobacillus plantarum

with anti-Candida activities." *Anaerobe* 10 (3): 165–9. doi:10.1016/j. anaerobe.2004.03.002. PMID 16701514.

17. Keeley J. 2004. "Good bacteria trigger proteins to protect the gut." Howard Hughes Medical Institute. Eurek Alert. Accessed January 9, 2007.

18. Denise Kelly[1], Jamie I Campbell[1], Timothy P King[1], George Grant[1], Emmelie A Jansson[2], Alistair G P Coutts[1], Sven Pettersson[2] & Shaun Conway[1] [1] Gut Immunology Group, Rowett Research Institute, Greenburn Road, Bucksburn, Aberdeen AB21 9SB, Scotland, UK. [2] Microbiology & Tumor Biology Center, Division of Molecular Pathology, Karolinska Institute, S-171 77 Stockholm, Sweden. "Commensal anaerobic gut bacteria attenuate inflammation by regulating nuclear-cytoplasmic shuttling of PPAR -Y and RelA", *Nature Immunology* 5, 104–112 (2003).

19. Gregory J. Velicer, Social strife in the microbial world: *Trends in Microbiology*, vol. 11, issue 7, 330–337. July 2003.

20. John A. Hamilton, Adrian Achuthan, "Colony stimulating factors and myeloid cell biology in health and disease: Trends in Immunology," vol. 34, issue 2, 81–89. Published online: September 24, 2012.

21. Van Kessel JC, Rutherford ST, Shao Y, Utria AF, Bassler BL. (2013) Individual and combined roles of the master regulators AphA and LuxR in control of the Vibrio harveyi quorum-sensing regulon. J Bacteriol 195:436-443.

22. Rutherford ST, Bassler BL. (2012) Bacterial quorum sensing: its role in virulence and possibilities for its control. In Cold Spring Harbor Perspectives. Bacterial Pathogens Eds Maloy S and Cossart P. Cold Spring Harbor Press.

23. Bassler BL (2010) "Cell-to-Cell Communication." Proc Am Philos Soc 154:307–314.

24. McGraw-Hill Dictionary of Scientific and Technical Terms, 63: 2003, McGraw-Hill Co. Inc.

25. Cho, I, Yamanishi, S, Cox, L, Methé, BA, Zavadil, J, Li, K, Gao, Z, Mahana, D, Raju, K, Teitler, I, Li, H, Alekseyenko, AV, Blaser, MJ (2012). "Antibiotics in early life alter the murine colonic

microbiome and adiposity." *Nature* 488 (7413): 621–6. doi:10.1038/nature11400. PMC 3553221. PMID 22914093.

26. Guarner, Francisco, Malagelada, Juan-R (2003). "Role of bacteria in experimental colitis." Best Practice & Research Clinical Gastroenterology 17 (5): 793–804. doi: 10.1016/S1521-6918(03)00068-4. PMID 14507589.

27. Kim, Eun-Hee, Hong, Hua, Choi, Ki-Seok, Han, Young-Min, Kangwan, Napapan, Cho, Young Chae, Hahm, Ki Baik (April 2012). "High Concentrated Probiotics Improve Inflammatory Bowel Diseases Better than Commercial Concentration of Probiotics." *Journal of Food & Drug Analysis* 20: 292–5.

Chapter 5

1. J. Julie Wu, Jie Liu, Edmund B. Chen, Jennifer J. Wang, Liu Cao, Nisha Narayan, Marie M. Fergusson, Ilsa I. Rovira, Michele Allen, Danielle A. Springer, Cory U. Lago, Shuling Zhang, Wendy DuBois, Theresa Ward, Rafael deCabo, Oksana Gavrilova, Beverly Mock, Toren Finkel. "Increased Mammalian Lifespan and a Segmental and Tissue-Specific Slowing of Aging after Genetic Reduction of mTOR Expression," *Cell Reports*, volume 4, issue 5, 913–920, 29 August 2013.

2. Owen O.E., P. Felig, A. P. Morgan, J. Wahren, and G.F. Cahill Jr., 1969. "Liver and Kidney Metabolism during Prolonged Starvation." *J. Clin. Invest.* 48: 574–583.

3. Owen O. E., A. P. Morgan, H. G. Kemp, J. M. Sullivan, G. M. Herrera, and G. F. Cahill Jr. 1967: "Brain Metabolism During Fasting." *J. Clin. Invest.* 46: 1589–1595.

4. A. J. Garber, P. H. Menzel, G. Boden, O. E. Owen, "Hepatic Ketogenesis and Glucogenesis in Humans." *J. Clin. Invest.* Vol 54–4, 1974, 54 – (4) 981–989.

5. Robert C Johnson, Susan K Young, Richard Cotter, Lawrence Lin, and W Bruce Rowe (1990). "Medium-chain-triglyceride lipid emulsion: metabolism and tissue distribution." *Am J Clin Nutr* 52 (3): 502–8.

6. Marshall, William J., Bangert, Stephen K. (2008). "Clinical biochemistry: metabolic and clinical aspects." Elsevier Health Sciences. 67–80. ISBN 978-0-443-10186-1.

7. Hartman AL, Vining EP (January 2007). "Clinical aspects of the ketogenic diet." Epilepsia 48 (1): 31–42. doi: 10.1111/j.1528-1167.2007.00914.x. PMID 17241206.

8. Taboulet, P., Deconinck, N., Thurel, A., Haas, L., Manamani, J., Porcher, R., Schmit, C., Fontaine, J., Gautier, J. (2007). "Correlation between urine ketones (acetoacetate) and capillary blood ketones (3-beta-hydroxybutyrate) in hyperglycaemic patients." *Diabetes & Metabolism* 33 (2): 135–139. doi:10.1016/j.diabet.2006.11.006.

9. Sekizawa, A, Sugito, Y, Iwasaki, M, Watanabe, A, Jimbo, M, Hoshi, S, Saito, H, Okai, T (2001). "Cell-free fetal DNA is increased in plasma of women with hyperemesis gravidarum." *Clinical Chemistry* 47 (12): 2164–5. PMID 11719487.

10. Burbos, Nikolaos, Shiner, Alice M., Morris, Edward (2008). "Severe metabolic acidosis as a consequence of acute starvation in pregnancy." Archives of Gynecology and Obstetrics 279 (3): 399–400. doi:10.1007/s00404-008-0715-3. PMID 18592261.

11. Phinney, Stephen D. (2004). "Ketogenic diets and physical performance." *Nutrition & Metabolism* 1 (1): 2. doi:10.1186/1743-7075-1-2. PMC 524027. PMID 15507148.

12. McClellan, Walter S., Du Bois, Eugene F. (February 13, 1930). "The Effects on Human Beings of a Twelve Months' Exclusive Meat Diet" (PDF). *Journal of the American Medical Association*.

13. Cordain, L., J. B. Miller, S. B. Eaton, N. Mann, S. H. Holt, and J.D. Speth (2000). "Plant-Animal Subsistence Ratios and Macronutrient Energy Estimations in Worldwide Hunter-Gatherer Diets." *American Journal of Clinical Nutrition,* 71 (3): 682–92.

14. Andreas Eenfeldt, MD. "The Carb Controversy", Published 2013, Ancestral Health Symposium, 2012.

15. "Eurekalart study finds, Routine periodic fasting is good for health and your heart," April 3, 2011. *British Journal of Nutrition* 2013 Oct., 110 (8): 1534–47.

16. Seyfried B T, Kiebish M, Marsh J, Mukherjee P. "Targeting Energy Metabolism in Brain Cancer through Calorie Restriction and the Ketogenic Diet. J Can Res Ther 2009, 5:7–15.

Chapter 6

1. Gray, Pickering and Howden, *Gray's Anatomy: The Liver.* 930–942, Ann Arbor Media, 2003.
2. Maton, Anthea, Jean Hopkins, Charles William McLaughlin, Susan Johnson, Maryanna Quon Warner, David LaHart, Jill D. Wright (1993). *Human Biology and Health.* Englewood Cliffs, New Jersey, USA: Prentice Hall. ISBN 0-13-981176-1. OCLC 32308337.
3. Dieter Häussinger, ed. (2011). *Liver Regeneration.* Berlin: De Gruyter. 1. ISBN 9783110250794.
4. Poehlman, Eric T. (1998). *Abdominal Obesity: The Metabolic Multi-Risk Factor* 9 (8). 469–471.
5. Carey, David G.P. (February 1998). *Abdominal Obesity,* 35–40. Retrieved 6 April 2012.
6. Jewell, A.P. (2005). "Is the liver an important site for the development of immune tolerance to tumours?" *Medical Hypotheses* 64 (4): 751–4. doi:10.1016/j.mehy.2004.10.002. PMID 15694692.
7. Malik VS, Popkin BM, Bray GA, Després JP, Willett WC, Hu FB (2010). "Sugar-sweetened beverages and risk of metabolic syndrome and type 2 diabetes: a meta-analysis." *Diabetes Care* 33 (11): 2477–83. doi:10.2337/dc10-1079. PMC 2963518. PMID 20693348.
8. Nakagawa T, Hu H, Zharikov S, Tuttle KR, Short RA, Glushakova O, Ouyang X, Feig DI, Block ER, Herrera-Acosta J, Patel JM, Johnson RJ (2006). "A causal role for uric acid in fructose-induced metabolic syndrome." *Am J Phys Renal Phys* 290 (3): F625–F631. doi:10.1152/ajprenal.00140.2005. PMID 16234313.
9. Hallfrisch J (1990). "Metabolic effects of dietary fructose." FASEB J 4 (9): 2652–2660. PMID 2189777.
10. Reiser S, Powell AS, Scholfield DJ, Panda P, Ellwood KC, Canary JJ (1989). "Blood lipids, lipoproteins, apoproteins, and uric acid in men fed diets containing fructose or high-amylose cornstarch." *Am J Clin Nutr* 49 (5): 832–839. PMID 2497634.

11. Bremer, AA, Mietus-Snyder, M, Lustig, RH. (2012 Mar,). "Toward a unifying hypothesis of metabolic syndrome." *Pediatrics.* 129 (3): 557–70. doi:10.1542/peds.2011-2912. PMID 22351884.

12. Hotamisligil GS. (June 1999). "The Role of TNF-alpha and TNF receptors in Obesity and Insulin Resistance." *Journal of Internal Medicine* 245 (6): 621–625. doi:10.1046/j.1365-2796.1999.00490.x. PMID 10395191.

13. Fukuchi S, Hamaguchi K, Seike M, Himeno K, Sakata T, Yoshimatsu H. (1 June 2004). "Role of Fatty Acid Composition in the Development of Metabolic Disorders in Sucrose-Induced Obese Rats." *Exp Biol Med* 229 (6): 486–493. PMID 15169967.

14. Whitney, Ellie and Ralfes, R. Sharon. 2011. *Understanding Nutrition.* Wadsworth Cengage Learning: Belmont, CA

15. Marchesini G[1], Marzocchi R, Agostini F, Bugianesi E., "Nonalcoholic fatty liver disease and the metabolic syndrome." *Curr Opin Lipidol.* 2005 Aug, 16(4):421–7.

Chapter 7

1. Chicago, June 27 (Ascribe Newswire) Samuel S. Epstein, MD, professor emeritus of environmental and occupational medicine at the University of Illinois at Chicago School of Public Health and Chairman of the Cancer Prevention Coalition. Commentary, Hormonal Milk Poses Greater Risks Than Just Twinning. "What's in Your Milk?" by Samuel Epstein, MD Epstein Tue Jun 27 09:05:47 2006 2011 May 11, 59(9):5125-32. Epub 2011 Apr 15.

2. Dr. Kaazla T. Daniel, *The Whole Soy Story, The Dark Side of America's Favorite Health Food.* New Trends Pub, 2005.

3. Azzouz A, Jurado-Sánchez B, Souhail B, Ballesteros E. Department of Physical and Analytical Chemistry, EPS of Linares, University of Jaén, Linares, Jaén, Spain. J of Agric Food Chem. May 2011 59(9) 5125 – 32 / EPub 2010 Apr 15, "Simultaneous determination of 20 pharmacologically active substances in cow's milk, goat's milk, and human breast milk by gas chromatography-mass spectrometry."

4. Alendini A, Green PH, Sander HW, Hays AP, Gamboa ET, Fasano A, Sonnenberg M, Lewis LD, Latov N, Department of

Neurology and Neuroscience, Cornell University, 525 E. 68th St. LC-807, New York, NY. 10021, USA Ara 2004 @medcornell.edu. J of Neuroimmunology 2002 June, 127(1–2): 145–8, Ganglioside Reactive Antibodies in the Neuropathy Associated with Celiac Disease.

5. Not T, Horvath K, Hill ID, Partaner J, Hammed A, Magazzu G, Fasano A, Dept. of Pediatrics University of Maryland at Baltimore 21201-1595, USA. Scand J. Gastroenterol May 1998, 33(5): 494 – 8, Celiac Disease in the USA, High Presence of Antiendomysium Antibodies in healthy blood donors.

6. University of Maryland Center for Celiac Research, 001-800-4925538, wwwceliaccenter.org.

7. Gluten-Free Diets, www.inside-story.com .

8. Knowles JA. J. Pediatrics 1965 Jun, 66: 1068–82 Excretion of Drugs in Milk: A Review.

9. John Chisholm, "Healthy Milk Has Its Own Immunity." *Lib. Wellness,* Oct. 31, 2010

10. Benachour N, Seralini G-E. 2009. "Glyphosate formulations induce apoptosis and necrosis in human umbilical, embryonic, and placental cells." *Chem Res Toxicol* 22:97–105.

11. Arbuckle TE, Lin Z, Mery LS. 2001. "An exploratory analysis of the effect of pesticide exposure on the risk of spontaneous abortion in an Ontario farm population." *Environ Health Perspect* 109:851–57.

12. Savitz DA, Arbuckle T, Kaczor D, Curtis KM. 1997. "Male pesticide exposure and pregnancy outcome." *Am J Epidemiol* 146(12):1025–36.

13. Yousef MI. 1995. "Toxic effects of carbofuran and glyphosate on semen characteristics in rabbits." *J Environ Sci Health B* 30(4):513–34.

14. *Medical News Today* May 4, 2012, "Exposing Fetus to Plant Estrogens May Lead to Infertility in Women."

15. Jefferson WN, Padilla-Banks E., Phelps JY., Cantor AM, Williams CJ, Reproductive Medical Group Laboratory of Reproductive and Environmental Toxicology, National Institute of Environmental Health Sciences, National Institute of Health, Research Triangle Park, North Carolina. "Abstract" Neonatal Phytoestrogen Exposure

Alters Oviduct Mucosal Immune Response to Pregnancy and Affects Pre-implantation and Embryo Development in Mouse."

16. American Academy of Pediatrics Vol 97 No. 3 Mar 1, 1996, 413–416 with re-affirmation statement to, Abstract, "Aluminum Toxicity in Infants and Children." Re Affirmation J. Pediatrics 2004, 114-4 1126, doi 10.1542 / peds. 2004–1516.

17. Michelle Zeager DO, MPH, Alen Woolf MD, MPH, Rose H Goldman MD, MPH. – J Pediatrics vol. 129 No. 1, Jan. 2012 e142–e147 (doi 10. 1542 / peds. 2010 – 3481), "Wide Variation of Reference Values for Aluminum Levels in Children."

18. Kenneth DR Setchell PHD, Linda Zimmer- Nechemias MS, Jinnan Cai MS, James E. Heubi MD. "Exposure of Infants to Phyto-Estrogens from Soy-Based Infant Formula." *Lancet* vol. 350, issue 9070, 23–27 July 1997.

19. Rosendale, R. MD., Designs for Health Institute's Boulder Fest Seminar, Aug 1999: "Insulin and Its Metabolic Effects."

20. Anderson JW, Johnstone BM, Cook-Newell ME. "Meta-analysis of the effects of soy protein intake on serum lipids." *N Engl J Med.* 1995,333(5):276–282.

21. Sacks FM, Lichtenstein A, Van Horn L, Harris W, Kris-Etherton P, Winston M. Soy Protein, Isoflavones, and Cardiovascular Health. An American Heart Association Science Advisory for Professionals, From the Nutrition Committee. Circulation. 2006, 113(7):1034-1044.

Chapters 8 and 9

1. Farooqui, AA, Farooqui T, Panza F, Frisardi V. (2012). "Metabolic syndrome as a risk factor for neurological disorders," *Cell Mol Life Sci.* 69 (5): 741–62. doi: 10.1007/s00018-011-0840-1. PMID 21997383.

2. Berthoud, H. R., Neuhuber, W. L. (2000). "Functional and chemical anatomy of the afferent vagal system." *Autonomic Neuroscience* 85 (1–3): 1–17. doi: 10.1016/S1566-0702(00)00215-0. PMID 11189015.

3. "Exploring the Mind-Body Orgasm," *Wired.* 2007-01-10.

4. Komisaruk, B.R, Whipple, B., Crawford, A., Grimes, S., Liu, W-C., Kalin, A., & Mosier, K. (2004). "Brain activation during

vaginocervical self-stimulation and orgasm in women with complete spinal cord injury: MRI evidence of mediation by the Vagus nerves."

5. http://www.utdallas.edu/news/2011/1/13-8021_Findings-Show-Promise-in-Battle-Against-Tinnitus_article.html

6. Vibhuti N, Singh, Monika Gugneja (2005-08-22). "Supraventricular Tachycardia." eMedicineHealth.com. Retrieved 2008-11-28.

7. Parrinello, et al. (2010) EphB signaling directs peripheral nerve regeneration through Sox2-dependent Schwann cell sorting. Cell: 143,145–155. DOI 10.1016/j.cell.2010.08.039. University College London (UCL): Life Sciences, Medicine, Health, Scientific Research, Biotechnology, Coordination, Cooperation.

8. Renaud Desgraz, Claire Bonal, Pedro L. Herrera, "β-Cell regeneration: the pancreatic intrinsic faculty:" *Trends in Endocrinology & Metabolism*, vol. 22, issue 1, 34–43. Published online: November 9, 2010.

9. Gordana Vunjak-Novakovic, David T. Scadden, Biomimetic Platforms for Human Stem Cell Research: Cell Stem Cell, vol. 8, issue 3, 252–261, Published in issue: March 04, 2011

10. Hartmut Geiger, K. Lenhard Rudolph, Aging in the lympho-hematopoietic stem cell compartment: Trends in Immunology, vol. 30, issue 7, 360–365. Published online: June 19, 2009.

11. Elizabeth Gould, Patima Tanapat, Nicholas B. Hastings, Tracey J. Shors, "Post-natal origin of microneurones in the rat brain," *Trends in Cognitive Sciences*, vol. 3, issue 5, 186–192. Published in issue: May 01, 1999.

12. Narveen Jandu, "Microbiology for the masses: teaching concepts and skills for a general audience," *Trends in Microbiology*, vol. 20, issue 10, 459–460. Published online: August 17, 2012.

13. Pamela A. Carpentier, Theo D. Palmer, "Immune Influence on Adult Neural Stem Cell Regulation and Function," *Neuron*, vol. 64, issue 1, 79–92. Published in issue: October 15, 2009.

14. Yaniv Ziv, Michal Schwartz, "Orchestrating brain-cell renewal: the role of immune cells in adult neurogenesis in health and disease," *Trends in Molecular Medicine*, vol. 14, issue 11, 471–478. Published online: October 23, 2008.

15. Kartik Chandran, Max L Nibert, "Animal cell invasion by a large nonenveloped virus: reovirus delivers the goods," *Trends in Microbiology*, vol. 11, issue 8, 374–382. Published in issue: August 2003.

16. M. William Lensch, Christine L. Mummery, "From Stealing Fire to Cellular Reprogramming: A Scientific History Leading to the 2012 Nobel Prize," *Stem Cell Reports*, vol. 1, issue 1, 5–17. Published in issue: June 04, 2013.

17. Amy Duckmanton, Anoop Kumar, Young-Tae Chang, Jeremy P. Brockes, "A Single-Cell Analysis of Myogenic Dedifferentiation Induced by Small Molecules," *Chemistry & Biology*, vol. 12, issue 10, 1117–1126. Published in issue: October 2005.

18. Irit Meivar-Levy, Sarah Ferber, "New organs from our own tissues: liver-to-pancreas transdifferentiation," *Trends in Endocrinology & Metabolism*, vol. 14, issue 10, 460–466. Published in issue: December 2003.

19. Stavros C. Manolagas, A. Michael Parfitt, "What old means to bone," *Trends in Endocrinology & Metabolism*, vol. 21, issue 6, 369–374. Published online: March 10, 2010.

20. Arumugam, Manimozhiyan, Raes, Jeroen, Pelletier, Eric, Le Paslier, Denis, Yamada, Takuji, Mende, Daniel R., Fernandes, Gabriel R., Tap, Julien, Bruls, Thomas, Batto, Jean-Michel, Bertalan, Marcelo, Borruel, Natalia, Casellas, Francesc, Fernandez, Leyden, Gautier, Laurent, Hansen, Torben, Hattori, Masahira, Hayashi, Tetsuya, Kleerebezem, Michiel, Kurokawa, Ken, Leclerc, Marion, Levenez, Florence, Manichanh, Chaysavanh, Nielsen, H. Bjørn, Nielsen, Trine, Pons, Nicolas, Poulain, Julie, Qin, Junjie, Sicheritz-Ponten, Thomas, Tims, Sebastian (2011). "Enterotypes of the human gut microbiome." *Nature* 473 (7346): 174–80. doi:10.1038/nature09944. PMC 3728647. PMID 21508958.

21. Wu, G. D., Chen, J., Hoffmann, C., Bittinger, K., Chen, Y.-Y., Keilbaugh, S. A., Bewtra, M., Knights, D., Walters, W. A., Knight, R., Sinha, R., Gilroy, E., Gupta, K., Baldassano, R., Nessel, L., Li, H., Bushman, F. D., Lewis, J. D. (2011). "Linking Long-Term Dietary Patterns with Gut Microbial Enterotypes." *Science* 334 (6052): 105–8. doi: 10.1126/science.1208344. PMC 3368382. PMID 21885731.

22. Zimmer, Carl (April 20, 2011). "Bacteria Divide People Into 3 Types, Scientists Say." *New York Times*. Retrieved April 21, 2011. "A group of scientists now report just three distinct ecosystems in the guts of people they have studied."

23. Alberts B, Johnson A, Lewis J, et al.; Molecular Biology of The Cell; 4th ed.: New York: Garland Science; 2002.

Chapters 10 and 11

1. Food and Nutrition Board (2005). A Report of the Panel on acronutrients, Subcommittees on Upper Reference Levels of Nutrients and Interpretation and Uses of Dietary Reference Intakes, and the Standing Committee on the Scientific Evaluation of Dietary Reference Intakes. Dietary Reference Intakes for Energy, Carbohydrate, Fiber, Fat, Fatty Acids, Cholesterol, Protein, and Amino Acids (Macronutrients). The National Academies Press, Washington, DC. ISBN 0-309-08537-3.

2. Bilsborough, Shane, Neil Mann (2006). "A Review of issues of Dietary Protein Intake in Humans." *International Journal of Sport Nutrition and Exercise Metabolism* (16): 129–152. Retrieved 6 December 2012.

3. Tarnopolsky MA, Atkinson SA, MacDougall JD, Chesley A, Phillips S, Schwarcz HP (1992). "Evaluation of protein requirements for trained strength athletes." *Journal of Applied Physiology* 73 (5): 1986–95. PMID 1474076.

4. "Dietary reference intakes: macronutrients" (PDF). Institute of Medicine. Retrieved 18 May 2008.

5. Born Steve. "Fueling for endurance: ten mistakes endurance athletes make and how you can avoid them." *UltraCycling Magazine.*

6. Elliott, Paul, Stamler, Jeremiah, Dyer, Alan R., Appel, Lawrence, Dennis, Barbara, Kesteloot, Hugo, Ueshima, Hirotsugu, Okayama, Akira, Chan, Queenie, Garside, Daniel B., Beifan, Zhou (2006). "Association between protein intake and blood pressure: the INTERMAP Study." Archives of Internal Medicine 166 (1): 79–87. doi: 10.1001/archinte.166.1.79. PMID 16401814. Retrieved 21 January 2013.

7. Spirin V, Gelfand M, Mironov A, Mirny L (June 2006). "A metabolic network in the evolutionary context: Multiscale structure and modularity." Proc Natl Acad Sci USA 103 (23): 8774–9. Bibcode:2006PNAS..103.8774S. do i:10.1073/pnas.0510258103. PMC 1482654. PMID 16731630.

8. McConville M, Menon A (2000). "Recent developments in the cell biology and biochemistry of glycosylphosphatidylinositol lipids (review)." Mol Membr Biol 17 (1): 1–16. doi: 10.1080/096876800294443. PMID 10824734.

9. "Identification of casein as the major allergenic and antigenic protein of cow's milk – Docena–2007–Allergy–Wiley Online Library." Campbell, T.C. and Campbell, T.M. 2006. The China Study. Benbella Books.

10. J. Pearce (1983). "Fatty acid synthesis in liver and adipose tissue." Proceedings of the Nutrition Society, 42, 263–271. Doi: 10.1079/PNS19830031.

11. Karmen, Arthur, Whyte, Malcolm, Goodman, DeWitt S. (July 1963). "Fatty acid esterification and chylomicron formation during fat absorption: 1. Triglycerides and cholesterol esters." *The Journal of Lipid Research* 4: 312–321. PMID 14168169. Retrieved 24 August 2013.

12. Lichtenstein AH, Jones PJ. Lipids: absorption and transport. In: Bowman BA, Russel RM, eds. Present Knowledge in Nutrition. 8th ed. Washington, D. C.: ILSI Press, 2001:93–103.

13. Muskiet FA, Fokkema MR, Schaafsma A, Boersma ER, Crawford MA. "Is docosahexaenoic acid (DHA) essential? Lessons from DHA status regulation, our ancient diet, epidemiology and randomized controlled trials. *J Nutr.* 2004, 134(1):183–186.

14. Cunnane SC. "Problems with essential fatty acids: time for a new paradigm?" *Prog Lipid Res.* 2003, 42(6):544–568.

15. Stillwell W, Wassall SR. "Docosahexaenoic acid: membrane properties of a unique fatty acid." *Chem Phys Lipids.* 2003, 126(1):1–27.

16. Innis SM. "Perinatal biochemistry and physiology of long-chain polyunsaturated fatty acids." *J Pediatr.* 2003, 143(4 Suppl): S1–8.

17. Fedorova I, Hussein N, Baumann MH, Di Martino C, Salem N, Jr. "An n-3 fatty acid deficiency impairs rat spatial learning in the Barnes maze." *Behav Neurosci.* 2009, 123(1):196–205.

18. Fedorova I, Salem N, Jr. "Omega-3 fatty acids and rodent behavior." Prostaglandins Leukot Essent Fatty Acids. 2006, 75(4–5):271–289.

19. Koletzko B, Lien E, Agostoni C, et al. "The roles of long-chain polyunsaturated fatty acids in pregnancy, lactation and infancy: review of current knowledge and consensus recommendations." *J Perinat Med.* 2008, 36(1):5–14.

20. Kris-Etherton PM, Harris WS, Appel LJ. "Fish consumption, fish oil, omega-3 fatty acids, and cardiovascular disease." *Circulation.* 2002, 106(21):2747–2757.

21. Calder PC. "Dietary modification of inflammation with lipids." *Proc Nutr Soc.* 2002, 61(3):345–358. http://www.ncbi.nlm.nih. gov/entrez/query.fcgi?cmd=Retrieve&db=PubMed&list_uids= 12296294&dopt=Abstract: "Symptoms of DHA deficiency is seen in skin reactions (rashes and scaling) similar to immune response. May be coupled with the formation of Sulfa and lipids in the skin."

22. Jeppesen PB, Hoy CE, Mortensen PB. "Essential fatty acid deficiency in patients receiving home parenteral nutrition." *Am J Clin Nutr.* 1998, 68(1):126–133.

23. Smit EN, Muskiet FA, Boersma ER. "The possible role of essential fatty acids in the pathophysiology of malnutrition: a review." Prostaglandins Leukot Essent Fatty Acids. 2004,71(4):241–250.

24. Mascioli EA, Lopes SM, Champagne C, Driscoll DF. "Essential fatty acid deficiency and home total parenteral nutrition patients." *Nutrition.* 1996, 12(4):245–249.

25. Steggink LD, Freeman JB, Wispe J, Connor WE. "Absence of the biochemical symptoms of essential fatty acid deficiency in surgical patients undergoing protein sparing therapy." *Am J Clin Nutr.* 1977, 30(3):388–393.

26. Jeppesen PB, Hoy CE, Mortensen PB. "Deficiencies of essential fatty acids, vitamin A and E and changes in plasma lipoproteins in patients with reduced fat absorption or intestinal failure." *Eur J Clin Nutr.* 2000, 54(8):632–642.

27. Lepage G, Levy E, Ronco N, Smith L, Galeano N, Roy CC. "Direct transesterification of plasma fatty acids for the diagnosis of essential fatty acid deficiency in cystic fibrosis." *J Lipid Res.* 1989,30(10):1483–1490.

28. Koletzko B, Lien E, Agostoni C, et al. "The roles of long-chain polyunsaturated fatty acids in pregnancy, lactation and infancy: review of current knowledge and consensus recommendations." *J Perinat Med.* 2008, 36(1):5–14. http://www.ncbi.nlm.nih.gov/entrez/query.fcgi?cmd=Retrieve&db=PubMed&dopt=Citation&list_uids=18184094

29. Leaf A, Xiao YF, Kang JX, Billman GE. "Prevention of sudden cardiac death by n-3 polyunsaturated fatty acids." *Pharmacol Ther.* 2003,98(3):355–377. http://www.ncbi.nlm.nih.gov/entrez/query.fcgi?cmd=Retrieve&db=pubmed&dopt=Abstract&list_uids=12782244&query_hl=60

30. Kris-Etherton PM, Harris WS, Appel LJ. "Omega-3 fatty acids and cardiovascular disease: new recommendations from the American Heart Association." *Arterioscler Thromb Vasc Biol.* 2003,23(2):151–152. http://www.ncbi.nlm.nih.gov/entrez/query.fcgi?cmd=Retrieve&db=pubmed&dopt=Abstract&list_uids=12588750&query_hl=57

31. Fortin PR, Lew RA, Liang MH, et al. "Validation of a meta-analysis: the effects of fish oil in rheumatoid arthritis." *J Clin Epidemiol.* 1995, 48(11):1379–1390.

32. Goldberg RJ, Katz J. "A meta-analysis of the analgesic effects of omega-3 polyunsaturated fatty acid supplementation for inflammatory joint pain." *Pain.* 2007, 129(1–2): 210–223.

33. Lorenz R, Weber PC, Szimnau P, Heldwein W, Strasser T, Loeschke K. "Supplementation with n-3 fatty acids from fish oil in chronic inflammatory bowel disease—a randomized, placebo-controlled, double-blind cross-over trial." *J Intern Med Suppl.* 1989, 225(731):225–232. http://www.ncbi.nlm.nih.gov/entrez/query.fcgi?cmd=Retrieve&db=PubMed&list_uids=2650694&dopt=Abstract

34. Lorenz-Meyer H, Bauer P, Nicolay C, et al. "Omega-3 fatty acids and low carbohydrate diet for maintenance of remission

in Crohn's disease. A randomized controlled multicenter trial. Study Group Members (German Crohn's Disease Study Group)." *Scand J Gastroenterol.* 1996, 31(8):778–785. http://www.ncbi.nlm.nih.gov/entrez/query.fcgi?cmd=Retrieve&db=PubMed&list_uids=8858747&dopt=Abstract.

35. Aslan A, Triadafilopoulos G. "Fish oil fatty acid supplementation in active ulcerative colitis: a double-blind, placebo-controlled, crossover study." *Am J Gastroenterol.* 1992, 87(4):432–437.

36. Stenson WF, Cort D, Rodgers J, et al. "Dietary supplementation with fish oil in ulcerative colitis." *Ann Intern Med.* 1992, 116(8): 609–614. http://www.ncbi.nlm.nih.gov/entrez/query.fcgi?cmd=Retrieve&db=PubMed&list_uids=1312317&dopt=Abstract

37. Hudgins LC, Hellerstein M, Seidman C, Neese R, Diakun J, Hirsch J. "Human fatty acid synthesis is stimulated by a eucaloric low fat, high carbohydrate diet." *J Clin Invest.* 1996, 97(9):2081–91.

38. United States Department of Agriculture. U.S. Food Supply – Food Supply Database. http://65.216.150.148/ifs/Query.htm. Accessed October 20, 2009.

39. Holman RT. "Autoxidation of fats and related substances. In: Progress in the chemistry of fats and other lipids." Academic Press, 1954, Dayton S, Pearce ML, Hashimoto S, Dixon WJ, Tomiyasu U. "A Controlled Clinical Trial of a Diet High in Unsaturated Fat in Preventing Complications of Atherosclerosis." Circulation. 1969, 40(1): Suppl 2:1–63.

40. Mata P, Odabella V, Alonso R, Lahoz C, de Oya M, Badimon L. "Monounsaturated and Polyunsaturated n-6 Fatty Acid-Enriched Diets Modify LDL Oxidation and Decrease Human Coronary Smooth Muscle Cell DNA Synthesis." *Arterioscler Thromb Vasc Biol.* 1997, 17(10):2088–95.

41. J J Kabara, *The Pharmacological Effects of Lipids,* J J Kabara, ed, The American Oil Chemists' Society, Champaign, IL, 1978, 1–14, L A Cohen, et al, J Natl Cancer Inst, 1986, 77:43.

42. B A Watkins and others. "Importance of Vitamin E in Bone Formation and in Chrondrocyte Function." Purdue University, Lafayette, IN, AOCS Proceedings, 1996, B A Watkins, and M F Seifert. *Food Lipids and Bone Health. Food Lipids and Health.* R

E McDonald and D B Min, eds, Marcel Dekker, Inc. New York, NY, 101.

43. J F Mead and others. *Lipids: Chemistry, Biochemistry and Nutrition,* Plenum Press, 1986, New York.

44. L D Lawson and F Kummerow. "B-Oxidation of the Coenzyme A Esters of Vaccenic, Elaidic and Petroselaidic Acids by Rat Heart Mitochondria." *Lipids,* 1979, 14:501–503.

45. Goerke J. "Pulmonary surfactant: functions and molecular composition." Biochim Biophys Acta. 1998, 1408(2–3): 79–89.

46. Data compiled from European Cardiovascular Disease Statistics, 2005 Edition, www.heartstats.org/uploads/documents%5CPDF.pdf.

47. Dreon, MD and others. *American Journal of Clinical Nutrition,* 2000 (71:1611–1616).

48. Hernandez ML. "Dietary cholesterol provided by eggs and plasma lipoproteins in healthy populations." *Curr Opin Clin Nutr Metab Care.* 2006,9(1):8–12.

49. Engelberg, Hyman, Lancet, Mar 21, 1992, 339: 727–728, Wood, W G, et al, Lipids, Mar 1999, 34(3):225–234.

50. He K, Rimm EB, Merchant A, et al. "Fish consumption and risk of stroke in men." *JAMA.* 2002, 288(24):3130–3136. (PubMed).

51. He K, Song Y, Daviglus ML, et al. "Fish consumption and incidence of stroke: a meta-analysis of cohort studies." *Stroke.* 2004, 35(7):1538–1542. (PubMed).

52. Tanaka K, Ishikawa Y, Yokoyama M, et al. "Reduction in the recurrence of stroke by eicosapentaenoic acid for hypercholesterolemic patients: subanalysis of the JELIS trial." *Stroke.* 2008, 39(7):2052–2058. (PubMed).

53. Austin MA, Hokanson JE, Edwards KL. "Hypertriglyceridemia as a cardiovascular risk factor." *Am J Cardiol.* 1998, 81(4A):7B–12B. (PubMed).

54. Harris WS. "N-3 fatty acids and serum lipoproteins: human studies." *Am J Clin Nutr.* 1997, 65(5 Suppl):1645S–1654S. (PubMed).

55. Iso H, Kobayashi M, Ishihara J, et al. "Intake of fish and n3 fatty acids and risk of coronary heart disease among Japanese: the Japan

Public Health Center-Based (JPHC) Study Cohort I." *Circulation*. 2006, 113(2):195–202. (PubMed).

56. Nakamura Y, Ueshima H, Okamura T, et al. "Association between fish consumption and all-cause and cause-specific mortality in Japan: NIPPON DATA80, 1980–99." *Am J Med*. 2005, 118(3):239–245. (PubMed).

57. Helland IB, Smith L, Saarem K, Saugstad OD, Drevon CA. "Maternal supplementation with very-long-chain n-3 fatty acids during pregnancy and lactation augments children's IQ at 4 years of age." *Pediatrics*. 2003, 111(1):e39–44. (PubMed).

58. Dunstan JA, Simmer K, Dixon G, Prescott SL. "Cognitive assessment of children at age 2(1/2) years after maternal fish oil supplementation in pregnancy: a randomised controlled trial." *Arch Dis Child Fetal Neonatal Ed*. 2008, 93(1):F45–50. (PubMed).

59. Judge MP, Harel O, Lammi-Keefe CJ. "Maternal consumption of a docosahexaenoic acid-containing functional food during pregnancy: benefit for infant performance on problem-solving but not on recognition memory tasks at age 9 mo." *Am J Clin Nutr*. 2007, 85(6):1572–1577.

60. Szajewska H, Horvath A, Koletzko B. "Effect of n-3 long-chain polyunsaturated fatty acid supplementation of women with low-risk pregnancies on pregnancy outcomes and growth measures at birth: a meta-analysis of randomized controlled trials." *Am J Clin Nutr*. 2006, 83(6):1337–1344.

61. European Commission Directorate General for Health and Consumer Protection. "Eurodiet: Nutrition and Diet for Healthy Lifestyles in Europe." 2001. Available at: http://ec.europa.eu/health/ph_determinants/life_style/nutrition/report01_en.pdf/. Accessed 3/9/09.

62. Hamazaki T, Okuyama H. The Japan Society for Lipid Nutrition recommends, "To reduce the intake of linoleic acid. A review and critique of the scientific evidence." *World Rev Nutr Diet*. 2003, 92:109–132. (PubMed).

63. Loren Cordain, Janette Brand Miller, S Boyd Eaton, Neil Mann, Susanne HA Holt, and John D Speth. "Plant-animal subsistence ratios and macronutrient energy estimations in worldwide

hunter-gatherer diets1, 2," 2000 American Society for Clinical Nutrition.

64. Robert C Johnson, Susan K Young, Richard Cotter, Lawrence Lin, and W Bruce Rowe (1990). "Medium-chain-triglyceride lipid emulsion: metabolism and tissue distribution." *Am J Clin Nutr* 52 (3): 502–8.

65. World Rev Nutr Diet. 2011, 102:124–36. doi: 10.1159/000327834. Epub 2011 Aug 5.

66. Okuyama H[1], Hamazaki T, Ogushi Y, "New Cholesterol Guidelines for Longevity (2010)," Committee on Cholesterol Guidelines for Longevity, the Japan Society for Lipid Nutrition.

67. Simopoulos AP (ed): "Healthy Agriculture, Healthy Nutrition, Healthy People." *World Rev Nutr Diet*. Basel, Karger, 2011, vol. 102, 124–136. (DOI:10.1159/000327834)

68. University of Copenhagen Facility of Health and Medical Sciences, healthsciences.ku.dk. "High Fat Diet and Brain Aging."

69. Alberts B, Johnson A, Lewis J, et al; Molecular Biology of The Cell, 4th ed. New York: Garland Science; 2002.

Chapter 12 References

1. Noakes TD, Wilson G, Gray DA, Lambert MI, Dennis SC (October 2001). "Peak rates of diuresis in healthy humans during oral fluid overload." *S. Afr. Med. J.* 91 (10): 852–7. PMID 11732457.

2. Almond CS, Shin AY, Fortescue EB, et al. (April 2005). "Hyponatremia among runners in the Boston Marathon." *N. Engl. J. Med.* 352 (15): 1550–6.

3. Moreau, David (Ed.). *Fluids and Electrolytes Made Incredibly Easy* (4th ed.). Lippincott Williams & Wilkins.

4. Timbrell, John (2005). *The Poison Paradox: Chemicals as Friends and Foes.* OUP Oxford. ISBN 978-0-19-280495-2.

5. "Research debunks health value of guzzling water." Reuters, April 2008.

6. H. Valtin, "Drink at least eight glasses of water a day. Really? Is there scientific evidence for 8 × 8?" *Am J Physiol Regul Integr Comp Physiol* 283: R993–R1004, 2002.

7. Negoianu, Dan, Goldfarb, Stanley (2008). "Just add water." *J. Am. Soc.* Nephrol 19 (6): 1041–1043. doi: 10.1681/ASN.2008030274. PMID 18385417

8. Noakes TD, Goodwin N, Rayner BL, et al. (1985). "Water intoxication: a possible complication during endurance exercise." *Med Sci Sports Exerc* 17 (3): 370–375. PMID 4021781.

9. Duhigg, Charles (2009-12-16). "That Tap Water Is Legal but May Be Unhealthy." *New York Times*.

10. Biological Water Filters says: "Pharmaceuticals in the Water Supply: Is this a threat? Water Matters—State of the Planet." Blogs. ei.columbia.edu. Retrieved 2011-12-05.

11. Crawford T, Crawford MD, "Prevalence of Pathological Changes of Ischemic Heart- Disease in a Hard-Water and in a Soft-Water Area." *Lancet*. 1967, 1: 229–232.

12. "Treatment Systems for Household Water Supplies." Distillation. Russell Derickson. Extension Associate in Water and Natural Resources. South Dakota. ww.ag.ndsu.edu/pubs/h2oqual/watsys/ae1032.pdf.

13. Y. Takahashi, D. M., and W. H. Daughaday, "Growth Hormone Secretion during Sleep." Washington University School of Medicine, Department of Medicine, Metabolism Division, St. Louis, Missouri 63110. *J Clin Invest*. Sep 1968, 47(9): 2079–2090. doi: 10.1172/JCI105893.

14. Hunter, W. M., J. A. R. Friend, and J. A. Strong, 1966. "The diurnal pattern of plasma growth hormone: concentration in adults." *J. Endocrinol*. 34:139.

15. Hunter, W. M., and W. M. Rigal. 1966. "The diurnal pattern of plasma growth hormone concentration in children and adolescents." *J. Endocrinol*. 34:147.

16. Quabbe, H-J., E. Schilling, and H. Helge. "1966: Pattern of growth hormone secretion during a 24-hour fast in normal adults." *J. Clin. Endocrinol*. 26:1173.

17. Dement, W., and N. Kleitman. 1957. "Cyclic variations in EEG during sleep and their relation to eye movements, body motility, and dreaming." *Electroencephalog*, Clin. Neurophysiol. 9:673.

18. Rick Nauert PhD, John M. Grohol, PsyD: "REM Sleep Disorder as Early Warning of Neurologic Impairment," *Psychotherapy News*, July 29, 2010.

19. Eric J. Olson, Bradley F. Boeve and Michael H. Silber: Department of Neurology, Mayo Clinic, Rochester, Minnesota, USA, "Rapid eye movement sleep behaviour disorder: demographic, clinical and laboratory findings in 93 cases," August 26, 1999.

20. Accepted National Institute of Neurological Disorders and Stroke National Institutes of Health: "Sleep, a Dynamic Activity, Dreaming and REM Sleep, What Does It Do For Us and How Much Do We Need?" Bethesda, MD 20892, NIH Publication No.06-3440-c, Last updated December 5, 2013.

21. UAB Neurology Sleep Services Director Jennifer L. DeWolfe, DO. "Sleep Problems. All in Your Head?" UAB Insight on Neurosciences, 2011.

22. Patlak, Joe, Gibbons, Ray (2000-11-01). "Electrical Activity of Nerves." *Aps in Nerve Cells*. Retrieved 2009-06-20.

23. National Institute of Health, "Understanding Neurology, Neurons, Brain Chemistry and Neurotransmission." 2010 BSCS and Videodiscovery Inc.

24. Dr. Chi Pang Wen MD, Jackson Pui Man Wai PhD, Min Kuang Tsai MS, Yi Chen Yang MS, Ting Yuan David Cheng MS, Meng-Chih Lee MD, Hui Ting Chan MS, Chwen Keng Tsao BS, Shan Pou Tsai PhD, Xifeng Wu MD, "Minimum amount of physical activity for reduced mortality and extended life expectancy: a prospective cohort study," *Lancet*, Volume 378, issue 9798, 1244–1253, 1 October 2011. Doi:10.1016/S0140-6736(11)60749-6.

25. Kanaley JA, Weltman JY, Veldhuis JD, Rogol AD, Hartman ML, Weltman A (November 1997). "Human growth hormone response to repeated bouts of aerobic exercise." *J. Appl. Physiol.* 83 (5): 1756–61. PMID 9375348.

26. Bowen R, "Overview of Hypothalamic and Pituitary Hormones: Colorado State. Edu: 1998.

27. Jung Eun Kim, Baik Kee Cho, Dae Ho Cho, and Hyun Jeong Park (2013). "Expression of Hypothalamic-Pituitary-Adrenal Axis in Common Skin Diseases: Evidence of its Association with

Stress-related Disease Activity." National Research Foundation of Korea. Retrieved 4 March 2014.

28. Theologides A (1976). "Anorexia-producing intermediary metabolites." *Am J Clin Nutr* 29 (5): 552–8. PMID 178168.

29. US CDC NCHS Data brief No. 241 April 2016.

30. American Foundation for Suicide Prevention Statistics, 2016.

31. Mercola Library, "Suicides are Surging May 2016, Teen Depression Linked to Sleep Habits," January 2010.

Chapter 13

1. Hiskias G Keizer, "The Mevalonate hypothesis: a cholesterol-independent alternative for the etiology of atherosclerosis," *Lipids Health Dis.* 2012, 11: 149. Published online 2012 November 5. doi: 10.1186/1476-511X-11-149. PMCID: PMC3496605.

2. Maria C. de Beer, Ailing Ji, Anisa Jahangiri, Ashley M. Vaughan, Frederick C. de Beer, Deneys R. van der Westhuyzen, Nancy R. Webb, "ATP binding cassette G1-dependent cholesterol efflux during inflammation," *J Lipid Res.* 2011 February, 52(2): 345–353. doi: 10.1194/jlr.M012328. PMCID: PMC3023555.

3. Sankaranarayanan S., Oram J. F., Asztalos B. F., Vaughan A. M., Lund-Katz S., Adorni M. P., Phillips M. C., Rothblat G. H. 2009. "Effects of acceptor composition and mechanism of ABCG1-mediated cellular free cholesterol efflux." *J. Lipid Res.* 50: 275–284.

4. Xiaoyan Zhang, Jonathan Hurng, Debra L. Rateri, Alan Daugherty, Geert W. Schmid-Schönbein, Hainsworth Y. Shin, "Membrane cholesterol modulates the fluid shear stress response of polymorphonuclear leukocytes via its effects on membrane fluidity," *Am J Physiol Cell Physiol.* 2011 August, 301(2): C451–C460. Published online 2011 April 27. doi: 10.1152/ajpcell.00458.2010. PMCID:PMC3154559.

5. Laurent Yvan-Charvet, Carrie Welch, Tamara A. Pagler, Mollie Ranalletta, Mohamed Lamkanfi, Seongah Han, Minako Ishibashi, Rong Li, Nan Wang, Alan R. Tall, "Increased inflammatory gene expression in ABC transporter deficient macrophages: free cholesterol accumulation, increased signaling via Toll-like receptors

and neutrophil infiltration of atherosclerotic lesions," *Circulation*. Author manuscript, available in PMC 2009 October 28., Published in final edited form as: *Circulation*. 2008 October 28, 118(18): 1837–1847. Published online 2008 October 13. doi: 10.1161/ CIRCULATIONAHA.108.793869.PMCID: PMC2756536.

6. R Scharff, R W Hendler, N Nanninga, and A.H Burgess, "Respiration and Protein Synthesis in Escherichia Coli Membrane-Envelope Fragments IV/Chemical and Cytological Characterization And Biosynthetic Capabilities of Fragments Obtained by Mild Procedures," From the Section on Cellular Physiology, Laboratory of Biochemistry, National Heart and Lung Institute, National Institutes of Health, Bethesda, Maryland 20014,and the Laboratory for Electron Microscopy, University of Amsterdam, Netherlands Pub. 1972.

7. O'Brian J, Sampson EL, Division of Chemical Pathology and Medicine, University of Southern California School of Medicine, "Lipid Composition of The Normal Human Brain: Gray Matter, White Matter, and Myelin." *J Lipid Research*, 1965, 6: 537–544.

8. Kummerow, F.A., Kummerow, J.M., "Cholesterol is not the culprit," Spacedoc Media LLC, 2014.

9. Kwiterovich Jr, P. O. (2000). "The metabolic pathways of high-density lipoprotein, low-density lipoprotein, and triglycerides: a current review." *The American Journal of Cardiology* 86 (12A): 5L–10L. doi: 10.1016/S0002-9149(00)01461-2. PMID 11374859.

10. Kummerow Fa, Przybylski R, Wasowicz E, "Changes in Arterial Membrane Composition May Procede Growth Factor Influence in the Pathogenesis of Atherosclerosis," *Artery*. 1994, 21: 63–75."

11. Grundy SM, Harvel R, Howard E. "The Evolution of Lipoprotein Analysis." *J Clin Invest*. 2004, 114: 1034–1037.

12. Christopher A Ross, Christopher A. Ross is in the Division of Neurobiology, Department of Psychiatry, and Departments of Neurology and Neuroscience, and Michelle A. Poirier is in the Division of Neurobiology, Department of Psychiatry, Johns Hopkins University School of Medicine, Ross Research Building, 720 Rutland Avenue, Baltimore, Maryland 21205, USA., Disulfide Bonds: *Nature Medicine* 10, S10–S17 (2004).

13. Kamio A, Kummerow FA, Taura S, Tokuyasu K, Cleveland JC, "Ultrastructure of Human Aorta: Cellular Composition of Diffuse Intimal Thickening." Med. Bull. Fukuoka University. 1976, 4: 15–28.

14. Zhou Qiao Lei, Hong Ping Xiang, Yong Jian Yuan, Min Zhi Rong, and Ming Qiu Zhang, Key Laboratory for Polymeric Composite and Functional Materials of Ministry of Education, GD HPPC Lab, School of Chemistry and Chemical Engineering, Sun Yat-Sen University, Guangzhou 510275, P. R. China: "Room-Temperature Self-Healable and Remoldable Cross-linked Polymer Based on the Dynamic Exchange of Disulfide Bonds." Chem. Mater., 2014, 26 (6), 2038–2046. DOI: 10.1021/cm4040616. Publication Date (Web): February 20, 2014. Copyright 2014 American Chemical Society.

15. CM Karch, DR Borchelt, "A limited role for disulfide cross-linking in the aggregation of mutant SOD1 linked to familial amyotrophic lateral sclerosis," Journal of Biological Chemistry, 2008, ASBMB.

16. Kummerow FA, Olinescu EM, Fleischer L, Handler B, Shinkareva SV, "The Relationship of Oxidized Lipids to Coronary Artery Stenosis," Atherosclerosis. 2000, 149: 181–190.

17. Lande KE, Sperry WM, Human Atherosclerosis in Relation to the Cholesterol Content of the Blood Serum," Arch. Pathol. 1936, 22: 301–312.

18. Thornton JM. "Disulphide bridges in globular proteins." 1981. J Mol Biol 151 (2): 261–87. doi: 10.1016/0022-2836(81)90515-5. PMID 7338898.

19. Thannhauser TW, Konishi Y, Scheraga HA. (1984). "Sensitive quantitative analysis of disulfide bonds in polypeptides and proteins." Anal. Biochem 138 (1): 181–8. doi: 10.1016/0003-2697(84)90786-3. PMID 6547275.

20. Ellgaard, Lars, Ruddock, Lloyd W. (2005). "The human protein disulphide isomerase family: substrate interactions and functional properties," EMBO Reports 6 (1): 28–32. doi: 10.1038/sj.embor.7400311. PMC 1299221. PMID 15643448.

21. Moore KL (2003). "The biology and enzymology of protein tyrosine O-sulfation." J. Biol. Chem. 278 (27): 24243–6. doi:10.1074/jbc.R300008200. PMID 12730193.

22. Enig, M and Sally Fallon, "The Skinny on Fats," The Weston A. Price Foundation, [xxiii] Lackland, D T, et al, J Nutr, Nov 1990, 120:11S:1433–1436. [xxiv] *Nutr Week*, Mar 22, 1991, 21:12:2–3.

23. Stryer L, Berg JM, Tymoczko JL (2007). *Biochemistry* (6th ed.). San Francisco: W.H. Freeman. ISBN 0-7167-8724-5. "Lipid By-layers: Microbiol Rev." Dec 1990, 54(4): 432–449. PMCID: PMC372788.

24. Van Meer G, Voelker DR, Feigenson GW (2008). "Membrane lipids: where they are and how they behave." *Nature Reviews Molecular Cell Biology* 9 (2): 112–24. doi: 10.1038/nrm2330. PMC 2642958. PMID 18216768.

25. Feigenson GW (2006). "Phase behavior of lipid mixtures." *Nature Chemical Biology* 2 (11): 560–63. doi: 10.1038/nchembio1106-560. PMC 2685072. PMID 17051225.

26. Zhou Q, Jimi S, Smith TL, Kummerow FA, "The Effect of 25-hydroxycholesterol on Accumulation of Intracellular Calcium. Cell Calcium," 1991, 12:467–476.

27. Alberts B, Johnson A, Lewis J, et al. Molecular Biology of the Cell. 4th edition. New York: Garland Science, 2002. The Lipid Bilayer. Available from: http://www.ncbi.nlm.nih.gov/books/NBK26871/.

28. Róg T[1], Pasenkiewicz-Gierula M, Vattulainen I, Karttunen M. "Ordering effects of cholesterol and its analogues," *Biochim Biophys Acta.* 2009 Jan, 1788(1):97–121. Doi: 10.1016/j.bbamem.2008.08.022. Epub 2008 Sep. 10.

29. Flis VV[1], Daum G. "Lipid transport between the endoplasmic reticulum and mitochondria," *Cold Spring Harb Perspect Biol.* 2013 Jun. 1, 5(6). pii: a013235. Doi: 10.1101/cshperspect.a013235.

30. Monnard PA, Deamer DW, "Membrane self-assembly processes: steps toward the first cellular life." *Astrobiology.* 2002 Winter, 2(4):371–81. *Anat Rec.* 2002 Nov 1, 268(3):196–207.

31. Deamer D[1], Dworkin JP, Sandford SA, Bernstein MP, Allamandola LJ, "The first cell membranes," *Proc Natl Acad Sci* USA. 2012 Apr 17, 109(16):5942–7. doi: 10.1073/pnas.1120327109. Epub 2012 Apr 2.

32. Prete PE[1], Gurakar-Osborne A, Kashyap ML, "Synovial fluid lipids and apolipoproteins: a contemporary perspective," *Adv Exp Med Biol.* 1991, 285:341–51. Biorheology. 1995 Jan–Feb, 32(1):1–16.

33. Chung BH[1], Segrest JP. "Cytotoxicity of remnants of triglyceride-rich lipoproteins: an atherogenic insult?" *Adv Exp Med Biol.* 1991, 285:341–51. Review. PMID: 1858566.

34. Marzolo MP[1], Rigotti A, Nervi F. "Secretion of biliary lipids from the hepatocyte," *Hepatology.* 1990 Sep, 12 (3 Pt. 2):134S–141S, discussion 141S–142S.

35. Zhou Q, Smith TL, Kummerow FA, "Cytology of Oxysterols on Cultured Smooth Muscle Cells, from Human Umbilical Arteries," *Proc Soc Exp Bio Med.* 1993, 202: 75–80.

36. Hessler JR, Morel DW, Lewis LJ, Chisolm GM, "Lipoprotein Oxidation and Lipoprotein-Induced Cytixicity," *Arteriosclerosis.* 1983, 3: 215–222.

37. Holvoet P, Sassen JM, Van Cleemput J, Collen D, Vanhaecke J, "Oxidized Low Density Lipoproteins in patients with transplant—Associated Coronary Artery Disease," *Aterioscler Thromb Vasc Biol.* 1998, 18: 100–107.

38. Mahfouz MM, Kummerow FA, "Oxysterols and TBARS Are Among the LDL Oxidation Products Which Enhance Thromboxane A2 Synthesis by Platelets," *Prostaglandins Other Lipid Mediat.* 1998, 56: 197–217.

39. Tolleter D[1], Jaquinod M, Mangavel C, Passirani C, Saulnier P, Manon S, Teyssier E, Payet N, Avelange-Macherel MH, Macherel D, "Structure and function of a mitochondrial late embryogenesis abundant protein are revealed by desiccation," *Plant Cell.* 2007 May, 19(5):1580–9. Epub 2007 May 25.

40. Ossoli A, Gomaraschi M, Franceschini G, Calabresi L, "Genetic Determinants of HDL Metabolism," *Curr Med Chem.* 2014 Mar 3. [Epub ahead of print].

41. Schenkel LC, Bakovic M, "Formation and Regulation of Mitochondrial Membranes," *Int J Cell Biol.* 2014, 2014:709828. Epub 2014 Jan 22.

42. Osamu Handa, Jancy Stephen, Gediminas Cepinskas, "Role of endothelial nitric oxide synthase-derived nitric oxide in activation and dysfunction of cerebrovascular endothelial cells during early onsets of sepsis," *American Journal of Physiology—Heart and*

Circulatory Physiology, Published 1 October 2008, vol. 295no. H1712–H1719DOI: 10.1152/ajpheart.00476.2008.

43. Naito C, Kawamura M, Yamamoto Y, "Lipid Perioxidesas the Initiating Factor of Atherosclerosis," *Ann N Y Acad Sci.* 1993, 676: 27–45.

44. Zhou Q, Wasowicz E, Handler B, Flischer L, Kummerow FA, "An Excess Concentration of Oxysterols in the Plasma is Cytotoxic to cultured Endothelial Cells," *Atherosclerosis.* 2000, 149: 191–197.

45. Smith TL, Kummerow FA, "Effect of Dietary Vitamin E on Plasma Lipids and atherogenesis in Restricted Ovulator Chickens," *Atherosclerosis.* 1989, 75: 105–109.

46. Smith TL, Kummerow FA, "Induction of Serum Lipid Perioxidation in Chickens," *Artery.* 1986, 14: 30–34.

47. Kummerow Fa, Pan HP, Hickman H, "The Effect of Dietary Fat on the Reproductive Performance and the Mixed Fatty Acid Composition of Fat-deficient Rats." *J Nutr.* 1952, 46:489–498.

48. Kummerow Fa, "The Negative Effects of Hydrogenated Trans-Fats and What to do About Them," *Atherosclerosis.* 2009, 205: 458–65.

49. Zalewaski S, Kummerow FA, "Rapeseed Oil in Two-Component Margarine base stock," *JAOCS.* 1968, 45: 87–92.

50. Kummerow Fa, Zhou Q, Mahfouz MM, Smiricky MR, Grieshop CM, Schaeffer DJ, "Trans Fatty Acids in Hydrogenated Fat Inhibited the Synthesis of the Polyunsaturated Fatty Acids in the Phospholipid of Arterial Cells," *Life Sci.* 2004, 74 (22): 2707–23.

51. Mosley EE, Wright AL, McGuire MK, McGuire MA, "Trans Fatty Acids in Milk Produced by Women in the United States," *Am J Clin Nutr.* 2005, 82: 1292 –1297.

52. Stary HC, Chandler AB, Dinsmore RE, et al, "A Definition of advanced types of Atherosclerotic Lesions and a Histological Classification of Atherosclerosis. A report from the committee on vascular lesions of the council on arteriosclerosis," American Heart Association. *Thromb Vasc Biol.* 1995, 15: 1512–1531.

53. Kummerow FA, Zhou Q, Mahfouz MM, "Effects of Trans Fatty Acids on Calcium Influx into Human Arterial Endothelial Cells." *A. J. Clin. Nutr.* 1999, 70: 832–838.

54. Stücker, M., A. Struk, P. Altmeyer, M. Herde, H. Baumgärtl & D.W. Lübbers (2002). "The cutaneous uptake of atmospheric oxygen contributes significantly to the oxygen supply of human dermis and epidermis." *Journal of Physiology* 538(3): 985–994. doi: 10.1113/jphysiol.2001.013067.

55. Blache D, Becchi M, Davignon J., "Occurrence and biological effects of cholesteryl sulfate on blood platelets," *Biochim Biophys Acta.* 1995 Dec 7, 1259(3):291–6.

56. Strott, C.A., "Cholesterol Sulfate in human physiology: What's it all about?" *J. Lipid Res.* 2003, 44, 1268–1278.

57. Dr. Mercola Interview with Dr. S. Seneff Senior Research Scientist MIT, "Could This Be The Hidden Factor Behind Obesity, Heart Disease, and Chronic Fatigue?" Mercola.com, Mercola Library, Sept. 2011.

58. Stephanie Seneff, Ann Lauritzen, Robert Davidson and Laurie Lentz-Marino, "Is Endothelial Nitric Oxide Synthase a Moonlighting Protein Whose Day Job is Cholesterol Sulfate Synthesis? Implications for Cholesterol Transport, Diabetes and Cardiovascular Disease." *Entropy* 2012, 14, 2492–2530, doi: 10.3390/e14122492.

59. Stephanie Seneff, Robert Davidson, and Luca Mascitelli, "Might cholesterol sulfate deficiency, contribute to the development of autistic spectrum disorder?" *Medical Hypotheses,* 8, 213–217, 2012.

60. Ziwei Huang, "The Chemical Biology of Apoptosis: Exploring Protein-Protein Interactions and the Life and Death of Cells with Small Molecules," *Chemistry & Biology,* vol. 9, issue 10, 1059–1072. Published in issue: October 2002.

61. Heymsfield S, Waki M, Kehayias J, Lichtman S, Dilmanian F, Kamen Y, Wang J, Pierson R (1991). "Chemical and elemental analysis of humans in vivo using improved body composition models." *Am J Physiol* 261 (2 Pt 1): E190–8. PMID 1872381.

62. Pacher P, Beckman JS, Liaudet L (2007). "Nitric oxide and Peroxynitrite in health and disease." *Physiol. Rev.* 87 (1): 315–424. doi: 10.1152/physrev.00029.2006. PMC 2248324. PMID 17237348.

63. Shafer EJ, McNamara JR, Parice H, D'Agostino R, Wilson P, Otvos J. "Low-Density Lipoprotein Particle Number, Size, and Subspecies in Assessing Cardiovascular Risk," Results of the Framingham Offspring Study. *Circulation* 2004, 110:III-777.

64. Executive Summary of The National Cholesterol Education Program Expert Panel (NCEP) on Detection, Education and Treatment of High Blood Cholesterol in Adults (ATPIII). *JAMA.* 2001, 285:2486-2497.

Chapter 14.

1. Crane FL. "Biochemical functions of coenzyme Q10." *J Am Coll Nutr.* 2001, 20(6):591-598.

2. Overvad K, Diamant B, Holm L, Holmer G, Mortensen SA, Stender S. "Coenzyme Q10 in health and disease," *Eur J Clin Nutr.* 1999,53(10):764-770.

3. Weber C. "Dietary intake and absorption of coenzyme Q." In: Kagan VE, Quinn PJ, eds. *Coenzyme Q: Molecular Mechanisms in Health and Disease.* Boca Raton: CRC Press, 2001:209-215.

4. Rustin P, Munnich A, Rotig A. "Mitochondrial respiratory chain dysfunction caused by coenzyme Q deficiency." *Methods Enzymol.* 2004, 382:81-88. http://www.ncbi.nlm.nih.gov/pubmed/15047097

5. Kalen A, Appelkvist EL, Dallner G. "Age-related changes in the lipid compositions of rat and Tran UC," Clarke CF (June 2007). "Endogenous Synthesis of Coenzyme Q in Eukaryotes." *Mitochondrion* 7 (Suppl): S62-71. doi:10.1016/j.mito.2007.03.007. PMC 1974887. PMID 17482885.

6. Bentinger M, Tekle M, Dallner G (May 2010). "Coenzyme Q—biosynthesis and functions." *Biochem. Biophys. Res. Commun.* 396 (1): 74-9. doi:10.1016/j.bbrc.2010.02.147. PMID 20494114.

7. Carmen Espinós, Vicente Felipo, Francesc Palau (1 August 2009). "Inherited Neuromuscular Diseases: Translation from Pathomechanisms to Therapies," Springer. 122–. ISBN 978-90-481-2812-9. Retrieved 4 January 2011.human tissues. Lipids. 1989, 24(7):579-584.

8. Bhagavan, Hemmi N., Chopra, Raj K. (2006). "Coenzyme Q_{10}: Absorption, tissue uptake, metabolism and pharmacokinetics." *Free Radical Research* 40 (5): 445–53. doi: 10.1080/10715760600617843. PMID 16551570.

9. Ochiai A, Itagaki S, Kurokawa T, Kobayashi M, Hirano T, Iseki K (August 2007). "Improvement in intestinal coenzyme Q_{10} absorption by food intake," *Yakugaku Zasshi* 127 (8): 1251–4. doi: 10.1248/yakushi.127.1251. PMID 17666877.

10. Kishi, H., Kanamori, N., Nisii, S., Hiraoka, E., Okamoto, T., Kishi, T. (1964). "Metabolism and Exogenous Coenzyme Q_{10} in vivo and Bioavailability of Coenzyme Q_{10} Preparations in Japan," *Biomedical and Clinical Aspects of Coenzyme Q*. Amsterdam: Elsevier. 131–42.

11. Ozawa, Y, Mizushima, Y, Koyama, I, Akimoto, M, Yamagata, Y, Hayashi, H, Murayama, H (1986). "Intestinal absorption enhancement of coenzyme Q_{10} with a lipid microsphere." *Arzneimittel-Forschung* 36 (4): 689–90. PMID 3718593.

12. Trevisson E, Dimauro S, Navas P, Salviati L (October 2011). "Coenzyme Q deficiency in muscle." *Curr. Opin. Neurol.* 24 (5): 449–56. doi:10.1097/WCO.0b013e32834ab528. PMID 21844807.

13. Hyson HC, Kieburtz K, Shoulson I, et al. (September 2010). "Safety and tolerability of high-dosage coenzyme Q_{10} in Huntington's disease and healthy subjects." *Mov. Disord.* 25 (12): 1924–8. doi: 10.1002/mds.22408. PMID 20669312.

14. Hathcock JN, Shao A (August 2006). "Risk assessment for coenzyme Q_{10} (Ubiquinone)," *Regul. Toxicol. Pharmacol.* 45 (3): 282–8. doi:10.1016/j.yrtph.2006.05.006. PMID 16814438.

15. Quiles, J, Ochoa, JJ, Huertas, JR, Mataix, J (2004). "Coenzyme Q supplementation protects from age-related DNA double-strand breaks and increases lifespan in rats fed on a PUFA-rich diet." *Experimental Gerontology* 39 (2): 189–94. doi: 10.1016/j.exger.2003.10.002. PMID 15036411.

16. Pravst, Igor, Zmitek, Katja, Zmitek, Janko (2010). "Coenzyme Q_{10} Contents in Foods and Fortification Strategies." *Critical Reviews in Food Science and Nutrition* 50 (4): 269–80. doi: 10.1080/10408390902773037. PMID 20301015.

17. Kenneth H. Nealson, Fumio Inagaki, Ken Takai, "Hydrogen-driven subsurface lithoautotrophic microbial ecosystems (SLiMEs): do they exist and why should we care?" *Trends in Microbiology,* vol. 13, issue 9, 405–410. Published in issue: September 2005.

18. Beal MF. "Therapeutic effects of coenzyme Q10 in neurodegenerative diseases," *Methods Enzymol.* 2004, 382:473–87.

19. Belardinelli R, Mucaj A, Lacalaprice F, et al., "Coenzyme Q10 and exercise training in chronic heart failure." *Eur Heart J.* 2006, 27(22):2675–81.

20. Dhanasekaran M, Ren J. "The emerging role of coenzyme Q-10 in aging, neurodegeneration, cardiovascular disease, cancer and diabetes mellitus," *Curr Neurovasc Res.* 2005, 2(5):447–59.

21. De Bustos F, Molina JA, Jimenez-Jimenz FJ, Garcia-Redondo A, Gomez-Escalonilla C, Porta-Etessam J, et al. "Serum levels of coenzyme Q10 in patients with Alzheimer's disease," *J Neural Transm.* 2000, 107(2):233–239.

22. Khan M, Gross J, Haupt H, et al., "A pilot clinical trial of the effects of coenzyme Q10 on chronic tinnitus aurium," *Otolaryngol Head Neck Surg.* 2007, 136(1):72–7.

23. Khatta M, Alexander BS, Krichten CM, Fisher ML, Freudenberger R, Robinson SW et al. "The effect of coenzyme Q10 in patients with congestive heart failure," *Ann Int Med.* 2000, 132(8):636–640.

24. Palan PR, Connell K, Ramirez E, Inegbenijie C, Gavara RY, Ouseph JA, Mikhail MS. "Effects of menopause and hormone replacement therapy on serum levels of coenzyme Q10 and other lipid-soluble antioxidants," *Biofactors.* 2005, 25(1–4):61–6.

25. Quinzii CM, Dimauro S, Hirano M. "Human coenzyme q(10) deficiency," *Neurochem Res.* 2007, 32(4–5):723–7.

26. Raitakari OT, McCredie RJ, Witting P, Griffiths KA, Letter J, Sullivan D, Stocker R, Celermajer DS. "Coenzyme Q improves LDL resistance to ex vivo oxidation but does not enhance endothelial function in hypercholesterolemic young adults," *Free Radic Biol Med.* 2000, 28(7):1100–1105.

27. Shults CW, Haas R. "Clinical trials of coenzyme Q10 in neurological disorders," *Biofactors.* 2005, 25(1–4):117–26.

28. Shults CW. Therapeutic role of coenzyme Q (10) in Parkinson's disease," *Pharmacol Ther.* 2005, 107(1):120–30.

29. Singh U, Devaraj S, Jialal I. "Coenzyme Q10 supplementation and heart failure," *Nutr Rev.* 2007, 65(6 Pt 1):286–93.

30. Rhodes C.J. (2000). "An overview of the role of free radicals in biology and of the use of electron spin resonance in their detection," *Toxicology of the Human Environment—The Critical Role of Free Radicals:* London: Taylor and Francis. ISBN 0-7484-0916-5.

Chapter 15

1. Rosado JO, Salvador M, Bonatto D., "Importance of the trans-sulfuration pathway in cancer prevention and promotion," *Mol Cell Biochem.* 2007 Jul, 301(1–2):1–12. Epub 2006 Dec 16.

2. Braga PC, Ceci C, Marabini L, Nappi G., "The antioxidant activity of sulphurous thermal water protects against oxidative DNA damage: a comet assay investigation," *Drug Res (Stuttg).* 2013 Apr, 63(4):198–202. doi: 10.1055/s-0033-1334894. Epub 2013 Feb 27.

3. Visagie M, Mqoco T, Joubert A., "Sulphamoylated estradiol analogue induces antiproliferative activity and apoptosis in breast cell lines," *Cell Mol Biol Lett.* 2012 Dec, 17(4):549–58. Epub 2012 Aug 29.

4. Jackson MR, Melideo SL, Jorns MS., "Human sulfide: quinone oxidoreductase catalyzes the first step in hydrogen sulfide metabolism and produces a sulfane sulfur metabolite," *Biochemistry.* 2012 Aug 28, 51(34):6804–15. Epub 2012 Aug 20.

5. Finkelstein JD., "Inborn errors of sulfur-containing amino acid metabolism," *J Nutr.* 2006 Jun, 136(6 Suppl):1750S-1754S.

6. Stipanuk MH., "Metabolism of sulfur-containing amino acids," *Annu Rev Nutr.* 1986, 6:179–209.

7. Waring R.H., Klovrza L.V., "Sulphur Metabolism in Autism." *Journal of Nutritional and Environmental Medicine* 10, 25–32 (2000)

8. Bauchart-Thevret C, Stoll B, Burrin DG., "Intestinal metabolism of sulfur amino acids," Department of Pediatrics, Baylor College of Medicine, USDA/ARS Children's Nutrition Research Center, Houston, Texas 77030, USA.

9. Fang Z, Yao K, Zhang X, Zhao S, Sun Z, Tian G, Yu B, Lin Y, Zhu B, Jia G, Zhang K, Chen D, Wu D., "Nutrition and health relevant regulation of intestinal sulfur amino acid metabolism: Key Laboratory for Animal Disease Resistance," Nutrition of the Ministry of Education of China, Animal Nutrition Institute, Sichuan Agricultural University, Ya'an, 625014, People's Republic of Chin., fangzhengfeng@hotmail.com

10. Shimada T, Kato H, Iwanaga S, Iwamori M, Nagai Y., "Activation of factor XII and prekallikrein with cholesterol sulfate," *Thromb Res.* 1985 Apr 1, 38(1):21–31.

11. Michael Merten, MD, Jing Fei Dong, MD, PhD, Jose A. Lopez, MD, Perumal Thiagarajan, MD. The Department of Internal Medicine, University of Texas Health Science Center (MM, PT), and the Department of Medicine, Baylor College of Medicine (JFD, JAL), Houston, Tex. In Correspondence to Perumal Thiagarajan, MD, University of Texas at Houston Medical School, 6431 Fannin, MSB 5.284, Houston, TX 77030. Email Perumal.Thiagarajan@uth.tmc.edu, "Cholesterol Sulfate, A New Adhesive Molecule for Platelets," Ahajournals.org/content/103/16/2032.full.

12. Fernandes I, Hampson G, Cahours X, Morin P, Coureau C, Couette S, Prie D, Biber J, Murer H, Friedlander G, Silve C., "Abnormal sulfate metabolism in vitamin D-deficient rats," *J Clin Invest.* 1997 Nov 1, 100(9):2196–203. Inserm U 426, Faculté Xavier Bichat and Université Paris VII, France.

13. Lippard, S. J., Berg, J. M. (1994). *Principles of Bioinorganic Chemistry.* University Science Books. ISBN 0-935702-73-3.

14. Pronk JT, Meulenberg R, Hazeu W, Bos P, Kuenen JG (1990). "Oxidation of reduced inorganic sulphur compounds by acidophilic thiobacilli." *FEMS Microbiology letters* 75 (2–3): 293–306.

15. Oz HS, Chen TS, Neuman M (2008). "Methionine deficiency and hepatic injury in a dietary steatohepatitis model." *Digestive Diseases and Sciences* 53 (3): 767–776. doi: 10.1007/s10620-007-9900-7. PMC 2271115. PMID 17710550.

16. Voet, Donald, Voet, Judith, Pratt, Charlotte. "Proteins: Three-Dimensional Structure." Fundamentals of Biochemistry, 158. Retrieved 2010-10-01. "Fibrous proteins are characterized by a

single type of secondary structure: a keratin is a left-handed coil of two a helices."

17. Schweizer J, Bowden PE, Coulombe PA, et al. (July 2006). "New consensus nomenclature for mammalian keratins." *J. Cell Biol.* 174 (2): 169–74. doi:10.1083/jcb.200603161. PMC 2064177. PMID 16831889.

18. Barnhill JG, Fye CL, Williams DW, Reda DJ, Harris CL, Clegg DO (2006). "Chondroitin product selection for the glucosamine/chondroitin arthritis intervention trial." *J Am Pharm Assoc* (Wash DC) 46 (1): 14–24. PMID 16529337.

19. Y Furukawa, R Fu, HX Deng, "Disulfide cross-linked protein represents a significant fraction of ALS-associated Cu, Zn-superoxide dismutase aggregates in spinal cords of model mice," Proceedings of the 2006 National Acad Sciences.

20. Terasawa H, Nishimura K, Suzuki H, Matsuura T, Yomo T., "Coupling of the fusion and budding of giant phospholipid vesicles containing macromolecules," *Proc Natl Acad Sci* USA. 2012 Apr 17, 109(16):5942–7. doi: 10.1073/pnas.1120327109. Epub 2012 Apr 2. PMID: 22474340.

21. Silbert JE, Sugumaran G (2002). "Biosynthesis of chondroitin/dermatan sulfate." *IUBMB Life* 54 (4): 177–86. doi: 10.1080/15216540214923. PMID 12512856.

22. Reichenbach S, Sterchi R, Scherer M, Trelle S, Bürgi E, Bürgi U et al. (2007). "Meta-analysis: chondroitin for osteoarthritis of the knee or hip," *Ann Intern Med* 146 (8): 580–90. doi: 10.7326/0003-4819-146-8-200704170-00009. PMID 17438317. Review in: ACP J Club. 2007 Sep–Oct, 147(2):44.

23. Moher D, Cook DJ, Eastwood S, Olkin I, Rennie D, Stroup DF (1999). "Improving the quality of reports of meta-analyses of randomised controlled trials: the QUOROM statement. Quality of Reporting of Meta-analyses," *Lancet* 354 (9193): 1896–900. doi: 10.1016/S0140-6736(99)04149-5. PMID 10584742.

24. Bruyere O, Reginster JY (2007). "Glucosamine and chondroitin sulfate as therapeutic agents for knee and hip osteoarthritis." *Drugs Aging* 24 (7): 573–80. doi: 10.2165/00002512-200724070-00005. PMID 17658908.

25. Clegg DO, Reda DJ, Harris CL, Klein MA, O'Dell JR, Hooper MM et al. (2006). "Glucosamine, chondroitin sulfate, and the two in combination for painful knee osteoarthritis." *N Engl J Med* 354 (8): 795–808. doi:10.1056/NEJMoa052771. PMID 16495392. Review in: *Evid Based Med.* 2006 Aug,11(4):115 *Review in: ACP J Club.* 2006 Jul–Aug,145(1):17

26. F. R. Bettelheim, "Tyrosine-O-sulfate in a peptide from fibrinogen," *J. Am. Chem. Soc.*, 1954, 76 (10), pp 2838–2839, doi:10.1021/ja01639a073

27. Moore KL (2003). "The biology and enzymology of protein tyrosine O-sulfation." *J. Biol. Chem.* 278 (27): 24243–6. doi: 10.1074/jbc.R300008200. PMID 12730193.

28. Hoffhines AJ, Damoc, E, Bridges, KG, Leary, JA, Moore, KL (2006). "Detection and purification of tyrosine-sulfated proteins using a novel anti-sulfotyrosine monoclonal antibody." *J. Biol. Chem.* 281 (49): 37877–87. doi: 10.1074/jbc.M609398200. PMC 1764208. PMID 17046811.

29. Jackson, D. S., Williams, G. (1956). "Nature of Reticulin," *Nature* 178 (4539): 915–916. doi: 10.1038/178915b0.

30. Osamu Handa, Jancy Stephen, Gediminas Cepinskas, "Role of endothelial nitric oxide synthase-derived nitric oxide in activation and dysfunction of cerebrovascular endothelial cells during early onsets of sepsis," *American Journal of Physiology, Heart, and Circulatory Physiology* Published 1 October 2008 vol. 295 no. H1712-H1719 DOI: 10.1152/ajpheart.00476.2008.

31. Alireza Minagar, Departments of Neurology, Psychiatry and Anesthesiology, Louisiana State University Health Sciences Center and J Steven Alexander, Departments of Molecular and Cellular Physiology, Louisiana State University Health Sciences Center, Shreveport, LA 71130, "Blood-brain barrier disruption in multiple sclerosis: Blood-brain barrier leakage may lead to progression of temporal lobe epilepsy," *Brain*, February 1, 2007 130: 521–534.

32. Hui-Ming Gao, Jau-Shyong Hong, "Why neurodegenerative diseases are progressive: uncontrolled inflammation drives disease progression," *Trends in Immunology*, vol. 29, issue 8, 357–365, Published in issue: August 2008.

33. Floyd, R. A., (1999). "Neuro-inflammatory processes are important in neurodegenerative diseases: A hypothesis to explain the increased formation of reactive oxygen and nitrogen species as major factors involved in neurodegenerative disease development," *Free Radical Biology and Medicine*, 26(9–10), 1346–1355. doi:10.1016/ S0891-5849(98)002937.

34. Merry J. G. Bolt, Wenhua Liu, Guilin Qiao, Juan Kong, Wei Zheng, Thomas Krausz, Gabriella Cs-Szabo, Michael D. Sitrin, Yan Chun Li, "Critical role of vitamin D in sulfate homeostasis: regulation of the sodium-sulfate co-transporter by 1,25-dihydroxyvitamin D_3, *American Journal of Physiology, Endocrinology, and Metabolism* Published 1 October 2004 vol. 287 no. E744-E749DOI: 10.1152/ ajpendo.00151.2004.

Chapter 16

1. McPhee S J, Papadakis M A, *Current Medical Diagnosis and Treatment*, McGraw Hill 2010 Dehydration 514,1172: Heat Exposure 1047: EDTA and Lead Poisoning 846, 1438.

2. Chapra D, Trivieri L, Anderson J W, *Alternative Medicine: The Definitive Guide: Detoxification Therapies:* Inovision Health Care 2002: 168–198.

3. Clarke NE, Clark CN, Mosher RE, "The 'in vivo' dissolution of metastatic calcium: An approach to atherosclerosis," *Am J Med Sci* 1955, 229:142–149.

4. Lamar CP, "Chelation therapy of occlusive atherosclerosis," *J Am Geriatr Soc*, 1966, 14:272–293.

5. Casdorph HR, Farr CH "EDTA chelation therapy III: Treatment of peripheral arterial occlusion, an alternative to amputation," *J Holistic Med* 1983, 5(1):3–15.

6. Altman J, Wakim KG and Winkelmann RK: "Effects of edathamil disodium on the kidney," *J Invest Derm* 38:215–218, 1962.

7. Angle CR and McIntire MS, "Lead poisoning during pregnancy. Fetal tolerance of calcium disodium edetate," *Am J Dis Child* 108:436, 1964.

8. Bessman SP, Ried H and Rubin M, "Treatment of lead encephalopathy with calcium disodium versenate," *Ann Med Soc DC* 21:312, 1952.

9. Birk RE and Rupe CE, "The treatment of systemic sclerosis with disodium EDTA, pyridoxine and reserpine," *Henry Ford Hosp Med Bull* 14:109, 1966.

10. Blumer W and Cranton EM, "Ninety percent reduction in cancer mortality after chelation therapy with EDTA," *J Adv Med* 2:183 1989.

11. Bolick LE and Blankenhor, DH, "A quantitative study of coronary arterial calcification," *Am J Path* 39:511, 1961.

12. Gutteridge JMC, "Ferrous-salt promoted damage to deoxyribose and benzoate, the increased effectiveness of hydroxyl-radical scavengers in the presence of EDTA." *Biochem J* 243:709, 1987.

13. Gutteridge JMC, "Ferrous-salt promoted damage to deoxyribose and benzoate, the increased effectiveness of hydroxyl-radical scavengers in the presence of EDTA," *Biochem J* 243:709, 1987.

14. Gutteridge JMC: "Ferrous-salt promoted damage to deoxyribose and benzoate, the increased effectiveness of hydroxyl-radical scavengers in the presence of EDTA," *Biochem J* 243:709, 1987.

15. Urschel HC, Finney JW, Balla GA, et al. "Protection of the ischemic heart with DMSO alone or with hydrogen peroxide," *Ann NY Adad. Sci.* 1967, 151: 231–241.

16. Gorren AC, Dekker H, Wever R, "Kinetic investigations of the reaction of cytochrome C oxidase by hydrogen peroxide," *Biochem Biophys Acta* 1986, 852(1):81–92.

17. Nathan CF, Cohn ZA, "Antitumor effects of hydrogen peroxide in vivo," *J Exp Med* 1981, 154:1539–1553.

18. Manakata T, Semba U, Shibuya Y, et al. "Induction of interferon-gamma production by human natural killer cells stimulated by hydrogen peroxide." *J Immunol* 1985, 134(4):2449–2455.

19. Oliver TH, Cantab BC, Murphy DV, "Influenzal pneumonia: the intravenous injection of hydrogen peroxide," *Lancet* 1920, 1: 432–433.

20. Urschel HC, Finney JW, Morale AR, et al. "Cardiac resuscitation with hydrogen peroxide," *Circ* 1965, 31 (suppl II), II–210.

21. Urschel HC, Finney JW, Balla GA, et al. "Protection of the ischemic heart with DMSO alone or with hydrogen peroxide," *Ann NY Adad. Sci.* 1967, 151:231–241.

22. Manakata T, Semba U, Shibuya Y, et al. "Induction of interferon-gamma production by human natural killer cells stimulated by hydrogen peroxide," *J Immunol* 1985, 134(4):2449–2455.

23. Lebedev LV, Levin AO, Romankova MP, et al. "Regional oxygenation in the treatment of severe destructive forms of obliterating diseases of the extremity arteries," *Vestn Khir* 1984, 132:85–88.

24. Bates GW, Billups C and Saltman P, "The kinetics and mechanism of iron (III) exchange between chelates and transferrin. II. The presentation and removal with ethylenediaminetetraacetate," *J Biol Chem* 242:2816, 1967.

25. Casdorph HR and Farr CH, "EDTA chelation therapy III: treatment of peripheral arterial occlusion, an alternative to amputation," *J Holistic Med* 5:3, 1983.

26. Chen IW, Park HM, King LR, Bahr GK and Goldsmith RE, "Radioimmunoassay of parathyroid hormone: peripheral plasma immunoreactive parathyroid hormone response to ethylenediaminetetraacetate," *J Nucl Med* 15:763, 1974.

27. Cranton EM, "The current status of EDTA chelation therapy," *J Holistic Med* 7:3, 1985.

28. Cranton EM, "Protocol of the American College of Advancement in Medicine for the safe and effective administration of EDTA chelation therapy," *J Adv Med* 2:269, 1989. Cranton EM, "A textbook on EDTA chelation therapy," *J Adv Med* 2:1–416, 1989.

29. Cranton EM and Frackelton JP, "Current status of EDTA chelation therapy in occlusive arterial disease," *J Holistic Med* 1:24, 1982.

Chapter 17

1. Panel on Micronutrients, Subcommittees on Upper Reference Levels of Nutrients and of Interpretation and Use of Dietary Reference Intakes, and the Standing Committee on the Scientific Evaluation of Dietary Reference Intakes (2001). "Dietary Reference Intakes for Vitamin A, Vitamin K, Arsenic, Boron, Chromium,

Copper, Iodine, Iron, Manganese, Molybdenum, Nickel, Silicon, Vanadium, and Zinc," Washington DC: National Academy Press. ISBN 0-309-07279-4.

2. Azoulay A, Garzon P, Eisenberg MJ. "Comparison of the mineral content of tap water and bottled waters," *J Gen Intern Med* 2001, 16:168–75. [PubMed abstract].

3. Fine KD, Santa Ana CA, Porter JL, Fordtran JS. "Intestinal absorption of magnesium from food and supplements," *J Clin Invest* 1991, 88:396–402. [PubMed abstract].

4. US Department of Agriculture, Agricultural Research Service, "USDA National Nutrient Database for Standard Reference," Release 25. Nutrient Data Laboratory Home Page, 2012.

5. Ranade VV, Somberg JC. "Bioavailability and pharmacokinetics of magnesium after administration of magnesium salts to humans," *Am J Ther* 2001, 8:345–57.

6. Firoz M, Graber M (2001). "Bioavailability of US commercial magnesium preparations." *Magnes Res* 14 (4): 257–62. PMID 11794633.

7. Lindberg JS, Zobitz MM, Poindexter JR, Pak CY (1990). "Magnesium bioavailability from magnesium citrate and magnesium oxide." *J Am Coll Nutr* 9 (1): 48–55. doi: 10.1080/07315724.1990.10720349. PMID 2407766.

8. Walker AF, Marakis G, Christie S, Byng M (2003). "Mg citrate found more bioavailable than other Mg preparations in a randomised, double-blind study," *Magnes Res* 16 (3): 183–91. PMID 14596323.

9. M. J. Bolland, A. Grey, A. Avenell, G. D. Gamble, I. R. Reid. (2011). "Calcium supplements with or without vitamin D and risk of cardiovascular events: reanalysis of the Women's Health Initiative limited access dataset and meta-analysis," *BMJ*, 342:d2040 DOI: 10.1136/bmj.d2040

10. Beall DP, Henslee HB, Webb HR, Scofield RH (2006). "Milk-alkali syndrome: a historical review and description of the modern version of the syndrome." *Am. J. Med. Sci.* 331 (5): 233–42. doi:10.1097/00000441-200605000-00001. PMID 16702792.

11. Picolos MK and Orlander PR (2005). "Calcium carbonate toxicity: The updated milk-alkali syndrome, report of 3 cases and review

of the literature." *Endocrine Practice* 4 (11): 272–80. doi:10.4158/ EP.11.4.272. PMID 16006300.

12. Jonanthan W. MD, Director Tahoma Clinic, Renton Washington, "Nutritional Therapy and Guide to Healing With Nutrition," *Mercola Newsletter,* Interview 6/14.

13. Singh, N., Singh, P., Hershman, J. (2000). "Effect of calcium carbonate on the absorption of levothyroxine." *JAMA,* 283 (21): 2822–2825. doi:10.1001/jama.283.21.2822. PMID 10838651.

14. Lockless, S. W., Zhou, M., MacKinnon, R. (2007). "Structural and thermodynamic properties of selective ion binding in a K+ channel." *PLoS Biol* 5 (5): e121. doi:10.1371/journal.pbio.0050121. PMC 1858713. PMID 17472437.

15. Slonim, Anthony D., Pollack, Murray M. (2006). "Potassium." *Pediatric Critical Care Medicine.* Lippincott Williams & Wilkins. 812. ISBN 978-0-7817-9469-5.

16. Visveswaran, Kasi (2009). "Hypokalemia." *Essentials of Nephrology* (2nd ed.). BI Publications. 257. ISBN 978-81-7225-323-3.

17. Potts, W. T. W., Parry, G. (1964). *Osmotic and Ionic Regulation in Animals.* Pergamon Press.

18. Lans, H. S., Stein, I. F., Meyer, KA (1952). "The relation of serum potassium to erythrocyte potassium in normal subjects and patients with potassium deficiency." *American Journal of Medical Science* 223 (1): 65–74. doi 10.1097/00000441-195201000-00011. PMID 14902792.

19. Fang Z, Yao K, Zhang X, Zhao S, Sun Z, Tian G, Yu B, Lin Y, Zhu B, Jia G, Zhang K, Chen D, Wu D., "Nutrition and health relevant regulation of intestinal sulfur amino acid metabolism," Key Laboratory for Animal Disease Resistance Nutrition of the Ministry of Education of China, Animal Nutrition Institute, Sichuan Agricultural University, Ya'an, 625014, People's Republic of China, fangzhengfeng@hotmail.com.

20. Seelig MS, Heggveit HA, "Magnesiu, Interrelationships in Ischemic Heart Disease: a review," *Am J Clin Nutr.* 1974, 27: 59–79.

21. Schroeder HA, Kraemer LA, "Cardiovascular Mortality, Municipal Water, and Corrosion," *Arch Environ Health,* 1974, 28: 303–311.

22. Visagie M, Mqoco T, Joubert A., "Sulphamoylated estradiol analogue induces antiproliferative activity and apoptosis in breast cell lines," *Cell Mol Biol Lett.* 2012 Dec, 17(4):549–58. Epub 2012 Aug 29.

23. Linus Pauling Institute, Oregon State University, Linus Pauling Science Center, Micronutrient Studies and Information Center, "Minerals, Calcium, Sodium, Magnesium, potassium and phosphorous," Update Dec. 2010.

24. Thompson R. MD., Barnes K, *The Calcium Lie,* In Tuuth Press, 2008.

Chapter 18.

1. Bowen R, "Overview of Hypothalamic and Pituitary Hormones," Colorado State .Edu: 1998.

2. Jung Eun Kim, Baik Kee Cho, Dae Ho Cho, and Hyun Jeong Park (2013). "Expression of Hypothalamic-Pituitary-Adrenal Axis in Common Skin Diseases: Evidence of its Association with Stress-related Disease Activity." National Research Foundation of Korea. Retrieved 4 March 2014.

3. Theologides A (1976). "Anorexia-producing intermediary metabolites." *Am J Clin Nutr* 29 (5): 552–8. PMID 178168.

4. Osamu Handa, Jancy Stephen, Gediminas Cepinskas, "Role of endothelial nitric oxide synthase-derived nitric oxide in activation and dysfunction of cerebrovascular endothelial cells during early onsets of sepsis," *American Journal of Physiology—Heart and Circulatory Physiology* Published 1 October 2008vol. 295no. H1712-H1719DOI: 10.1152/ajpheart.00476.2008.

5. Alireza Minagar, Departments of Neurology, Psychiatry and Anesthesiology, Louisiana State University Health Sciences Center and J Steven Alexander, Departments of Molecular and Cellular Physiology, Louisiana State University Health Sciences Center, Shreveport, LA 71130, "Blood-brain barrier disruption in multiple sclerosis: Blood-brain barrier leakage may lead to progression of temporal lobe epilepsy," *Brain,* February 1, 2007 130: 521–534.

6. Stéphane Uroz, Christophe Calvaruso, Marie-Pierre Turpault, Pascale Frey-Klett, "Mineral weathering by bacteria: ecology, actors and mechanisms," *Trends in Microbiology*, vol. 17, issue 8, 378–387. Published online: August 5, 2009.

7. van Kessel JC, Rutherford ST, Shao Y, Utria AF, Bassler BL. (2013) "Individual and combined roles of the master regulators AphA and LuxR in control of the Vibrio harveyi quorum-sensing regulon," *J Bacteriol*, 195:436–443.

8. Rutherford ST, Bassler BL. (2012) "Bacterial quorum sensing: its role in virulence and possibilities for its control." In Cold Spring Harbor Perspectives. *Bacterial Pathogens*, Eds Maloy S and Cossart P. Cold Spring Harbor Press.

9. Bassler BL (2010), "Cell-to-Cell Communication," *Proc Am Philos Soc* 154:307–314.

10. Maria Høyer-Hansen, Sasja Pauline Schultz Nordbrandt, Marja Jäättelä, "Autophagy as a basis for the health-promoting effects of vitamin D," *Trends in Molecular Medicine*, vol. 16, issue 7, 295–302. Published online: May 19, 2010.

11. Bischoff-Ferrari HA, Giovannucci E, Willett WC, Dietrich T, Dawson-Hughes B. "Estimation of optimal serum concentrations of 25-hydroxyvitamin D for multiple health outcomes." *Am J Clin Nutr.* 2006 Jul, 84(1):18–28. Review.

12. Nesby-O'Dell S, Scanlon KS, Cogswell ME, Gillespie C, Hollis BW, Looker AC, Allen C, Doughertly C, Gunter EW, Bowman BA. "Hypovitaminosis D prevalence and determinants among African American and white women of reproductive age," Third National Health and Nutrition Examination Survey, 1988–1994. Am J Clin Nutr. 2002 Jul, 76 (1):187–92.

13. Rovner AJ, O'Brien KO. "Hypovitaminosis D among healthy children in the United States: a review of the current evidence," *Arch Pediatr Adolesc Med.* 2008 Jun, 162(6):513–9.

14. Michos ED, Melamed ML. "Vitamin D and cardiovascular disease risk," *Curr Opin Clin Nutr Metab Care.* 2008 Jan, 11(1):7–12.

15. Melamed ML, Michos ED, Post W, Astor B. "25-hydroxyvitamin D levels and the risk of mortality in the general population," *Arch Intern Med.* 2008 Aug 11, 168(15):1629–37.

16. White JH, "Vitamin D signaling, infectious diseases, and regulation of innate immunity," *Infect Immun.* 2008 Sep; 76(9):3837–43.

17. Bikle DD. "Vitamin D and the immune system: role in protection against bacterial infection," *Curr Opin Nephrol Hypertens.* 2008 Jul, 17(4):348–52.

18. Cannell JJ, Vieth R, Umhau JC, Holick MF, Grant WB, Madronich S, Garland CF, Giovannucci E. "Epidemic influenza and vitamin D," *Epidemiol Infect.* 2006 Dec, 134(6):1129–40.

19. Lappe JM, Travers-Gustafson D, Davies KM, Recker RR, Heaney RP. "Vitamin D and calcium supplementation reduces cancer risk: results of a randomized trial," *Am J Clin Nutr.* 2007 Jun, 85(6):1586–91.

20. Moan J, Porojnicu AC, Dahlback A, Setlow RB. "Addressing the health benefits and risks, involving vitamin D or skin cancer, of increased sun exposure," *Proc Natl Acad Sci USA.* 2008 Jan 15, 105(2):668–73.

21. Giovannucci E, Liu Y, Rimm EB, Hollis BW, Fuchs CS. Stampfer MJ, Willett WH. "Prospective study of predictors of vitamin D status and cancer incidence and mortality in men," *JNCI* 2006, 98:451–9.

22. Schwalfenberg, G., "Not enough vitamin D: health consequences for Canadians," *Can Fam Physician*, 2007. 53(5): 841–54.

23. Stumpf WE, "Vitamin D and the digestive system," *Eur J Drug Metab Pharmacokinet.* 2008 Apr–Jun, 33(2):85–100.

24. Cannell JJ, Hollis BW. "Use of vitamin D in clinical practice," *Altern Med Rev.* 2008 Mar, 13(1):6–20.

25. Cherniack EP, Florez H, Roos BA, Troen BR, Levis S. "Hypovitaminosis D in the elderly: from bone to brain," *J Nutr Health Aging.* 2008 Jun–Jul, 12(6):366–73.

26. DeLuca HF. "The vitamin D story: a collaborative effort of basic science and clinical medicine," *FASEB J.* 1988 Mar 1, 2(3):224–36. Review.

27. Holick MF (March 2006). "High prevalence of vitamin D inadequacy and implications for health." *Mayo Clin. Proc.* 81 (3): 353–73. doi: 10.4065/81.3.353. PMID 16529140.

28. Calvo MS, Whiting SJ, Barton CN (February 2005). "Vitamin D intake: a global perspective of current status." *J. Nutr.* 135 (2): 310–6. PMID 15671233.

29. Norman AW (August 2008). "From vitamin D to hormone D: fundamentals of the vitamin D endocrine system essential for good health." *Am. J. Clin. Nutr.* 88 (2): 491S–499S. PMID 18689389.

30. Ribaya-Mercado JD., "Influence of dietary fat on beta-carotene absorption and bioconversion into vitamin A," *Nutr Rev.* 2002 Apr, 60(4):104–10.

31. McEvoy, G.K. (ed.), "Beta-carotene is well tolerated," American Hospital Formulary Service. AHFS Drug Information. American Society of Health-System Pharmacists, Bethesda, MD. 2006, 3555.

32. "A. Drug Thomson Warnings: Pregnancy risk category: X / CONTRAINDICATED IN PREGNANCY. Studies in animals or humans, or investigational or post-marketing reports, have demonstrated positive evidence of fetal abnormalities or risk which clearly outweights any possible benefit to the patient. /Parenteral vitamin A: Micromedex," Drug Information for the Health Care Professional. 24th ed. volume 1. Plus Updates. Content Reviewed by the United States Pharmacopeial Convention, Inc. Greenwood Village, CO. 2004. 2842.

33. Ribaya-Mercado JD[1], Maramag CC, Tengco LW, Dolnikowski GG, Blumberg JB, Solon FS, "Carotene-rich plant foods ingested with minimal dietary fat enhance the total-body vitamin A pool size in Filipino schoolchildren as assessed by stable-isotope-dilution methodology," *Am J Clin Nutr.* 2007 Apr, 85(4):1041–9.

34. Groff JL, *Advanced Nutrition and Human Metabolism.* 2nd ed. St. Paul: West Publishing, 1995.

35. Ross AC. "Vitamin A and retinoids," In: Shils M, Olson JA, Shike M, Ross AC. ed. *Modern Nutrition in Health and Disease.* 9th ed. Baltimore: Lippincott Williams & Wilkins, 1999, 305–327.

36. Semba RD. "The role of vitamin A and related retinoids in immune function," *Nutr Rev.* 1998, 56 (1 Pt. 2): S38–48.

37. McCullough, F. et al. "The effect of vitamin A on epithelial integrity," *Nutr Soc.* 1999, volume 58: 289–293.

38. Jang JT, Green JB, Beard JL, Green MH. "Kinetic analysis shows that iron deficiency decreases liver vitamin A mobilization in rats," *J Nutr.* 2000, 130(5):1291–1296.

39. Field CJ, Johnson IR, Schley PD. "Nutrients and their role in host resistance to infection," *J Leukoc Biol.* 2002, 71(1):16–32.

40. West CE. "Vitamin A and measles," *Nutr Rev.* 2000, 58(2 Pt 2): S46–54.

41. Feskanich D, Singh V, Willett WC, Colditz GA. "Vitamin A intake and hip fractures among postmenopausal women," *JAMA*, 2002, 287(1):47–54.

42. Rohde CM, DeLuca H. "Bone resorption activity of all-trans retinoic acid is independent of vitamin D in rats," *J Nutr.* 2003, 133(3):777–783.

43. Penniston KL, Tanumihardjo SA, "The acute and chronic toxic effects of vitamin A," *Am J Clin Nutr.* 2006, 83(2):191–201.

44. Chan A, Hanna M, Abbott M, Keane RJ. "Oral retinoids and pregnancy," *Med J Aust.* 1996, 165(3):164–167.

45. Sibrian-Vazquez M, Escobedo JO, Lim S, Samoei GK, Strongin RM (January 2010). "Homocystamides promote free-radical and oxidative damage to proteins." *Proc. Natl. Acad. Sci. USA* 107 (2): 551–4. doi: 10.1073/pnas.0909737107. PMC 2818928. PMID 20080717.

46. Leklem JE. Vitamin B_6. In: Machlin L, ed. *Handbook of Vitamins.* New York: Marcel Decker Inc, 1991:341–378.

47. Leklem JE. Vitamin B_6. In: Shils M, Olson JA, Shike M, Ross AC, eds. *Modern Nutrition in Health and Disease.* 9th ed. Baltimore: Williams & Wilkins, 1999: 413–422.

48. Meydani SN, Ribaya-Mercado JD, Russell RM, Sahyoun N, Morrow FD, Gershoff SN. "Vitamin B-6 deficiency impairs interleukin 2 production and lymphocyte proliferation in elderly adults," *Am J Clin Nutr.* 1991, 53(5):1275–1280.

49. Riggs KM, Spiro A, 3rd, Tucker K, Rush D. "Relations of vitamin B-12, vitamin B-6, folate, and homocysteine to cognitive performance in the Normative Aging Study," *Am J Clin Nutr.* 1996, 63(3):306–314.

50. Bender DA. "Non-nutritional uses of vitamin B6," *Br J Nutr.* 1999, 81(1):7–20.

51. Hansen CM, Leklem JE, Miller LT. "Vitamin B-6 status of women with a constant intake of vitamin B-6 changes with three levels of dietary protein," *J Nutr.* 1996, 126(7):1891–1901.

52. Williams AL, Cotter A, Sabina A, Girard C, Goodman J, Katz DL. "The role for vitamin B-6 as treatment for depression: a systematic review," *Fam Pract.* 2005, 22(5):532–537.

53. Kretsch MJ, Sauberlich HE, Skala JH, Johnson HL. "Vitamin B-6 requirement and status assessment: young women fed a depletion diet followed by a plant- or animal-protein diet with graded amounts of vitamin B-6," *Am J Clin Nutr.* 1995, 61(5):1091–1101.

54. Hansen CM, Shultz TD, Kwak HK, Memon HS, Leklem JE. "Assessment of vitamin B-6 status in young women consuming a controlled diet containing four levels of vitamin B-6 provides an estimated average requirement and recommended dietary allowance," *J Nutr.* 2001, 131(6):1777–1786.

55. Fu CS, Swendseid ME, Jacob RA, McKee RW. "Biochemical markers for assessment of niacin status in young men: levels of erythrocyte niacin coenzymes and plasma tryptophan," *J Nutr.* 1989, 119(12):1949–1955.

56. Dantzer F, Santoro R. "The expanding role of PARPs in the establishment and maintenance of heterochromatin," *FEBS J.* 2013, 280(15):3508–3518.

57. El Ramy R, Magroun N, Messadecq N, et al. "Functional interplay between Parp-1 and SirT1 in genome integrity and chromatin-based processes," *Cell Mol Life Sci.* 2009, 66(19):3219–3234.

58. Negri E, Franceschi S, Bosetti C, et al. "Selected micronutrients and oral and pharyngeal cancer," *Int J Cancer.* 2000, 86(1):122–127.

59. Seybolt SE. "Is it time to reassess alpha lipoic acid and niacinamide therapy in schizophrenia?" *Med Hypotheses.* 2010, 75(6):572–575.

60. Zell M, Grundmann O. "An orthomolecular approach to the prevention and treatment of psychiatric disorders," *Adv Mind Body Med.* 2012, 26(2):14–28.

61. Voutilainen S, Rissanen TH, Virtanen J, Lakka TA, Salonen JT. "Low dietary folate intake is associated with an excess incidence of acute coronary events: The Kuopio Ischemic Heart Disease Risk Factor Study," *Circulation.* 2001, 103(22):2674–2680.

62. "Dose-dependent effects of folic acid on blood concentrations of homocysteine: a meta-analysis of the randomized trials," *Am J Clin Nutr.* 2005, 82(4):806–812.

63. Scholl TO, Johnson WG. "Folic acid: influence on the outcome of pregnancy," *Am J Clin Nutr.* 2000, 71(5 Suppl.): 1295S–1303S.

64. Eskes TK. "Open or closed? A world of difference: a history of homocysteine research," *Nutr Rev.* 1998, 56(8):236–244.

65. Gerhard GT, Duell PB. "Homocysteine and atherosclerosis," *Curr Opin Lipidol.* 1999, 10(5):417–428.

66. Herbert V. Folic acid. In: Shils M, Olson JA, Shike M, Ross AC, eds. *Modern Nutrition in Health and Disease.* 9th ed. Baltimore: Lippincott Williams & Wilkins, 1999: 433–446.

67. Bailey LB. "Dietary reference intakes for folate: the debut of dietary folate equivalents," *Nutr Rev.* 1998, 56(10):294–299.

68. Ebly EM, Schaefer JP, Campbell NR, Hogan DB. "Folate status, vascular disease and cognition in elderly Canadians," *Age Ageing.* 1998, 27(4):485–491.

69. Snowdon DA, Tully CL, Smith CD, Riley KP, Markesbery WR. "Serum folate and the severity of atrophy of the neocortex in Alzheimer disease: findings from the Nun study," *Am J Clin Nutr.* 2000, 71(4):993–998.

70. Wang HX, Wahlin A, Basun H, Fastbom J, Winblad B, Fratiglioni L. "Vitamin B(12) and folate in relation to the development of Alzheimer's disease," *Neurology.* 2001, 56(9):1188–1194.

71. Apeland T, Mansoor MA, Strandjord RE. "Antiepileptic drugs as independent predictors of plasma total homocysteine levels," *Epilepsy Res.* 2001, 47(1–2):27–35.

72. Hendler SS, Rorvik DR, eds. *PDR for Nutritional Supplements.* Montvale: Medical Economics Company, Inc., 2001.

73. Zempleni J, Mock DM. "Human peripheral blood mononuclear cells, Inhibition of biotin transport by reversible competition with pantothenic acid is quantitatively minor," *J Nutr Biochem.* 1999, 10(7):427–432. (PubMed)

74. Briggs DR, Wahlqvist ML. *Food facts: the complete no-fads-plain-facts guide to healthy eating.* Victoria, Australia: Penguin Books, 1988.

75. Staggs CG, Sealey WM, McCabe BJ, Teague AM, Mock DM. "Determination of the biotin content of select foods using accurate and sensitive HPLC/avidin binding," *J Food Compost Anal.* 2004, 17(6):767–776.

76. Zempleni J, Mock DM. "Marginal biotin deficiency is teratogenic," *Proc Soc Exp Biol Med.* 2000, 223(1):14–21.

77. Pabuccuoglu A, Aydogdu S, Bas M. "Serum biotinidase activity in children with chronic liver disease and its clinical significance," *J Pediatr Gastroenterol Nutr.* 2002, 34(1):59–62.

78. Said HM, Ortiz A, McCloud E, Dyer D, Moyer MP, Rubin S. "Biotin uptake by human colonic epithelial NCM460 cells: a carrier-mediated process shared with pantothenic acid," *Am J Physiol.* 1998, 275(5 Pt. 1):C1365–1371.

79. Mock DM, Quirk JG, Mock NI. "Marginal biotin deficiency during normal pregnancy," *Am J Clin Nutr.* 2002, 75(2):295–299.

80. Mock DM. Biotin. In: Shils ME, Shike M, Ross AC, Caballero B, Cousins RJ, eds. *Modern Nutrition in Health and Disease.* 10th ed. Baltimore: Lippincott Williams & Wilkins, 2006:498–506.

81. Food and Nutrition Board, Institute of Medicine. Biotin. "Dietary Reference Intakes: Thiamin, Riboflavin, Niacin, Vitamin B_6, Vitamin B_{12}, Pantothenic Acid, Biotin, and Choline." Washington, D.C.: National Academy Press, 1998:374–389. (National Academy Press)

82. McCormick DB. "Two interconnected B vitamins: riboflavin and pyridoxine." *Physiol Rev.* 1989, 69(4):1170–1198.

83. Wacker J, Fruhauf J, Schulz M, Chiwora FM, Volz J, Becker K. "Riboflavin deficiency and preeclampsia," *Obstet Gynecol.* 2000, 96(1):38–44.

84. Tanphaichitr V, Thiamin. In: Shils M, Olson JA, Shike M, Ross AC, eds. "Modern Nutrition in Health and Disease," 9th ed. Baltimore: Williams & Wilkins, 1999:381–389.

85. Rindi G. Thiamin. In: Ziegler EE, Filer LJ, eds. "Present Knowledge in Nutrition, 7th ed." Washington, DC: ILSI Press, 1996:160–166.

86. Hutson SM, Sweatt AJ, Lanoue KF. "Branched-chain [corrected] amino acid metabolism: implications for establishing safe intakes," *J Nutr.* 2005, 135(6 Suppl.):1557S–1564S.

87. Brody T. *Nutritional Biochemistry.* 2nd ed. San Diego: Academic Press, 1999.

88. Donnino M., "Gastrointestinal beriberi: a previously unrecognized syndrome," *Ann Intern Med.* 2004, 141(11):898–899.

89. McDowell L, "Thiamin," *In Vitamins in Animal and Human Nutrition.* 2nd ed. Ames: Iowa State University Press, 2000: 265–310.

90. Yamasaki H, Tada H, Kawano S, Aonuma K. "Reversible pulmonary hypertension, lactic acidosis, and rapidly evolving multiple organ failure as manifestations of shoshin beriberi," *Circ J.* 2010, 74(9):1983–1985.

91. Gibson GE, Hirsch JA, Cirio RT, Jordan BD, Fonzetti P, Elder J, "Abnormal thiamine-dependent processes in Alzheimer's disease: Lessons from diabetes," *Mol Cell Neurosci.* 2013, 55:17–25.

92. Rodriguez-Martin JL, Qizilbash N, Lopez-Arrieta JM, "Thiamine for Alzheimer's disease," *Cochrane Review,* Cochrane Database Syst Rev. 2001, 2: CD001498.

93. Said HM, Ortiz A, McCloud E, Dyer D, Moyer MP, Rubin S. "Biotin uptake by human colonic epithelial NCM460 cells: a carrier-mediated process shared with pantothenic acid," *Am J Physiol.* 1998, 275(5 Pt. 1):C1365–1371.

94. Hendler SS, Rorvik DR, eds. *PDR for Nutritional Supplements.* Montvale: Medical Economics Company, Inc., 2001.

95. Flodin N, "Pharmacology of micronutrients," New York: Alan R. Liss, Inc., 1988.

96. Combs J, Gerald F. *The Vitamins,* 4 ed. Burlington: Elsevier Science, 2012.

97. Erdman JW, MacDonald I, Zeisel SH, International Life Sciences Institute. *Present Knowledge in Nutrition.* 10th ed. Ames, Iowa: International Life Sciences Institute, 2012.

98. Carr AC, Frei B. "Toward a new recommended dietary allowance for vitamin C based on antioxidant and health effects in humans," *Am J Clin Nutr.* 1999, 69(6):1086–1107.

99. Bruno RS, Leonard SW, Atkinson J, et al. "Faster plasma vitamin E disappearance in smokers is normalized by vitamin C supplementation," *Free Radic Biol Med.* 2006, 40(4):689–697.

100. Simon JA, Hudes ES, "Serum ascorbic acid and gallbladder disease prevalence among US adults: The Third National Health and Nutrition Examination Survey (NHANES III)," *Arch Intern Med.* 2000, 160(7): 931–936.

101. Levine M, Padayatty SJ, Espey MG, "Vitamin C: a concentration-function approach yields pharmacology and therapeutic discoveries," *Adv Nutr.* 2011, 2(2):78–88.

102. Goodman M, Bostick RM, Kucuk O, Jones DP. "Clinical trials of antioxidants as cancer prevention agents: past, present, and future," *Free Radic Biol Med.* 2011, 51(5):1068–1084.

103. Roswall N, Olsen A, Christensen J, Dragsted LO, Overvad K, Tjonneland A, "Micronutrient intake and breast cancer characteristics among postmenopausal women," *Eur J Cancer Prev.* 2010, 19(5):360–365.

104. Nagel G, Linseisen J, van Gils CH, et al., "Dietary beta-carotene, vitamin C and E intake and breast cancer risk in the European Prospective Investigation into Cancer and Nutrition (EPIC)," *Breast Cancer Res Treat.* 2010, 119(3):753–765.

105. Hutchinson J, Lentjes MA, Greenwood DC, et al, "Vitamin C intake from dairy recordings and risk of breast cancer in the UK Dietary Cohort Consortium," *Eur J Clin Nutr.* 2012, 66(5):561–568.

106. Vallance S, "Relationships between ascorbic acid and serum proteins of the immune system," *Br Med J.* 1977, 2(6084):437–438.

107. Kennes B, Dumont I, Brohee D, Hubert C, Neve P, "Effect of vitamin C supplements on cell-mediated immunity in old people," *Gerontology.* 1983, 29(5):305–310.

108. Panush RS, Delafuente JC, Katz P, Johnson J, "Modulation of certain immunologic responses by vitamin C. III. Potentiation of in vitro and in vivo lymphocyte responses," *Int J Vitam Nutr Res Suppl.* 1982, 23:35–47.

109. Jariwalla RJ, Harakeh S, "Antiviral and immunomodulatory activities of ascorbic acid," In: Harris JR (ed), *Subcellular*

Biochemistry. vol. 25: "Ascorbic Acid: Biochemistry and Biomedical Cell Biology," New York: Plenum Press, 1996:215–231.

110. Levy R, Shriker O, Porath A, Riesenberg K, Schlaeffer F, "Vitamin C for the treatment of recurrent furunculosis in patients with imparied neutrophil functions," *J Infect Dis.* 1996, 173(6):1502–1505.

111. Anderson R, Oosthuizen R, Maritz R, Theron A, Van Rensburg AJ, "The effects of increasing weekly doses of ascorbate on certain cellular and humoral immune functions in normal volunteers," *Am J Clin Nutr.* 1980, 33(1):71–76.

112. Alberts B, Bray D, Lewis J, Raff M, Roberts K, Watson JD. *Differentiated cells and the maintenance of tissues: Molecular Biology of the Cell,* 3rd Ed. New York: Garland Publishing, Inc., 1994:1139–1193.

113. Jariwalla RJ, Harakeh S, "Mechanisms underlying the action of vitamin C in viral and immunodeficiency disease," Packer L, Fuchs J, eds. *Vitamin C in Health and Disease.* New York: Marcel Dekker, Inc., 1997:309–322.

114. Pauling L. The immune system. *How to Live Longer and Feel Better,* 20th Anniversary ed. Corvallis: Oregon State University Press, 2006:105–111.

115. Dahl H, Degre M, "The effect of ascorbic acid on production of human interferon and the antiviral activity in vitro," *Acta Pathol Microbiol Scand B.* 1976, 84 B(5):280–284.

116. "Biotin." Micronutrient Information Center, Linus Pauling Institute, Oregon State University.

117. "Chromium." Micronutrient Information Center, Linus Pauling Institute, Oregon State University.

118. Food and Nutrition Board, Institute of Medicine, Folate. "Dietary Reference Intakes: Thiamin, Riboflavin, Niacin, Vitamin B$_6$, Folate, Vitamin B$_{12}$, Pantothenic Acid, Biotin, and Choline," Washington, DC: National Academy Press, 1998: 196–305. (National Academy Press)

119. Choi SW, Mason JB, "Folate and carcinogenesis: an integrated scheme," *J Nutr.* 2000, 130(2):129–132.

120. Bailey LB, Gregory JF, III, "Folate metabolism and requirements," *J Nutr.* 1999, 129(4):779–782.

121. Fiume, "Final report on the safety assessment of biotin." *International Journal of Toxicology.* 2001. 2: 45–61. PMID 11800048.

122. Zempleni J, Hassan YI, Wijeratne SS, "Biotin and biotinidase deficiency," *Expert Review of Endocrinology & Metabolism,* 2008. 3 (6): 715. doi: 10.1586/17446651.3.6.715.

123. Marquet A, Bui BT, Florentin D, "Biosynthesis of biotin and lipoic acid," *Vitamins & Hormones,* 2001. 61: 51–101. doi: 10.1016/S0083-6729(01)61002-1. ISBN 978-0-12-709861-6. PMID 11153271.

124. Zempleni J, Wijeratne SS, Hassan YI, "Biotin.," *BioFactors,* 2009. 35 (1): 36–46. doi: 10.1002/biof.8. PMID 19319844.

125. Hymes J, Fleischhauer K, Wolf B, "Biotinylation of histones by human serum biotinidase: assessment of biotinyl-transferase activity in sera from normal individuals and children with biotinidase deficiency," *Biochem Mol Med.* 1995. 56 (1): 76–83. doi: 10.1006/bmme.1995.1059. PMID 8593541.

126. Zempleni J, Mock DM, "Biotin biochemistry and human requirements": *J Nutr Biochem,* 1999. 10 (3): 128–138. doi: 10.1016/S0955-2863(98)00095-3. PMID 15539280.

127. Bowman BA, Russell RM, ed, "Biotin," *Present Knowledge in Nutrition, Ninth Edition,* vol 1. Washington, DC: International Life Sciences Institute. 2006. ISBN 978-1-57881-198-4.

128. Linus Pauling Institute, Oregon State University, Linus Pauling Science Center, "Microneutrient studies. Vitamins: A, B, C, D, and K," Dec. 2010.

129. Copra D, Trivieri L, Anderson J, "Alternative Medicine, The Definitive Guide," *Nutritional Medicine,* 393–405.

130. Chuck Hyman, Pediatrician, USA, Marvin Miller, Wright State University Boonshoft School of Medicine, USA, David Ayoub, Clinical Radiologists, SC, USA, "Evidence of Metabolic Bone Disease in Young Infants with Multiple Fractures Misdiagnosed as Child Abuse ASBMR 2010 Annual Meeting: Categories: Bone Acquisition and Pediatric Bone Disease (Clinical) Disorders of Bone and Mineral Metabolism (Genetic, Basic, and Trans.),"

Presentation Number: SA0023: October 16, 2010 Metro Toronto Convention Center.

131. Maria Efigênia de Queiroz Leite, John Lasekan, Geraldine Baggs, Tereza Ribeiro, Jose Menezes-Filho, Mariana Pontes, Janice Druzian, Danile Leal Barreto, Carolina Oliveira de Souza, Ângela Mattos and Hugo Costa-Ribeiro, "Calcium and fat metabolic balance, and gastrointestinal tolerance in term infants fed milk-based formulas with and without palm olein and palm kernel oils: a randomized blinded crossover study," *BMC Pediatrics* 2013, 13:215 doi: 10.1186/1471-2431-13-215.

132. Yu ZB, Han SP, Zhu C, Sun Q, Guo XR, "[Effects of infant formula containing palm oil on the nutrient absorption and defecation in infants: a meta-analysis]" [Article in Chinese] Zhonghua Er Ke Za Zhi. 2009 Dec, 47(12):904–10.

133. Koo WW[1], Hockman EM, Dow M, "Palm olein in the fat blend of infant formulas: effect on the intestinal absorption of calcium and fat, and bone mineralization," 2006 Apr, 25(2):117–22.

134. Ayoub DM[1], Hyman C, Cohen M, Miller M, "A critical review of the classic metaphyseal lesion: traumatic or metabolic?" *Am J Roentgenol*, 2014 Jan, 202(1):185–96. doi: 10.2214/AJR.13.10540.

135. Richard B. Weller, Medical Research Council Centre for Inflammation Research, University of Edinburgh. "Sunlight has Cardiovascular Benefits Independently of Vitamin D."

Chapter 19

1. Netherwood et al, "Assessing the survival of transgenic plant DNA in the human gastrointestinal tract," *Nature Biotechnology*, 22 (2004): 2.

2. Division of Food Chemistry and Technology and Division of Contaminants Chemistry, "Points to Consider for Safety Evaluation of Genetically Modified Foods: Supplemental Information," November 1, 1991, www.biointegrity.org

3. M. Malatesta, C. Caporaloni, S. Gavaudan, M. B. Rocchi, S. Serafini, C. Tiberi, G. Gazzanelli, "Ultrastructural Morphometrical and Immunocytochemical Analyses of Hepatocyte Nuclei from

Mice Fed on Genetically Modified Soybean," *Cell Struct Funct.* 27 (2002): 173–180

4. Jeffrey M. Smith, "Genetic Roulette: The Documented Health Risks of Genetically Engineered Foods," Yes! Books, Fairfield, IA USA, 2007.

5. Irina Ermakova, "Experimental Evidence of GMO Hazards," Presentation at Scientists for a GM Free Europe, EU Parliament, Brussels, June 12, 2007.

6. V.Ermakova, "Genetically Modified Organisms and Biological Risks," Proceedings of International Disaster Reduction Conference (IDRC), Davos, Switzerland August 27 – September 1, 2006: 168–172.

7. Irina Ermakova, "Genetically modified soy leads to the decrease of weight and high mortality of rat pups of the first generation. Preliminary studies," *Ecosinform* 1 (2006): 4–9.

8. Irina Ermakova, "Experimental Evidence of GMO Hazards," Presentation at Scientists for a GM Free Europe, EU Parliament, Brussels, June 12, 2007

9. Vazquez et al, "Intragastric and intraperitoneal administration of Cry1Ac protoxin from Bacillus thuringiensis induces systemic and mucosal antibody responses in mice," *Life Sciences*, 64, no. 21 (1999): 1897–1912, Vazquez et al, "Characterization of the mucosal and systemic immune response induced by Cry1Ac protein from Bacillus thuringiensis HD 73 in mice," *Brazilian Journal of Medical and Biological Research* 33 (2000): 147–155.

10. Vazquez et al, "Bacillus thuringiensis Cry1Ac protoxin is a potent systemic and mucosal adjuvant," *Scandinavian Journal of Immunology*, 49 (1999): 578–584. See also Vazquez-Padron et al., 147 (2000b).

11. Nagui H. Fares, Adel K. El-Sayed, "Fine Structural Changes in the Ileum of Mice Fed on Endotoxin Treated Potatoes and Transgenic Potatoes," *Natural Toxins* 6, no. 6 (1998): 219–233.

12. Arpad Pusztai, "Can Science Give Us the Tools for Recognizing Possible Health Risks for GM Food?" *Nutrition and Health,* 16 (2002): 73–84.

13. S. Leeson, "The Effect of Glufosinate Resistant Corn on Growth of Male Broiler Chickens," Department of Animal and Poultry Sciences, University of Guelph, Report No. A56379, July 12, 1996.

14. Malatesta, et al, "Ultrastructural Analysis of Pancreatic Acinar Cells from Mice Fed on Genetically Modified Soybean," *J Anat.* 2002 November, 201(5): 409–415.

15. M. Malatesta, M. Biggiogera, E. Manuali, M. B. L. Rocchi, B. Baldelli, G. Gazzanelli, "Fine Structural Analyses of Pancreatic Acinar Cell Nuclei from Mice Fed on GM Soybean," *Eur J Histochem,* 47 (2003): 385–388.

16. M. Green, et al., "Public health implications of the microbial pesticide Bacillus thuringiensis: An epidemiological study, Oregon, 1985–86," *Amer. J. Public Health* 80, no. 7 (1990): 848–852.

17. M.A. Noble, P.D. Riben, and G. J. Cook, "Microbiological and epidemiological surveillance program to monitor the health effects of Foray 48B BTK spray" (Vancouver, BC, Ministry of Forests, Province of British Columbia, Sep. 30, 1992).

18. G. A. Kleter and A. A. C. M. Peijnenburg, "Screening of transgenic proteins expressed in transgenic food crops for the presence of short amino acid sequences identical to potential, IgE-binding linear epitopes of allergens," *BMC Structural Biology* 2 (2002): 8–19.

19. Hye-Yung Yum, Soo-Young Lee, Kyung-Eun Lee, Myung-Hyun Sohn, Kyu-Earn Kim, "Genetically Modified and Wild Soybeans: An immunologic comparison," *Allergy and Asthma Proceedings* 26, no. 3 (May–June 2005): 210–216(7).

20. FLRAG, "Comments to ANZFA about Applications A346, A362 and A363," http://www.iher.org.au/ 88 Doug Gurian-Sherman, "Holes in the Biotech Safety Net, FDA Policy Does Not Assure the Safety of Genetically Engineered Foods," Center for Science in the Public Interest, http://www.cspinet.org/new/pdf/fda_report__final.pdf.

21. Bill Freese, "The StarLink Affair, Submission by Friends of the Earth to the FIFRA Scientific Advisory Panel considering Assessment of Additional Scientific Information Concerning StarLink Corn," July 17–19, 2001.

22. Manuela Malatesta, et al, "Ultrastructural Analysis of Pancreatic Acinar Cells from Mice Fed on Genetically Modified Soybean," *Journal of Anatomy* 201, no. 5 (November 2002): 409, see also M. Malatesta, M. Biggiogera, E. Manuali, M. B. L. Rocchi, B. Baldelli, G. Gazzanelli, "Fine Structural Analyses of Pancreatic Acinar Cell Nuclei from Mice Fed on GM Soybean," *Eur J Histochem* 47 (2003): 385–388.

23. Jeffrey M. Smith, *Genetic Roulette: The Documented Health Risks of Genetically Engineered Foods,* Yes! Books, Fairfield, IA USA 2007.

24. Steven M. Druker, "How the US Food and Drug Administration approved genetically engineered foods despite the deaths one had caused and the warnings of its own scientists about their unique risks," *Alliance for Bio-Integrity,* http://www.biointegrity.org/ext-summary.html.

25. "Statement of Policy: Foods Derived from New Plant Varieties," *Federal Register* 57, no. 104 (May 29, 1992): 22991.

26. Linda Kahl, Memo to James Maryanski about Federal Register Document "Statement of Policy: Foods from Genetically Modified Plants."

27. Alliance for Bio-Integrity (January 8, 1992) http://www.biointegrity.org

28. Netherwood T, Martin-Orue SM, O'Donnell AG, et al, "Assessing the survival of transgenic plant DNA in the human gastrointestinal tract," *Nat Bio technol.* Feb 2004, 22(2): 204–209.

29. Heritage J, "The fate of transgenes in the human gut," *Nat Bio technol,* Feb 2004, 22(2): 170–172.

30. Nordlee JA, Taylor SL, Townsend JA, Thomas LA, Bush RK., "Identification of a Brazil-nut allergen in transgenic soybeans," *N Engl J Med.* Mar 14 1996, 334(11): 688–692.

31. Aris A, Leblanc S. "Maternal and fetal exposure to pesticides associated to genetically modified foods in Eastern Townships of Quebec, Canada," *Reproductive Toxicology.* 2011, 31(4).

32. Dallegrave E, Mantese FD, Oliveira RT, Andrade AJM, Dalsenter PR, Langeloh A, "Pre- and postnatal toxicity of the commercial glyphosate formulation in Wistar rats," *Arch Toxicol,* 2007. 81:665–73.

33. USDA Economic Research Services, Data Sets 2000–2012, Inclusive.

34. J Mercola, Oct. 4, 2010, Interview Jeffery Smith, "This Supermarket Health Food Killed Baby Rats in 3 Weeks," "No GMO Researchers."

35. Michael Antoniou, Claire Robinson, John Fagan, "GMO Myths and Truths," June 2012. Open Earth Source.

Chapter 20

1. Braunwald, Fauci, Kasper, Hauser, Longo, & Jaameson, *Principles of Internal Medicine: Pathologic Consequences of Obesity, Cardiovascular Disease, Exercise & Cholesterol Management,* 15ᵗʰ ed., 2001.

2. Cline, Ma, Tintinalli, Kelen, Stapczynski, *Emergency Medicine, a Comprehensive Guide: Rhabdomylisis,* Fifth ed., 2000.

3. Paiva, Thelen, Van Coster, Smet, Kari, Laakso, Lehtmaki, Bergman, Lutjohann, & Laaksonen- with Merck Research laboratories & Tampere University Hospital research fund, "High Dose Statins and Skeletal Metabolism in Humans, a randomized controlled trial: Clinical Pharmacology and Therapeutics," 2005 (78) 60–68.

4. Wayne Hendrikson, Filippo Mancia, & Ming Zhou, Department of Physiology and Cellular Biopsychology—Colombia University, "Structural Biology," (www. physiology.colombia.edu/structural.html)

5. Linus Pauling Institute at Oregon State University, "Micronutrients for Older Adults," last update 11/07/08, Copyright 2008–2009.

6. M. Bloom, E. Evans, O. Mouritsen, Department of Physics, University of British Colombia "Physical Properties of the Fluid Lipid-bilayer Component of Cell Membranes," Mar 2001.

7. D. Brown, E. London, department of biochemistry and cell biology, State University of New York @ Stony Brook, "Functions of Lipid Rafts in Biological Membranes," 11794-5215, *Bio Info Bank Library,* 1997.

8. Eleanor Laise, Smart Money Publications, Dow Jones & CO. Inc. and Hearst SM Partnership, *The Lipitor Dilemma,* Nov. 2003.

9. SK. Rodal, G. Skretting, O. Garrad, F. Vihardt, B. Van Deurs, K. Sandvig, Institute for Cancer Research, The Norwegian Radium

Hospital, Montebello, Oslo, Norway, "Extraction of Cholesterol with Methyl-beta-cyclodextrin Perturbs Formation of Endocentric Vesicles," *Science Pub.* 2002 Apr. 19:296 (5567) 535–9.

10. S. Fallon, M. Enig, Scribd doc., "Dangers of Statin Drugs" 2005. (www.scribd.com/doc/5448407/dangers-of-statin-drugs?)

11. Beatrice A. Golomb MD, PHD, "Statin Drugs," Mar. 2002 (www.coloradohealthsite.org/topics/interviews/golomb.html)

12. S. Wahrle, P. Das, AC. Nyberg, "Cholesterol Dependent Y— Secretase Activity in Buoyant Cholesterol-Rich Membrane Micro Domains," *Neurobiological Discoveries*, 2002, 9:11–23 (pub med).

13. M. Maho, I. Yasuo, "Abstract Amyloid B Protein in Low-Density Membrane Domains," *Landes Bioscience*, copyright 2008.

14. Yannis, Chatzizisis, C. Vaslavas, G. Gannoglon, "Coenzyme Q- 10 Depletion, Idiopathic or Predisposing Factor in Statin Associated Myopathy?" *American Journal of Cardiology*, vol. 101, 7 Apr. 2008, 1071.

15. United States Food and Drug Administration, Joint Advisory Committee Meeting, NDA, 21—213, Jan. 13–14, 2005, Bethesda, MD.

16. National Center for Health Statistics (NCHS) National Vital Statistics Systems, "10 Leading Causes of Death in United States," 2007 Library of Congress catalog #76-641496, Washington, DC.

17. Jiang, Zaidi, Bean JL, & Michaelis ML, Department of Pharmacology and Toxicology, University of Kansas, Department of Biochemistry, Kansas City University School of Medicine & Bioscience, "Partitioning of the Plasma Membrane Ca++ AT Phase into Lipid Rafts in Primary Neurons: Effects of Ganglioside Depletion," Art. 6 Dec 2008.

18. Abbott, Wilson, Kannel, Castelli, National Heart Lung and Blood Institute, Bethesda, MD, "High Density Lipoprotein Cholesterol, Total Cholesterol Screening, and Myocardial Infarction.: The Framingham Study," Arteriosclerosis (Dallas, TX.) 8: 3,207–11 PubMed 3370018.

19. Abbot, Sharp, Burchfiel, Curb, Rodriguez, Hakim, & Yano, Division of Biostatistics, University of Virginia School of Medicine, Charlottesville, VA, "Abstract—Cross-sectional and Longitudinal

Changes in Total and High-Density-Lipoprotein Cholesterol Levels Over a 20-year Period in Elderly Men," The Honolulu Heart Program., *Annals of Epidemiology* 7: 6.417–24, Aug. 1997, PubMed 9279451/ 9678287.

20. Stemmermann, Chyou, Kagan, Nomura, & Yano, The Honolulu (Hawaii) Heart Program., "Serum Cholesterol and Mortality among Japanese-American Men," *Arch Internal Med.* May 1991, 151(5):969–72 (pub med) 2025146.